Voices of Classical Pilates

Collected Essays

28 Classical Pilates Teachers
Write About Their Lives and Work

Edited By

PETER FIASCA, Ph.D.

AMY BARIA BERGESEN, Ph.D.   SUZANNE MICHELE DIFFINE, M.A.

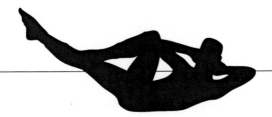

First American Edition 2013

Voices of Classical Pilates can be purchased through:
ClassicalPilates.net

Library of Congress Control Number: 2013901031

ISBN: 978-0-615-67238-0

Cover Art & Interior Layout: Joanna Libonati

Caution:

This book is not intended for treatment of any injuries.
Do not use as a replacement for medical care.
Obtain a physician's advice before starting any physical
fitness program.

Table of Contents

Table of Contents (cont.)

Dedication

This book is dedicated to Joseph and Clara Pilates, as well as to my primary teachers, Romana Kryzanowska and Jay Grimes, who have preserved the full spectrum of Contrology with love, wisdom, and a wonderful sense of humor. It is equally important to acknowledge all the loyal, exceptionally skilled professionals who share their knowledge of Joseph Pilates' traditional method with students and future generations of faithful instructors.

-PETER FIASCA

Foreword
by
Peter Fiasca, Ph.D.
Amy Baria Bergesen, Ph.D.   Suzanne Michele Diffine, M.A.

With great pleasure we present *Voices of Classical Pilates* and hope that you enjoy this wonderful collection of essays. We believe the lives, work, and ideas of these 28 well-respected Classical Pilates teachers are fascinating, fun, and truly inspiring. This project has been three years in the making. Although a greater number of teachers were asked to join the project, various circumstances precluded them from collaborating.

There are three reasons for collecting these essays into a single resource: (1) to help preserve Joseph Pilates' Classical Method of mental and physical conditioning; (2) to share intriguing ideas among individuals who are dedicated to Classical Pilates; (3) to help educate the public as well as various professionals about divergent perspectives within the ranks of those who share Joseph Pilates' traditional values and technique.

For clarity, we have categorized chapters into the following areas:

- Defining and Preserving Pilates
- On (Our) Teachers
- Methodology
- Athletic Applications for Pilates
- Pilates and Academia
- History and Apparatus

In *Voices of Classical Pilates*, you will find fascinating subjects, ranging from boxing, martial arts, and traditional apparatus, to changing careers, teaching in secondary schools, the experience of being an apprentice, understanding the integrated system, a history of Gratz Industries, as well as many other areas of interest. The process of gathering these deeply personal experiences and professional ideas from seasoned teachers has been deeply rewarding because their ideas and experiences have the potential to benefit everyone. We sincerely hope that *Voices of Classical Pilates* helps bring you to a deeper—even more positive—connection with Pilates, your life, and professional work.

Chapter 1

Defining and Preserving Pilates

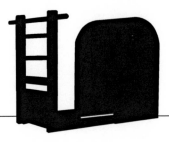

My Voyage Through the World of Pilates

By David Freeman

Injuries became a thing of the past....

My journey into the world of Pilates started early in the 1990s, before Pilates was a household name. It started a bit differently from most. I had no idea at that time that Pilates would be a major force in my life, ending in my becoming a certified Pilates instructor under the watchful eyes of Romana Kryzanowska, and subsequently a teacher trainer, owner of the Pilates Institute of Fort Lauderdale and one of the founders of The United States Pilates Association® Teacher Certification and Continuing Education Program.

I was not a young dancer, or exercise physiologist or physical therapist planning to use Pilates as a livelihood or as an aid in enhancing my professional skills. I was a 45-year-old attorney, and now I'm 67. I did not have a dancer's body; instead I was 5'8", 160 pounds of pure inflexible muscle. I was a workout fanatic who was about to have back surgery because, unbeknownst to me, the way I was working out was in reality making me more susceptible to injury. It was my belief, pounded into me by personal trainers, that bulk was good and stretching not that important. I don't think I ever heard the word "core" before I started Pilates. Looking back, I wish I had read the following quote from Joseph Pilates:

> Contrology is not a system of haphazard exercises designed to produce only bulging muscles...Nor does Contrology err either by over developing a few muscles at the expense of all others with resulting loss of grace and suppleness, or at a sacrifice of the heart or lungs. Rather, it was conceived to limber and stretch muscles and ligaments so that your body will be as supple as that of a cat and not muscular like that of the body of a brewery-truck horse or the muscle-bound body of the professional weight lifter you so much admire in the circus.[1]

Pilates was going to be my last step, a useless one I thought, before succumbing to the scalpel. This was especially true when I walked into my first Pilates studio, which looked more like a medieval torture chamber rather than a gym. Boy, was I in for a surprise. Three months later, after intensely working out three to four times a week under the tutelage of Carole Baker—whom I later learned was Romana's first teacher trainer—my sciatic pain was gone; and as an additional benefit, my body had changed in a very noticeable way. Not only did I look taller and thinner—this was brought to my attention by many people—but also I had an energy that I had never experienced in all my years of working out.

I felt good not only about the way I looked, but also about the way I moved and felt. Everything seemed easier: walking up steps, playing sports, and even in the bedroom. I later found out the phrase coined by Pilates himself, "Feel better in 10 sessions, look better in 20 sessions, and have a new body in 30 sessions, or get your money back,"[2] was really true!

Injuries became a thing of the past. My skiing trips, tennis matches, and baseball no longer ended with a strained hamstring or calf; and there was no need for me to stand on my tiptoes when having a picture taken. This crazy program with the weird-looking equipment had worked a miracle. I later learned from Romana, quite emphatically I might add, that Pilates equipment is called "apparatus" (instead of machines) because the person should be in control, not the equipment.

So I continued taking lessons for a few more years, reaping the benefits of this transformational exercise program. Pilates not only created a new body but it created a new spirit, a feeling of being almost invincible. I felt this way even before I read Joseph Pilates' book, *Return to Life Through Contrology*, where he said, "Contrology develops the body uniformly, corrects wrong postures, restores physical vitality, invigorates the mind, and elevates the spirit."[3]

Intrigued, I started to do some research, soon discovering that Joseph Pilates was a man after my own heart. He loved the pursuit of a fruitful and healthy life, innovation, vodka and cigars (although cigars were not for me, so I just doubled up on the vodka). He liked being ahead of the curve. I also started to discover more about Romana, who, from a certain point of view, appeared to be a primary—if not the primary—connecting link and torchbearer of this methodology. The first day I met Romana I decided that Pilates was going to be a part of my life forever. She was unlike any person in their 70s whom I had ever met. She expressed a love for life, she was a "lightning rod" of a person, and she was completely committed to this methodology. I wanted to learn everything I could from this woman—not only how to teach The Method, but how to use it for living life at a high level, with supreme vitality. And I would help transfer this feeling to whomever I taught.

At first Romana questioned my motivation for wanting to become certified; however, after a few conversations with her, she decided that we were "on the same page." She welcomed me with open arms, and on many social occasions there was an open bottle of champagne.

During my apprenticeship, while my mind and body continued to experience a transformation, I became more and more enthralled with what was happening to my psyche. I spent almost two years as an apprentice, staying as close to Romana as I could and soaking in every word and gesture. Her clients were total devotees, their breadth hanging on every Romana command: "Lead with the heels." "Stretch and strengthen." "Engage your powerhouse." I was not only learning the movements themselves but, more importantly, how she communicated the spirit of Pilates to her students. It was a welcome relief compared to the stress of my legal occupation. Again Joe Pilates had predicted this result: "Moreover, such a body free from nervous tension and fatigue is the ideal shelter provided by nature for housing a well-balanced mind that is always fully capable of successfully meeting all the complex problems of modern living."[4]

The stories about Joe and Clara were a major part of my apprenticeship as well as my time with Romana after becoming certified. I learned how they struggled so hard to get the general public to adopt Contrology and how they were disappointed when it did not catch on as much as they wanted. But now, I thought, I would not let this opportunity pass me by. I knew there would be a sacrifice because I took close to 1,000 hours out of my law practice to finish the teacher training program. But this would be my Fountain of Youth. And I could pass it on to many more people. It gave my life a new sense of accomplishment. While I helped people as a lawyer, Pilates would be different, much more visceral and rewarding. I truly believed I would be happier and, at the same time, spread the work.

There were clients in their 80s with the vitality of 40-year-olds; there were athletes, actors, business professionals, dancers, and everything in between. Although their bodies differed greatly, their lust for a more vibrant life was evident. It was this quest that propelled them forward. They made Pilates a part of their lives, not an exercise program, but a way of life, one designed to make them live longer and lead an active life. One need only look at Romana walking up the stairs to her apartment in Manhattan during her 70s as a prime example. I kept thinking *this is how I want to grow old and remain vitally alive.*

I worked and studied hard to become a certified instructor. I treated my apprenticeship as if I were studying for the Bar Exam because I knew that this could be the most important goal I could achieve to ensure a long and healthy life. Romana gave me high compliments when she said that people whom I had taught asked for me when I wasn't at the studio. Romana said these individuals liked the way I understood the mechanics of movement. Yet there was more. Because I was older than most apprentices, these people felt that I understood, appreciated, and communicated important nonphysical benefits of the work. For example, I conveyed how Pilates could make you feel more positive and how much more energy could be realized. There was a message that had to be spread, and Joe said it well: "To achieve the highest accomplishments within the scope of our capabilities in all walks of life, we must constantly strive to acquire strong, healthy bodies and develop our minds to the limits of our ability."[5]

Fast-forward 17 years after my first introduction to Pilates and 13 years after my certification. I ask myself, "Has the word been spread? Has the spirit of Joseph Pilates and his primary protégé, Romana Kryzanowska, been adequately disseminated? Have Pilates devotees carried on The Methodology as it was created by Joseph Pilates?" During my post-certification years, as I was teaching and becoming more familiar with the Pilates world—which had been fractured with the infamous Trademark lawsuit—I seriously questioned the focus and validity of different exercise styles called "Pilates" that were being taught in the world. It seemed like the physical benefits of Pilates were being touted, but not the spirit. A great many instructors had not read about Joseph Pilates.

Most teachers seemed uninterested in reading his books or communicating the message that Romana and other first generation teachers were trying to get across. And the majority of instructors had not seen Joseph Pilates' archival film footage, which demonstrated his strength, decisiveness, vigor, and zest.

There seems to be a lack of the "spirit" in current variations of Pilates being taught. Joseph wrote, "Contrology is complete coordination of body, mind, and spirit."[6] Although spirit has multiple interpretations, we might simply construe it as a ubiquitous presence, or energy, that is spaceless, timeless, formless in all living things. One important question to consider is how we, as instructors, incorporate that energy, that spirit, into The Methodology. How can we communicate the spirit of Contrology so that clients experience it fully? How can we inspire students to develop motivation and concentration to embrace The Methodology as a way of life? In an article titled "Romana Kryzanowska: Pilates Living Legend," Ms. Rosalind Davis referred to comments made by Jay Grimes, another distinguished former student of Joseph Pilates:

> Technically, nobody knows Joseph Pilates' work better than Romana Kryzanowska, and he believes she embodies the true Pilates spirit. Joe was like a missionary, a revival preacher; he was so adamant that he had found the secret to good health and longevity. Clara knew it too, but she was very quiet about it. They gave so much, each in their own way. It was their reward when they could take a broken-down body and turn it into a healthy, vital body. It permeated everything they did. Romana has this same spirit.[7]

The same spirit Jay Grimes talks about should be visible in the Pilates instructor. The Methodology is not comprised of rote teaching and counting. Pilates is so much more than describing and counting. So it is the instructor's responsibility to carry on the positive spirit and energy. Most apprentices do not enter a teacher training program with this spirit. As instructors, it is best to radiate the positive spirit and energy so these qualities become naturally part of students' lives. Romana was always pointing to the energy required by instructors in their training sessions. Yet sustaining energy can be challenging if someone is teaching too many hours. The energy that is so vital can be diminished or lost. If you keep reminding students how good concentration will pay off in making their lives more rewarding, it will happen. Regrettably, other considerations have come into play. For example, instructors are teaching too many hours and sapping themselves of the required energy. Classes are getting larger and larger, making it impossible to devote the attention required to individual clients. As a result, clients are missing out by not experiencing the spirit which, in my opinion, is the most vital element of the Pilates Methodology. Balance is key. It's important to replenish and share one's energy in any chosen profession. If instructors find creative ways to sustain a dynamic balance of positive energy and conviction, The Methodology will provide a means for students to accomplish realistic and very rewarding goals. Consider the description below from Joseph Pilates about the benefits of his work:

> This (Contrology) is the equivalent of an "internal shower." As the spring freshness born of the heavy rains and vast masses of melting snows on mountains in the hinterlands cause rivers to swell and rush turbulently onward to the sea, so too will your blood flow with renewed vigor as the direct result of your faithfully performing the Contrology exercises.[8]

The second trend that I have witnessed in the Pilates world is the "variations" that have been incorporated into The Methodology and the dilution of The Methodology for the usual reasons of money and power. Variations of the traditional method have potential, even beneficial effects, and they are based upon sound theories of exercise physiology. What I object to, however, is the use of the term "Pilates" to describe these variations and the lack of training that some instructors receive in getting their certifications. If a Pilates instructor is not fully trained, not only in the exercises but in the spirit and energy required to make these exercises more effective, the client will have difficulty realizing beneficial changes to his mind, body, and spirit that Joseph Pilates envisioned.

It is not my intent to go into each variation or each training program that I have seen and comment on them. In many cases I am not qualified to do so. I do not pretend to be the expert on Pilates. Yet I am a second generation instructor, and I do know what Romana taught me. I have also spoken to, and have been taught by, some of the remaining first generation teachers. So I have an idea of what they feel should be the message that the Pilates technique should deliver.

The questions I ask myself are: *Can the Methodology be effectively taught by a so-called instructor who is performing the exercises in front of 20 or 30 or more students who have various experiences in Pilates and have different physical limitations? Can an instructor be actually "certified" by going through a training program in only a few weekends? 100 hours? Can an instructor communicate the spirit of Pilates without having read Joseph's books? Are clients safe when there are so many different variations and levels of training? Will Pilates clients become disillusioned when their bodies and vitality do not change as promised?*

I remember reading an article in the *The Wall Street Journal*, of all places. That article was entitled, "Is Your Pilates Instructor a Health Hazard?" This article outlined tremendous growth in the Pilates industry and the simultaneous lack of trained instructors to accommodate consumer demand. This article points to a serious problem, a "red light" in the profession. Expansion has been too rapid to develop quality-controlled growth. Certification should be monitored. Pilates became popular because it worked, and injuries were kept to a minimum. If the current trend continues, will Pilates be questioned as a valid and safe program? Regrettably, the warning signs such as those written in *The Wall Street Journal* have not been taken to heart by professionals in the Pilates world. Business expansion, larger classes, and fast certification programs continue to be the norm. Clients in the various Pilates programs have not seen the difference in their bodies and in their spirit and are switching to other forms of exercise. More people are getting injured.

The result has been a decline in the popularity of Pilates. In 2010, a poll taken by the Sporting Goods Manufacturers Association revealed that Pilates, with 8.6 million clients, was the nation's fastest growing exercise activity. The poll showed participation up by 450% from 2000. This report, however, was misleading. American Sports Data Inc. reported that in 2004 there were 10.5 million Pilates clients. Therefore, participation went down from 2004 to 2010 by almost 2 million people.[9]

In addition, The American College of Sports Medicine published their worldwide survey of 2012 fitness trends. For the second year in a row, Pilates is out of the top 20 after having been in the top 10 in 2008, 2009, and 2010. As stated by Dr. Walter R. Thompson, a writer for the *American College of Sports Medicine's Fitness Journal*, in referring to the survey:

> Staying out of the top 20 was balance training, Pilates, and stability ball (or Swiss Ball). These three potential trends had shown remarkable strength in past years. Pilates was no. 9 on the list as recent as 2010 and appeared also as no. 7 in 2008 and 2009. Although Pilates had all of the characteristics of a trend in the industry, it may now be thought of as a fad (as supported by this current trend analysis).[10]

Is this what the exercise world is labeling Pilates? A fad? After more than 80 years, and after ascending to the top of the exercise world, Pilates has moved out of the mainstream of exercise. Is this what Joseph had in mind, or did he feel, as did I, that The Methodology was going to be a stalwart in the exercise world? In my opinion, the lack of popularity of Pilates is directly related to the dilution of The Methodology as discussed above.

The dilution of The Methodology has meant that clients have not been experiencing the positive results they had hoped for. Their bodies have not changed. Their energy and lust for life have not increased. Their motivation has not been properly channeled. What naturally follows is disillusionment and abandonment of The Methodology. In my mind that is precisely what is happening. Some of the Pilates community has been spoiled by the meteoric rise of the industry over a relatively short period of time. These individuals seem to believe that growth will continue independent of quality related to training and instruction. The future looks bleak with the lack of quality training and instruction as well as the growing number of technical modifications.

Ron Fletcher, who was a student of Joseph and Clara Pilates, also questioned the meteoric rise of the Pilates industry and, as a result, the uncertain quality of new instructors. When asked about this issue during an interview, Ron Fletcher replied:

I have mixed feelings. We have many more dedicated students from around the world, and we have many good teachers. Yet we need more true teachers instead of trainers or instructors. Many are becoming "teachers" before their time, before they complete their student process. You need more than four workshops and a piece of paper to teach Body Contrology. You need to study it.[11]

Fletcher made that comment in 2008. Apparently he foresaw the problems which have surfaced in the profession.

As we look into the future, what can we anticipate? We know that many individuals are dedicated to preserving and teaching Joseph Pilates' work as envisioned by the master as well as his protégés. Mindful of the idea that Contrology is much more than an exercise program, its practice and benefits are a profound source of health and vitality. Although there may never be a way to unify divergent approaches to Pilates in today's world, it seems beneficial to sustain the dialogue between us. We have been given a gift; it is up to us to take advantage of this gift by sharing knowledge and the positive spirit of this work. As Ron Fletcher has said about Pilates:

The trouble with this work, in general, is that people mistake it for an exercise regimen, and it's not. It's an art and it's a science and it's a study of movement. Many of the people who are so-called "doing Pilates" 10 years from now will still be doing the same thing they're doing now. They'll never get up to that point of saying, "Whee! Wow!" where you want to shout with joy at what you can do.[12]

Let's get to the point again where Pilates clients go, "Whee! Wow!"

About David

David is co-founder of the United States Pilates Association® (www.UnitedStatesPilatesAssociation.com) whose mission is to preserve the tradition of the Classical Pilates Methodology by offering teacher certification, continuing education, and archival seminars. Certified as a Pilates Instructor by Romana Kryzanowska in 1999, David owns the Pilates Institute of Ft. Lauderdale (www.ThePilates-Institute.net) and is teacher trainer for the U.S.P.A.® He graduated Georgetown Law Center in 1969 and practiced law over 40 years, including arguing before the U.S. Supreme Court. David has been a restaurateur and owner/operator of commercial real estate. He enjoys Pilates, swimming, traveling, golf and his grandchildren.

---

[1]Joseph H. Pilates and William John Miller, *Return to Life Through Contrology*. (Incline Village, NV: Presentation Dynamics, Inc., 1998), 14. Originally Published by J.J. Augustine, 1945.
[2]Advertisement by Joseph Pilates. Unknown origin.
[3]Pilates and Miller, 9.
[4]Pilates and Miller, 23.
[5]Pilates and Miller, 6.
[6]Pilates and Miller, 9.
[7]Rosalind Gray Davis, "Romana Kryzanowska: Pilates Living Legend," Ideafit.com/fitness-library/romana-kryzanowska-pilates. November 2007.
[8]Beatty, Sally, "Is Your Pilates Instructor a Health Hazard," *The Wall Street Journal*, March, 15 2005: 15D1 D4.
[9]Mary Monroe: "The Pilates Phenomenon: Where Do We Go From Here" Ideafit. com/fitness-library/the-pilates-phenomenon-where-do-we-go-from-here, July 2010.
[10]Walter R. Thompson, "Worldwide Survey of Fitness Trends for 2012," http://i2.cdn. turner.com/cnn/2011/images/12/16/fitness.trends.pdf November/December 2010.
[11]Elizabeth Larkham, "Fascinating Rhythm for First Generation Teacher Ron Fletcher, The Beat Goes On," *Pilates Style*, fletcherpilates.com/LiteratureRetrieve. aspx?ID=88513, July/August 2008.
[12]Alice Wignall, "Pilates is an Art," guardian.co.uk/lifeandstyle/2008/jun/10/healthandwellbeing.dance, June 9, 2008.

WORKS CONSULTED

Beatty, S. "Is Your Pilates Instructor a Health Hazard?" *The Wall Street Journal* (New York) 15 March, 2005: D1, D4. Print.

David, Rosalind. "Romana Kryzanowska: Pilates Living Legend." IDEA Health & Fitness Association. IDEA, n.d. Web. 27 Aug. 2012. <http:/www.ideafit.com/ fitness-library/romana-kryzanowska-pilates>.

Larkham, Elizabeth . "Fascinating Rhythm for First Generation Teacher Ron Fletcher." *Pilates Style*, n.d. Web. 27 Aug. 2012. http:// www.fletcherpilates.com/LiteratureRetrieve.aspx?ID=88513>.

Monroe, May. "The Pilates Phenomenon: Where Do We Go From Here?" IDEA Health & Fitness Association. IDEA, n.d. Web. 27 Aug. 2012. <http://www. ideafit.com/fitness-library/the-pilates-phenomenon-where-do-we-go-from-here.

Pilates, Joseph H., and William John Miller. Pilates' *Return to Life Through Contrology*. Incline Village, NV: Presentation Dynamics Inc. 1998. Print.

Thompson, William. "Worldwide Survey of Fitness Trends for 2012." *ACSM's Health & Fitness Journal*. ACSM, n.d. Web. 27 Aug. 2012. http:/i2.cdn.turner. com/cnn/2011/images/12/16/fitness.trends.pdf .

Wignall, Alice. "Pilates is an Art." *The Guardian*, 9 June 2008. Web. 27 August 2012. http:/http://www.guardian.co.uk/lifeandstyle/2008/jun/10/ healthandwellbeing. dance.

Wikipedia. "Spirit." *Wikipedia The Free Encyclopedia*. Wikipedia, n.d. Web. 27 Aug. 2012. http:/http://en.wikipedia.org/wiki/Spirit..

Flow in Pilates and Life

By Larry Gibas

> *...your brain and your body are*
> *working seamlessly together.*

Pilates stays interesting for me because fascinating aspects of the work spontaneously emerge. When they do, I'll emphasize a particular idea for a week or month in my teaching. Right now, the idea that's captured my attention is flowing movement. In Pilates, flow describes the state of being where things happen effortlessly. Time passes quickly because your brain and your body are working seamlessly together. The idea of flow is something that a lot of other exercise programs don't have. I know there's flow in certain styles of yoga, but in more traditional Western exercises, there's really not much involving the concept of flowing movement. When you create flow, transitions connecting the exercises become really important. Romana described them as pearls on a beautiful necklace, or links in a beautiful chain. I'm taken with the idea that connecting the exercises, and the way you keep them connected, becomes just as important, or even more important, as the exercises themselves.

Most articles that are written about Pilates describe it as the force of stretching to achieve muscle tone or to build strength, but they frequently write that Pilates is not a cardiovascular workout. This is completely untrue. Any normal, healthy individual can at least get a low-level cardio workout, equivalent to a light aerobic workout. This, again, goes back to the idea of flow.

With Pilates, you are continually moving. The definition of an aerobic workout is bringing the heart rate within a certain range; you can definitely do that in a Pilates workout that maintains flow. When we bring this element of flow into our teaching, we make people stronger. We make them more flexible. We give them a better sense of balance.

Although the cardiovascular component of Pilates is frequently overlooked, it is something I was taught by Romana. She wanted you to keep moving. She regularly encouraged students to maintain the movement, the energy, the flow. After Hurricane Katrina, I was not in good shape. At first, I lost a lot of weight, but I ended up gaining 50 pounds just from stress. I lived in a small trailer in my front yard for three years. I gained 50 pounds just from the stress of rebuilding my house.

During this period, I visited Romana in Dallas. Those days were a nice break from the reality of trying to recover from Katrina, but I learned some really interesting lessons. Being out of shape and trying to accomplish the same movements that I used to regularly practice gave me a new appreciation for all of the Pilates principles, especially flow. I'd be panting through my workout, and Romana would say, "Why are you making all that noise?" I'd answer, "Well, I'm winded." She responded, "Well, you shouldn't be." I kept thinking about her comment and decided she was right. I should be able to move through these exercises like before. That realization showed me what I had lost. I was still able to do most of the strength and flexibility moves, but I had no cardiovascular endurance.

To some degree, Pilates always defies description. It's hard to be concise at a cocktail party when someone asks, "I've always heard about Pilates, but I never tried it. What is it exactly?" Pilates is difficult to explain without either being too involved or too vague. But the cardiovascular aspect of the work is something I regularly teach and describe as important.

When we teach an exercise to a client, the idea of flow usually comes a little bit later because we're teaching them the mechanics of the exercise. Students first learn where to put their arms, where to put their legs, how to breathe, where to feel the exercise, and what the exercise is good for. Yet as soon as we enter the concept of flow, we're given an incredible opportunity. Students can show us how they move in a very real way. As instructors, we also observe clients as they walk in the studio. We naturally notice students as they put their coats away or put their purses away. We observe how they move, noting idiosyncrasies.

Instructors can see through a magnifying glass, so to speak. We get a chance to observe how students use their bodies. For example, when they step off the Reformer and walk to pick up the Long Box, this might be how they get out of bed in the morning. We can see how they bend to pick something up off the floor. Different transitions during the workout where students sit up and spin around, stand up and move to a different apparatus, sit down on another piece of apparatus, lie down on the floor, or come to a standing position may demonstrate exactly how they stand up from their computer chair to get a drink from the refrigerator. We can imagine how they might bend forward to look in the bottom shelf of their cupboard to get the cereal. In those moments when the client is unguarded and unaware, we truly get a glimpse into their daily physical world, the way they move in their lives to accomplish regular yet important activities.

Those little glimpses into the client's movement world are an incredible revelation. I emphasize this idea with all of my clients. I might say, "When you're bending over to pick up the box, you're mostly using your left arm instead of both arms equally." I educate students how to move in biomechanically better or more efficient ways, not just in the studio, not just within their Pilates routine, but in the real world. So the idea of watching and learning from transitions becomes a great tool for the teacher.

Ultimately, Pilates should help people become more aware of their movement in daily life. As people continue to concentrate on their Pilates exercises, those movements gradually become subconscious and more instinctual. Then their bodies automatically move in a certain way, in a very balanced way, from a strong central core. This, in turn, translates into how people move in their lives. With this shift, little things become integrated. Things like the way they do the laundry and pick up the laundry basket, and the way they lean over and fold the clothes, automatically happen in a balanced way.

Let's look at the analogy of driving a car. It's something that requires multitasking. I use that example because many people talk about how hard Pilates is because it requires you to think of several things at once: the way you hold your core; the way you breathe; the way you hold your spine, arms, and legs; even the way you move your fingers and toes. There are a lot of elements within each individual exercise.

Driving a car requires multitasking that people take for granted. They do it all the time. They drive from the house to the grocery store, to school to drop off the kids. Driving requires an awareness of your surroundings, as well as a certain anticipation of what could happen. You have to think about the car coming to an intersection. There are strong similiarities with Pilates.

When you're working with flow, not only are you in the moment, concentrating on what muscular effort and articulation is necessary to make an exercise happen, you're also listening to your teachers, feeling your body, making sure that your springs are correct, and anticipating what's going to happen next. In your mind, you're always one step ahead. This creates a sense of accomplishment that you rarely see in other exercise techniques. With Pilates, there's not just a physical feeling of accomplishment but also a mental feeling of achievement, not unlike the feeling you get from solving complicated math problems.

There is a satisfaction people derive from Pilates. That's the hook; that's the compelling part of it. There's a lot of brain chemistry that comes from a job well done, not just physically, but also mentally. I think this experience feeds people in a certain way. When you create and experience flow, you're training people's bodies, yet you're also training their minds. I always tell my clients, "Not only are we going to make you more flexible and stronger, and more fit, but we're going to make you smarter, too." I really feel that that's true; Pilates requires that people train their brains.

In Pilates, flow comes from that feeling of the mind and the body working together seamlessly. Your session just goes by, and it seems like only five minutes have elapsed, but you're already coming to the end. If we could incorporate flow into every aspect of our lives, what a happier planet this would be. It has positive ramifications that are staggering. If people could create flow at will, there would never be such a thing as labor or laboring. We'd have to get rid of those words because nothing would be laborious. Every activity would be part of a larger harmonious whole.

From the moment students walk into the studio, we encourage them to understand the principle of flowing movement. For both teacher and student, it takes a lot of work; it takes a lot of grounding. I start introducing flow relatively soon because it takes time to develop. It's best to impart essential concepts of the Pilates Method during early stages of training so that fundamental concepts are integrated into students' bodies and minds from the beginning.

Flow is beautiful. I love to watch people when they're doing something really, really well. I think that there's nothing more inspiring. For example, it could be an auto mechanic fixing a car. But when they're in that moment of flow, they're really concentrating on what they're doing, and they're totally in the moment with their tools, with the engine, with the car. It doesn't matter what profession it is; it's inspiring. It's sexy as hell. There's nothing more attractive than seeing somebody in their element like that.

Finding flow in my own life sometimes isn't easy. I don't think I'm any different than most people. We have multiple roles and wear different hats, so to speak. We often compartmentalize our lives, which is totally the opposite of what flow is about.

I do have moments of flow in various circumstances. As a Pilates instructor, I'm there with the client. I'm moving with them. I'm pulling my powerhouse in and up with them. The next client is coming in. I'm watching the new student walking in the studio while I'm still finishing up with the client that I have. I'm walking the client to the desk where they can get checked out, making sure that they're set up for their next appointment. For example, I'm trying to remember when they told me they were leaving for vacation. Then right away I start teaching my next client. I'm connecting with them, keeping my energy up, and keeping in mind what I observed about their movement when they walked in.

I'm pretty good at balancing multiple roles. My days go by; my time at the studio flows very nicely for the most part. Everybody has days when things seem a little jagged, or you have some random cancellations. Those times are difficult for me because it's hard for me to get out of my teaching mindset and into an administrative mindset. I even ask friends of mine to come and fill those spots, and I don't charge them. Filling those spots helps make my morning smooth and seamless, and I like that.

Flowing through a whole day remains a challenge. Think of the soccer mom who has kids of different ages who all have different activities, who volunteers at the homeless shelter, who has to look wonderful on her husband's arm at a business function, who then organizes an important charity event. She has many irons in the fire. These people are my clients, and I see the struggle that they have.

Our mutual struggle gives me another way of connecting to my clients. To create an entire day where my office and my home life flow together, where my mental, physical, intellectual, and spiritual needs all come together, is a tough thing. Despite this challenge, Pilates has given me more awareness of flow. I think I'm more fortunate than a lot of people that way. Most days, I'm able to experience flow for at least part of the day. Although I have not experienced flow throughout an entire day, Pilates will help me get there.

About Larry

As an instructor and teacher trainer, Larry has been a driving force in the Pilates community in New Orleans. In 1996, he began his studies in New York with the renowned master teacher Romana Kryzanowska. In 2001, he opened his own studio, Uncle Joe's Pilates, a full-service Pilates studio that reflects the traditional teachings of his world-famous mentor. Larry is a committed instructor who is dedicated to getting clients to realize their potential for a lean, strong physique. A certified group exercise instructor and personal trainer, he also danced with the New Orleans Ballet Ensemble.

Intuition: An Essential Element of the Pilates Method

By Ernesto Reynoso

...a call to consider and be aware of our intuitive spark and to respect the role that intuition plays and played in Pilates.

Joseph Pilates was reputed to have had a "healthy" ego. His vast knowledge, insight, and experience form the underpinning for The Method, but perhaps it was his ego that fueled the abiding confidence he had in his method, which was so far ahead of its time. I came to Pilates after having spent 20 years as a professional ballet dancer and, in that world, a healthy ego is a necessity. Thus, I respect the power that Joseph drew from his ego. Beyond his ego and his many talents, however, Joseph possessed a stunning level of intuition about how the human body works, how the mind and body are interrelated, and how to convey his method to others in a way that would produce results. It is that gift that fascinates me, both in the role it played in the development of The Method and in the role that it plays today, for each of us, as we learn, teach, understand, advance, and preserve The Method.

Joseph Pilates developed his approach with only a fraction of the scientific information we now have available about how and why the body, the mind, and exercise work as they do. He relied instead on available knowledge of anatomy, superb observation skills, a passion for his work, and an extraordinary level of intuition. He used what he had and let his intuition guide him as he developed his method, building on what worked and adding what he sensed and knew would work even better. I believe that his intuition is what kept him moving forward, revising and adding to his method until, powered by his passion and the confidence born of his ego, he created a masterpiece.

I am drawn to this examination because, as Joseph built his method by drawing on a number of tools—his ego, his varied training, and his hands-on experience—I drew on similar tools in my career as a dancer: the powerful ego to find the drive to keep moving forward; the training in which technique is acquired by learning one movement pattern in order to create more movement; and the hands-on approach, experiencing movement through movement. Like most dancers and, I surmise, like Joseph Pilates, I used all of these tools to learn, to perform, to teach, and to increase my level of confidence so that a movement could be done again and again in an ever-improving upward spiral. We improve, we keep learning, we try again, always reaching a little further. In dance, that is how one builds a single performance as well as an entire career. I think that is also the manner in which Joseph began developing his method.

Ultimately, however, whether in dance or in the genesis and teaching of Pilates, the factor that enables us to pull away from mere training and mere technique and to reach greater heights and truly profound levels of understanding—of movement, of people, of art—is the same thing that enabled Joseph to continue to believe in and refine his work. It is what provided the spark that moved Pilates beyond a collection of exercises into a profound fitness regimen. It is intuition.

Some might call intuition common sense, but it is more. The term intuition comes from the Latin "intueri," which Latin scholars have translated as "to look inside" or "to contemplate," and the word today refers to the ability to acquire knowledge without inference or the use of reason. In short, intuition takes over where our knowledge, and even our logic, ends. It is that "something" that has nothing to do with training or talent. We are born with it, but some heed it more effectively than others. It also operates separately from experience. Experience, of course, can strengthen intuition, if we stay attuned to it within the context of our experiences. Intuition kicks in to help us when we must make a decision, select an option, or develop a strategy. Perhaps it is a product of our survival skills, as it is a mechanism that cannot be turned off. It may be ignored, perhaps at peril, but can never be silenced. Most of us have noted that whenever we stop listening to the voice of our intuition and instead do what we think we are supposed to do or are expected to do, things do not always go well. With good training and a wealth of experience, one can avoid major problems, but it is intuition that creates great work and great moments. This is not to say one should disregard logic and reasoning, but, rather, it is a call to consider and be aware of our intuitive spark and to respect the role that intuition plays and played in Pilates.

Indeed, one of the central elements of the Pilates method is based upon Joseph's intuitive understanding of the importance of the spine: its alignment, the need to work the surrounding muscles to protect it, and its connection to the nervous system. This is what formed the core of his method. Further, his even more intuitive grasp of the mind-body connection and his awareness that it was not just a metaphor is part of why The Method continues to gain respect and to win dedicated practitioners, decades later. Joseph knew these things without the benefit of MRIs, CAT scans, or double-blind tests. Even today, there is very little formalized study of the Pilates method, yet the athletic and medical communities have known for decades that Pilates works. We trust in that awareness and in our own experience in seeing the success and effectiveness of Pilates.

Even beyond the fundamental components of Pilates, we see that intuition was at work in the manner in which Joseph would read his clients, knowing, for example, that one set of exercises would be appropriate for a dancer while a different approach, albeit drawn from the same fundamentals, would be required for a client with a different background. Through this intuitive understanding, Joseph imbued The Method with a focus on personalization of workouts, a concept that is so central to the work we do today. Joseph was known for loving the challenge presented by the specific issues associated with a new client, for whom he would create a program precisely tailored to that person's needs. Certainly, Joseph's knowledge and experience were at work here, but intuition taught him that the need for personalization, and intuition was triggered each time he sought to develop a program for a given client.

With every single day in our studio and with every client, my appreciation grows for Joseph's gift of intuition, and I strive to find and use my own. Like everyone in Romana's program, I studied, practiced, and observed for 600 hours to become a Pilates instructor. I had been involved with athletic pursuits all my life and had been a Pilates practitioner for years. So, upon completing my apprenticeship, armed with this knowledge and background, as well as a strong ego, I thought I knew all about Pilates: how it works, why it works, and how to teach it. I now know how little we know and how much we have to learn and I recognize, more and more, the central role that intuition plays in effective Pilates instruction.

Pilates is a continuous process of discovery, both as a whole and on a client-by-client basis. I believe that intuition plays a critical part in this process, just as it must have played a critical role in Joseph's original development of The Method. Thus, I write this essay less to impart insights than to start the discussion about an aspect of Pilates that I find particularly fascinating, which is the role of intuition.

The Role of Intuition in Pilates

In Pilates, we teach a collection of exercises. It is a method, and those of us trained in Romana's program teach the same basic techniques, sequences, and exercises. In addition, our bodies all are the same; we all have the same muscles, joints, and tendons. At the same time, however, every single person is different. In recognition of this, the Pilates method incorporates a flexibility that is part of its beauty. This one remarkably effective collection of exercises allows for substantial variation and modification to suit each client's needs, goals, and body. I believe that it is through this process of adaptation that we see the greatest results and instill the most powerful motivation in our clients, and I believe that it is our intuition which is the most effective guide for shaping the approach for each client.

Joseph took the challenge to use his skills, knowledge, and intuition to create a different approach for each specific client; and I believe that this is what we do day after day with each client, even if we have worked with that client for years. Joseph's legacy was the technique, and it is up to us to incorporate our intuition in using it, knowing when, why, and what to do with each client. To achieve this, it is essential to try to understand what the client feels; and this requires us to tap our intuition, just as Joseph did in developing and then in using his method. I do this with each client by asking myself these questions: How would it be to do this movement with this client's body, with these restrictions or limitations? Should this movement be modified to be safer or more effective? Is there another approach that would be better for this body with these issues? That, to me, is the greatest challenge of teaching Pilates and the greatest reward. It is this intuitive sense of the client that takes over where our knowledge stops. It is what tells us when to have patience, when to push, when to return to basics, and how to hold a client's interest so that he or she stays with the program and sees its value. In this way, intuition enables us to round out the training to make each session and the entire program effective for each client.

We hew to Joseph Pilates' technique, but we recognize that teaching and training clients in the Pilates method requires us to tap our intuition. Thus, Pilates is also a creative process. Within The Method as developed by Joseph and taught by Romana is a structure that allows each of us, working with each client, to use our own intuition and creativity in moving the client through the progression to achieve greater levels of fitness, strength, and flexibility. These are among the developments we need to examine, explore, and, above all, share with our colleagues as we continue to develop a greater understanding of the Pilates method.

How Intuition Maximizes the Effectiveness of Pilates

In Pilates, we work with each body as it comes to us. We start with the basics and build from there, adjusting the exercises as needed and adapting the program to each client's needs, using our intuition to guide the development of the strategic approach. In turn, each client's body adapts and adjusts, growing stronger and more flexible as we progress; and our intuition tells us those moments when we can take a client to a more advanced level. While we have been taught a specific sequence of exercises, the needs and issues presented by a client may require some deviation from the sequence or even from the traditional manner in which an exercise is taught. Those are the times when I believe it is essential for us to look inside, contemplate, and, while drawing, of course, on our technique and experience, let our intuition inspire us and guide us.

Using Romana's approach in our studio, we have been greatly satisfied to see the woman who could not hold her head up for the Hundred progress in a few months to a nearly perfect Teaser. And the man who was strong, but so tight that he could barely bend over, after six weeks of training, was able to execute a complete Tendon

Stretch on the Reformer. In each case, the instructor drew on intuition to read the client on a session-by-session and moment-by-moment basis, deciding how to progress, when to press, when to ease up, how much to explain, what modifications to make, and when to introduce more advanced moves. It is through such careful progression, attuned through intuition to the needs and abilities of each specific person, that we achieve the noticeable results that create dedicated and successful Pilates clients.

Incorporating Intuition in Training Sessions: Practical Concepts

The use of intuition in training starts the moment the client enters the studio. Factors such as the person's gait, posture, and even work-out attire begin to tell me what approach to take with that client's training. In the initial conversation, I, of course, gather information about any injuries the client may have and also about the client's experience, goals, and approach to exercise. At the same time, however, I note more subtle factors, such as the client's openness to advancement, ways of communicating, mode of learning, willingness to express feelings of discomfort, degree of curiosity, and level of patience.

It is from this initial reading of the client that I begin to know how much to explain, how rapidly to move through the exercises, and how to hold the client's interest. I develop a strategy of how to push that client to the maximum level of effectiveness in each session. This is what makes the difference between a client who becomes committed to the workout—and therefore achieves results—and a client who loses interest and drifts away.

Starting the session, I watch the facial expressions, especially with new clients, to gauge the client's level of comfort with the movements and also to ensure that the client maintains confidence in the safety of The Method. In these early stages, the client begins to convey a wealth of information beyond what he or she actually says. This process of "reading" the client continues throughout every session, getting easier, of course, as I begin to know and understand the client and the client's body. Then the function of intuition shifts as we move to more complicated maneuvers and advanced use of equipment.

As we teach the basic movements and refinements, ensuring the precision of movement that is so essential, we may vary the sequence of movements, sometimes even modifying an exercise itself to suit the particular client's situation. Most of my clients progress quickly, and I attribute much of the effectiveness of their training to the cues that my intuition provides. After learning the basics of the workout and developing strength and control through fundamentals on the apparatus, we move on to some of the more advanced moves, suitable for that particular client. Clients become so enthusiastic about the process that they view these advanced moves as rewards and bonuses. Careful addition of such exercises enhances the client's motivation. I rely on intuition and careful observation to know when to add more, when to back up and return to basics, and when to make a significant leap into something truly challenging for the client.

At every phase of training, but especially when advancing a client to new and more difficult moves, spotting is a critical skill; and intuition is essential to that task. To advance with the client, I want to take a client to the limits of an exercise without putting the client (or myself) at risk. It is a matter of feeling how far to go with an exercise in a way that achieves maximum movement but keeps the client safe. Through this, the instructor anticipates the actions and adjustments the client may attempt; and we thus are prepared to provide direction and, literally, support at crucial points. In dance, your partner counts on you for balance, support, focus, and strength, and the sense of integration, fusion, and trust; in teaching Pilates, the client counts on you in the same way, beyond the reliance upon you for instruction and insight.

Developing Intuition

How does one develop this intuition, this ability to read a client and have a sense of the client's body, motion, and mindset? For me, 20 years of experience as a classical ballet dancer, partnering ballerinas, has helped me develop an intuitive sense of what is happening with the other person's body. This sense of what is happening to the client is what enables an instructor to challenge clients to achieve greater and greater success. Instructors must constantly ask themselves what it feels like for each client to be performing each particular move, with that client's body, limits, and abilities. It is okay to ask the client, "What does this feel like?" and "Where do you feel that?" Such feedback, whether obtained directly from the client or from the instructor's intuition and awareness, is essential to maximizing the effects of the Pilates workout.

My goal with each client is to use my intuition to develop a sense of trust and integration, not just to reach his or her fitness goals, but to help the client develop the confidence that builds an awareness of one's own body and an independent relationship with the Pilates method. Focusing only on having the client become fit is like focusing only on making money. To me, the joy is found in connecting through intuition so that the client and I become teammates. This is achieved not just through winning the client's trust but also by making sure they know that you, in turn, trust them. With reciprocal trust comes teamwork. And intuition is essential in conveying the message of trust to a client. Words in this context are not particularly helpful. Rather, it is necessary to sense, for example, when a client can do more, when a client can proceed independently, and even when to let a client fail. It is intuition which gives us this knowledge. Intuition enables instructors to become teammates and colleagues with our clients, helping them not just to get fit, but, beyond that, to find their own intuition to create their own connections to The Method.

In a way, our goal as instructors is to help each client fall in love with The Method. We spark the client's interest and then help the client progress and, through intuition, we guide that client through The Method in the way that will lead to internalization of Pilates, making it a part of his or her life. Clients must know that they will not be and are not expected to be perfect in their execution, but still the instructor must provide motivation to always do better, to seek greater precision, and to do more in what becomes a lifelong journey of mind-body fitness and connection.

For this process and this connection, there is a word in Spanish that has no direct or effective translation in English. It is "complicidad." A rough translation in English sometimes is given as "complicity," but this English term carries only negative connotations, as when a person is complicit in a crime. Complicidad, by contrast, is a beautiful word which captures the idea of a joint effort and commitment that is more than teamwork, more than collaboration, more than partnership. It is a link in which people unite and connect on several levels in appreciation of something, working together for advancement, almost to the point of fusion. To create complicidad in any context, intuition is essential. As we instruct clients, we of course tap our training, skills, and technique; but it is intuition through which we attain complicidad and in turn enable the client to have his or her own relationship with and connection to the Pilates method. For me, the greatest achievement as an instructor is the moment that I see, having drawn on intuition, that I have found complicidad with a client, not only in pursuit of fitness, but in building the client's mind-body connection, quality of life, and enduring love for the Pilates method.

About Ernesto

Ernesto's 20-year career as a ballet dancer naturally transitioned into that of professional Pilates instructor and entrepreneur. It also marks a change in focus. As a dancer, he concentrated on building his own body, developing his "talent," perfecting his performance. Now, drawing on what he has learned through training, certification from Romana's Pilates, experience, teaching, and injuries, he focuses on helping others, relying on intuition when teaching. Ernesto strives to learn as much as possible and share broadly, promoting an awareness of and access to the traditional method of body conditioning.

Intuition, Positivity and Personal Responsibility

By Brooke Siler

We empower ourselves by acknowledging that we have all the tools already.

One of the main focuses of Pilates, in my mind, is personal responsibility. My belief comes from this line in *Your Health*[1]:

Pardon this thought, but is it not idiotic, figuratively speaking, to permit one's self to be led around by the nose by these wholly mercenary, unscrupulous and irresponsible exploiters who, through their misleading advertisements, fake references and unconscionable methods, prey upon the blind credulity of the public? Think it over, you saps!

It's as if Joseph Pilates is telling us, "Wake up and recognize the power that you have in YOU!" You don't need anyone to tell you about your body, about what you're feeling, about what's wrong with you or what you need to strengthen. You already know! You just need to own these things and then work on them!

When we coddle or we try to do for somebody, when what they really need is to do for themselves, we're actually taking away from their power. So, one of the things that has gotten stronger and stronger, both in my teaching and in my life, is my ability to take responsibility for myself. By doing that, I am actually helping those around me.

I can't be a burden on other people if I'm taking care of myself. And that's the way we make a society. It's our job to take care of ourselves so that other people don't have to. And it doesn't mean we don't nurture and love other people; it means that we nurture and love ourselves as well.

Obviously, this starts to get very philosophical and a little esoteric, but I believe Joe Pilates says it over and over again in his book:

> Were man to devote as much time and energy to himself as he has devoted to that which he has produced, what astounding and almost unbelievable progress he could make. It would be a success eclipsing all he has so far accomplished, miraculous as that is! Just think that over my friends.[2]

We empower ourselves by acknowledging that we have all the tools already. The ruby red slippers are on your feet all the time. You just click those heels, and you're there. You've been there the whole time. We have clients flooding into the studio who are looking for our help, our sage advice, all of the things that we know. It's our job to teach them that they have all of that already. It's already in them. There is not one person who doesn't know everything that we teach them. It's the truth. If they were in a room with a gun to their head and someone saying, "Find your abdominal muscles right now or else!" they're going to figure it out. Because they intuitively know how!

We have the innate knowledge already. Teachers are the people who bring that knowledge out of us. They inspire and motivate us. Romana was able to see beyond the technical and to tap into your inner power. It was an inspiration to be around her because she wanted you to be great. With her, it was, "Come on, honey. Look what you can accomplish!" And when you weren't great, you felt a bit of her sting because she didn't like that. She didn't like people to disempower themselves. I agree with her. We're very empowered beings, men and women. I feel it's my job to give people the message, "You are so strong, and you don't even know it. Show me. Let's prove it together. Let's prove together how strong you are."

I have a client, someone with whom I am incredibly close because I've been teaching her for 15 years. She originally came to me with a back that was in spasm all the time. She couldn't sleep in the bed with her husband. She had to sleep in a separate bed with pillows stuffed between her knees and under her head. She had adapted her life to suit her back. Within a short amount of time, I had her doing all the advanced work, not because it was about doing advanced work, but because I wanted to show her that she could do the advanced work.

Her problem had very little to do with her back—and much more to do with her perception of herself. I feel it's my job as a teacher to help that person help themself. If they are dependent on me, then I'm doing them no favors. Because I may not be here someday. So what are you going to do as a teacher? If I'm making you completely dependent on me, I'm wasting your time. You need to learn how to do these things for yourself, and that doesn't mean learning how to do the Single Straight Leg Stretch properly. It means learning how to be in your body and be responsible for yourself.

When we truly bring awareness to our bodies, to our movements, the whole world opens up to us. There is nothing we can't do. That's why I believe everything becomes Pilates, because Pilates is how we sit, how we stand, how we move, how we walk. It is a philosophy. It's a methodology of movement. It's not about just the exercises. Yes, of course, there's a sequence and it makes sense, and it's brilliant, but Joe wrote an entire book that had nothing to do with exercises at all. He doesn't have one exercise in *Your Health*. It's all about his philosophy of living. It's his manifesto! I love the idea of him saying, "Hey, wake up and look at yourself, and realize you are so powerful! There's nothing you can't do! You're the only one standing in your own way!"

After three or four years, people are doing the exercises by themselves. They don't need you. The reason they come to you is that you're still inspiring them in some way; it usually doesn't have a lot to do with exercise. I think it has to do with motivation. We, as humans, need this motivation and support. Joe Pilates led by showing us, "Hey, I stood up and did it for myself." We could all use a little of that in ourselves.

A Pilates teacher who hasn't read and reread Joseph Pilates' writings is missing a connection. It's like a yogi just doing a move without feeling its connection to a greater good. If you make the pretty pictures with your body but don't understand why, then there's no spiritual connection. And there is something very spiritual about where Joe was coming from, because he believed in what we could accomplish both in ourselves and as a part of a greater whole. There is a spirit within us that can be empowered and brought out, and that's what Joe was looking to do.

This system of exercises is the segue into discovering that power within ourselves. When I went into Pilates, I had not done very much of it. I had come from a personal training background. So I was more of the external type of thinker: you build your biceps, and you build your quads and you're looking for muscle, bulk and reps. But getting to the real core of Pilates, pun intended, changed the way I experienced life.

I had done the gym thing for years. There was nobody who could have said that I wasn't a strong person. But I wasn't strong, because until I really found Pilates, and Pilates found me, I don't think that what I had was strength. I think that it was superficial muscle alone. When I started doing Pilates, the challenge of it wasn't just the physical. It was embodying the movement. The word that always stuck with me, even before I went into the training program, was "empowered." That was what I felt. I felt empowered in my body. I had always felt bulky, and being almost 6'1", it's an uncomfortable thing for most women to feel. I never felt truly graceful or fast or that I had alacrity in my body. I just felt big and strong. That was it. I felt like a strong person. But after Pilates, I felt in control, and that's where the empowerment comes from. This is MY arm. This is MY leg. I will have it forever, and it is MINE. And until I develop some kind of relationship with it, I'll be disembodied. So, getting into my body and recognizing how much power I had there was an absolute game-changer. I felt superhuman.

Very early on in my career, I wrote an article where I said Pilates is "the difference between being Arnold Schwarzenegger or Bruce Lee."[3] I mean, scandals aside, whom would you rather embody? When I started Pilates, I unleashed my inner Bruce Lee. I felt the beauty of his movement, his control, his discipline. I felt that power.

So we need to empower ourselves and recognize, as Joe would say, "Health is a normal condition."[4] It's not anything that needs to be given to us. It's there already. We just have to learn how to use it. My job as a Pilates teacher is teaching personal responsibility. I'm going to get you started; then it's your job to listen to what's happening in your own body. We're too quick to pop a pill and run to a doctor. If you choose to do that with conscious attention, fine. That's one thing. But to do it because you don't think you can do anything else, that's not okay. We already have the tools to fix ourselves.

There are some people, I will admit, who keep to themselves. They don't want to break free from that mindset, their self-victimization. They're very comfortable letting other people do the work. Those people are just not as interesting to me. So, there's always a time limit on how long I will actually be with a client. If they want change, and they keep seeking it out, even if their progress is very slight, I'll stick it out. But when there's no progress, that's an energy I can't stick with because it truly pains me to see somebody who has all that innate power, not using it.

I definitely feel my role is to bring out the fierce warrior in you that knows your power in this world. The more I can do that, the more you help me. If I can get you to stand on your own two feet, then I don't have to do it for you. I can move on to the next person, and that is wonderful. And all the while I'm trying to get myself to do the same thing. I have to be an inspiration, too.

I think that the most faithful students of Pilates, if you were to interview them, would tell you that Pilates didn't just change their bodies but changed their lives too. In the same way, I think a lot of people would tell you that yoga changes lives. And I don't think it's about the movements in either one of those cases. What I have noticed is there's a lot of change that comes when we unleash that huge stream of power within us. There really is no end. I could give you specifics. People changed jobs, got out of bad marriages, or even became Pilates teachers.

When we realize we have choices, it's very empowering. And that's what I think Pilates gives you. It gives you choices. I am constantly saying to the participants in my training program, "I can't give you a definitive answer about how to do this exercise because it has many forms and there are many choices to be made. We need to see it on a body before we can tell what it looks like. A Stomach Massage for you looks very different than the Stomach Massage for me, and so on." That's the truth; it all depends on what we have to work with and the choices we make.

This is not a one-size-fits-all method, even though it gets boxed into a kit like that. I'm fairly guilty of that myself at times; just to get information out into the world we sometimes have to wrap it up in a pretty box. Not everyone can do a 700-hour course to learn Pilates, especially when there are programs out there who are feeding it to you for $50 in a 10-hour course.

There is a real difference between the traditional Pilates method as I learned it and other versions of The Method. It's not about whether you work with a "neutral spine" or "flat back"; I think it's about the energy from whom you were taught. Romana and Joe lived in a different era. It was a different mentality. It was a time of war. My father was exactly Romana's age and of that same time. Having gotten through World War I, there was a real sense of victory, relief and empowerment because of what we were able to achieve during that war. That sense very much carried over into how Romana taught; she taught us life lessons, not just Pilates lessons.

So, I feel that training with Romana (she herself having trained with Joe) changed who we are as teachers and where we are in the Pilates landscape. I don't think it's any mistake that, if you look around, there are many traditional teachers who have put a lot of important material out into the world. I think that our aim as traditional teachers became very clear, because it was an imperative. I feel it's an imperative to promote Pilates from the point of view of empowerment. That it has less to do with the way you're technically executing the exercises, although ultimately this is of course very important, and everything to do with the philosophy behind how you are taught.

When I have met people from nontraditional training programs, I have been saddened to see that they didn't know the philosophy behind their training. They had just come out of a certification program, and they didn't know why they were doing the exercises or where they came from. That is very sad to me because there is no tradition in that. Tradition means that the beliefs have been passed down. How can you tell a story that doesn't have a moral at the end? Or at the beginning? They don't know why they're doing the movement that way.

Yes, you feel your abs. Great. What is that feeling attached to? That's like isolating a floating atom in the air and saying that doesn't connect to anything. Where does it attach to the rest of the universe? The tradition that Romana brought to the work was that it's attached to something. It's attached to the person and to the world around them. That's why she would tell us to leave early, and go to the ballet, and go outside, and live our lives.

Romana always said Joe didn't want us stuck in a gym or studio all day. He wanted you to do Pilates so that you could empower and inspire yourself to do everything else. That way, there would be no limitations for you. The fact that Joe was sick as a child and was able to bring himself to that ideal level of physicality is a perfect example of this idea, and is exactly what the work is about.

Pilates can have very little to do with where the toes go on the footbar. That is a matter of physiology. We can argue that 'til the cows come home. We're all going to feel it somewhat differently because of how we're built, and that's great. We can play with that, and we can talk about the technicalities. But that is not what Pilates is about. Pilates is about the holistic quality of the work, the act of integrating it all.

I often describe the body as a baseball team or a sporting team. You can't have some of the guys sitting on the bench; everyone's got to be playing, or it doesn't work. One guy can't steal the show. Oftentimes when I teach, I humanize each body part: "Come on, move lefty," I'll say as I'm taking their left arm. "What's wrong with this guy? What's wrong with lefty? Come on lefty, get in the game. Get in the game, lefty." Because lefty is a part of the whole and without him the rest of the team must compensate. We don't reach back with just an arm to grab something without engaging the rest of the body, too. So there are a lot of muscles participating in any one action. We generally, organically, don't move in a segregated fashion.

Sometimes, when I watch people going about their workout, I see a constipation in their movement that makes me ask myself, *How do you move like that? That's not what you look like walking down the street, so stiff in your movement. There has to be some fluidity there.* This is why the Pilates ideal of seeing the body as a whole, using it as a fluid whole that has its initiation point in the center, is an enlightened philosophy for movement.

We don't move mechanically, we move organically in our bodies. The synergetic nature of the movements of Pilates and the movements of our life have to continually be recognized and worked on. This parallel between the Pilates system and daily life must be acknowledged over and over between teacher and client, so that the connection can become part of their belief system. Movement and life are inextricably linked. The syllogism that follows is: the more we learn one, the better we become at the other.

Joe Pilates said the movements should feel like the natural movements of your day because, guess what, they are. When we twist during the Stomach Massage, there's a direct correlation to sitting on your bed and turning to grab a drink from your nightstand. Pilates movements consciously made in a session teach us how to make sound movement choices in life. And soon enough conscious movement becomes second nature.

Since Pilates is dynamic, and we generally don't hold a position long enough to integrate every little nuance, we have to be pretty quick about how we're going to get all our muscles to fire, or let go, or whatever we need them to do at once. We are synthesizing a lot of information in an instant, which is much more in keeping with the way we move on a daily basis than holding a beautiful pose and having the luxury of being able to hone it while you're in it.

Pilates makes you think on your toes, and that's challenging for people. I'm a New Yorker, and thinking on your toes is what life's about here. I'm sure there are plenty of places in the world where people have more time to think about how they're going to move, but in New York you move fast or you lose your taxi!

I read a great article about Joe where he's in his studio, looking out the window at the pallid, gray New Yorkers shuffling about, and he says, "Just like all of them! Americans! They want to go 600 miles an hour, and they don't know how to walk!"[5] There is such irony to how much we try to accomplish externally when the very thing that we live in every day seems so beyond our control. The body is not beyond our control, but that's still what many people believe.

I happen to be a woman who has been through her share of bodily ordeals that might've been considered "out of my control." In 2009, I underwent an aortic surgery to repair an aneurysm from a syndrome called Loeys-Dietz. It is something that I went into with my eyes wide open and, other than the slight fear of putting my life into the doctor's hands, I felt 100% in control of things on my end. Because in the end that's really all we can control anyway, our end. It reminds me of one of my favorite expressions; "It'll all be okay in the end, and if it's not okay, it's not the end." I knew that I'd be fine because I know that about myself. Much of the reason I know that is because of the foundation Pilates has given me.

Because of Pilates, I recognize that our bodies are one of the few things that we really do have some control over, and I have formed a relationship with mine that is solid and respectful. My body respects me, and I respect it—most of the time. I truly do see myself as having a relationship with my body. It is mine to nurture and care for, or to know when I'm not nurturing and caring for it. In order to survive, you have to know you can. The Pilates method is one of the most positive means of learning this concept. I don't know a more positive, can-do technique. Again, perhaps this was due to my teacher. Way before Obama, Romana was all about "Yes, we can!"

For me, that positivity was another great connector to Pilates. I grew up with a father who was an incredibly positive man. And my mother, despite having multiple sclerosis for 30 years, had a great outlook on things. I grew up in a very positive household.

Romana reflected that back to me. It was very natural for me to go from my house to Romana's house. She really believed in living life, and she'd go out and champagne-it-up and come in to the studio first thing in the morning having danced all night. There's something to be said for that. When you're in your late 70s, you could easily give up and sit on the sidelines and watch. But not Romana.

I always loved when she would look over at a young apprentice, and you'd think she was being very compassionate, and she'd say, "Oh, you look tired dear. Are you tired?" Inevitably, one of them would reply, "Yes, I'm tired." And Romana would sniff, "Well you'll sleep when you're dead!" And she would turn on her heel and march away with a little twinkle in her eye. I loved that! She was right! This is the time to live. We're here now. We're alive. Let's make the most of it. Because of Romana, there's was so much positivity in the way we were taught Pilates.

That's something I hope that I pass on to my students, because that is, to me, empowering. We can always look at everything as what we can't do. I'm terrible at the Star, but so what? Really, in the broad scheme of things, you keep working until you get it. I had a client who said, "Do you think that I will ever be able to slim down my knees?" And I said, "Well, we won't know until we're nailing the coffin shut, will we?" We don't know what we can achieve until we've achieved it—or haven't achieved it. But the bottom line is that we just never know unless we try! I will never say, "Oh, no, that's just not possible." Never.

I know what my body was able to do back when I first started Pilates and what it's able to do now, and there's a difference. Back then, when I was Little-Miss-Superhuman, there were always things that were hard—that darn Star on the Reformer, for instance. But I never stopped doing it. I never left it out of my session; I just did it to my ability. Who's going to argue with that? Am I kicking up to the stars? No. But am I doing it? Yes. I'm a very positive person in that way. I'm a firm believer that if at first you don't succeed, try, try again.

I would bring my mom, who couldn't walk, down to the studio and put her onto the apparatus. I made stuff up, a lot of stuff, because it worked and she loved feeling that she could move. Being able to use the springs in a particular way to get her to move her leg, which didn't move on its own, was a phenomenal feeling for us both.

The work got her circulation flowing, which is exactly what Joe wanted it to do. He wanted you to have circulatory energy in your body so you could live your life with zest and zeal. That's the stuff of Pilates. I don't really care if you are in neutral spine. Sure, I have my opinions about it from a physiological standpoint, but I simply see a huge difference between the physiology of Pilates and the philosophy of Pilates.

Romana was not a technician, but not because she couldn't be. She knew those movements inside and out. But she realized at her age and after all those years of teaching that the technical aspect was not what was so vitally important about Pilates. What's vitally important about Pilates is getting it in your body, taking control, doing the absolute best you can do, and living that in your life. Get out. Go dance. Go live your life. That's what it's about, and you can't do that until you've learned that you can.

When you know that potential is there, that's the most positive motivator in the world. So I like to take people who always tell themselves that they can't do this or that, and have them do the Walkover or flip on the Cadillac. I take them there almost from the get-go. Hey, I'm tall and strong and confident in my hands, so why not? I don't even tell them what we're doing beause I don't want them to psych themselves out. It's one of my favorite things to do because it knocks "I can't" right out of the studio.

After that, it's such a pleasure sending them out into the world. I always say, "As you walk around the city today, I want you to remember that you did a flip on the Cadillac. I want you to remember that because, when you look around at the other people on the street, you'll know that nobody else did what you did this morning. Be proud of that!" That's the kind of empowerment I like people to feel. Did they perform it well? Who cares? Did they do it? Yes. I've got my hands on them; they're safe. I know to whom to give the exercise and whom not to, and I know how to push people past their comfort zone.

Ironically sometimes pushing "past the comfort zone" can mean actually reining people in. I like taking students who are "advanced" and pulling them back to a place where they can't be the racehorse that goes all out. They may chomp at the bit but I'm challenging them.

Teaching a new generation about Pilates is challenging, too. What an enormous responsibility. I've got Romana on one shoulder and Joe on the other! I try to make sure that the students understand that teaching Pilates is not a formula of what to wear, and what to say. It's about really seeing the person in front of you, figuring out how best to work with them, and giving them exactly what they need. And to do that takes a lot of work!

I began my training program in 2005. Every year I wax a little more esoteric about it. I think becoming a Pilates teacher is a very profound process. There's a big difference between an instructor and a teacher, and my program has a sort of breakdown/breakthrough process whereby you realize, *I might be good at doing Pilates or even instructing it, but teaching it is a whole different story!*

For that reason I don't take many participants. I usually only have about four to six people in the program at a time. That's a lot, if you ask me. It's a lot of energy. Teaching is sharing. Sharing your passion and your knowledge about this art and science and philosophy of

Contrology with your students. There are clients who are very rigid in how they think and how they do things, and they don't want to be pulled out of that comfort zone and so we, as teachers, have to learn to be adaptable. My hope for the trainees is that they'll learn to really hold and direct a session with positivity and passion. That they can empower without being overpowering. That they learn to teach sessions that are not about them but about the person they're teaching.

As teachers, we must leave our issues at the door. Drop your story. Drop your stuff at the door. You can pick it up on the way out if you want it. When we're here, when we're teaching, it's not about us.

Those kinds of things are hard to teach. I can teach anybody how to do the Footwork. I can teach anybody how to do the Elephant. But being able to teach someone to teach from a place of caring and knowing, without over-thinking, is really tough.

I show videos of Romana teaching and doing. I show videos of Joe Pilates teaching and doing. I want the students to know from whence this method came. I think that most people come into Pilates programs thinking it's about learning the exercises, and they discover that it's about interacting with another human being and being able to teach them on a very profound level. That sometimes it has less to do with the execution of the movements than the spirit in which they are delivered.

You never know what people are going to do with the training once they graduate; you can only give them the foundation, help hone their intuition and hope that they carry Pilates on in a way that is reflective of what you taught them. I can only do what I can do. And, of course, hope for the best.

About Brooke

Brooke began her Pilates training in 1994 under the masterful tutelage of Romana Kryzanowska, spending over a decade basking in her wisdom. She was chosen to sit alongside Romana on the inaugural board of the Pilates Guild and currently sits on the board of the Authentic Pilates Union.

Brooke opened her award-winning NYC studio, re:AB Pilates, in 1997 and in 2000 penned *New York Times'* best-seller *The Pilates Body* followed by *The Pilates Body Kit, Your Ultimate Pilates Body Challenge* and *Element Pilates for Weight Loss*. Brooke's Pilates Teacher Training program began in 2005 and was labeled "The Gold Standard" by *Time Out* magazine.

REFERENCES

[1] Joseph Pilates, *Your Health*. (Incline Village, NV: Presentation Dynamics, Inc., 1998), 16. Originally published in 1934 by Joseph Pilates.
[2] Pilates, 118.
[3] Tracey Pepper. "Journey to the Center." Naturalhealthmag.com/fitness/journey-center?page=2
[4] Pilates, 16.
[5] Robert Wernick. "To Keep in Shape: Act Like An Animal." *Sports Illustrated*, February 12, 1962.

Keeping It Real

By Greg Webster

> *...a flexibility and a strength that I hadn't known before.*

I had a very smart boxing coach who had heard about Pilates and asked me to come check it out. So, I walked into a studio in Chicago where Romana happened to be teaching one day. She was teaching a master class, one of her seminars, and I came in and took a lesson. As Romana is known to do, she just stopped the teacher who was teaching me, grabbed me, took me over to the Wunda Chair and tried to have me do a Pull-Up. I couldn't move the pedal.

Here I was, this big, muscle-bound boxer, and I got really frustrated and upset. Romana, of course, was laughing playfully. I said, "What's the trick to this thing?" She said, "There's no trick, darling. You're just weak." Then she walked away and continued with her teaching. That experience made me so mad that I dedicated myself to learning more.

I'm not sure if it's true, but after Max Schmeling beat Joe Louis in the 1936 Olympics, the story goes that Louis came to see Joe Pilates. Supposedly, Joe Louis said, "I know you trained this guy. How do I beat him?" Louis knew that Pilates was a fighter and had done some boxing training. Pilates said, "Well, you've got to buckle his body. You've got to hit him in his midsection and travel up his spine because I've made his spine like steel."

That story really interested me, because in boxing you're taking very powerful hits and trying to absorb or deflect them. You're getting hit really hard. The object in boxing is to hit someone square in the jaw, so that you cause them to black out. That's what you're trying to do.

So with Pilates, I found immediately that the strength and the power started to return to my spinal column. My ability to take punches got significantly better, and I found a flexibility and a strength that I hadn't known before. Joseph Pilates' idea of the powerhouse, finding internal power to allow the limbs to be an extension of the center of the body, fits perfectly with what you're trying to do in boxing.

The more I discovered about Pilates, the more I started to feel my skills flowing from the center of my body. My arms were an extension of my powerhouse, and I could move quickly with flexibility and power. That was of great use to me as a fighter. It took me to Golden Gloves in Chicago.

My interest grew, and I dove into the archival aspects of Pilates. I started to understand the practical applications that Pilates had for prize fighting. Fighting is an exercise in being totally present. There's nothing quite like being in a boxing ring, having 3,000 people cheering for your blood. Lord knows that's an experience. It's the closest thing, that I can think of, to going to war.

So, like boxing, Pilates is about being present in your body at all times. Through every inch, every second, of Joe's work, from the moment you walk into the studio to when you sit down on a Reformer or other piece of equipment, you have to be completely present and in dialogue with what you do.

For people who don't know what they're looking at, it seems that a punch is actually flying from your upper body, and you're punching from your arm and shoulder. You're not punching from your arm and your shoulder; you're punching from your powerhouse. Your arms need to be totally relaxed for your punches to actually work with speed.

If you watch a fighter's body while he's warming up in the dressing room, his hands are really relaxed. He's flowing. He's bobbing. He's weaving. He's doing all the things that Pilates has put into his work. Pilates exercises employ principles that you use while you're boxing. Pilates and boxing teach relaxation and power.

So often when I coached women, I found that women were naturally better boxers than men because women didn't have the kind of tension in their upper bodies that men have. Therefore, women found it easier to tap into their center. The problem for men, because of what we've been taught, is getting caught up in a huge muscular structure. In the end, you have to allow the muscular structure to be relaxed in relation to the center of your body. So when I punch someone or a bag, the center of my body is tightening while my arms are relaxing. My arms are an extension of the center of my body. That's the only way you can deliver power.

When I was first training with Romana, she told me a great story about when Joe first opened up his place. She said to me, "You know, when this place opened in 1928, it was filled with boxers and strippers, and it was wild." But with the men all going off to war, Joe Pilates had to shift the mantle of his work to a population where he could survive, which was women. The connection to the masculine aspect of Pilates got lost somewhat. The dancers did a very good job keeping Pilates alive, but they also took it in a very particular direction and made it very feminine. And Joe Pilates was a guy's guy. A tough guy.

So part of the work that I started doing in Chicago was to apply Pilates to guys. But what I saw happening was that the work got somehow delicate, feminine. No man would want to go in and do it unless, of course, he was being taught by one of the master teachers. Romana and Juanita Lopez were not delicate. They were excellent teachers.

So I opened a studio with Dave Englund, who also trained with Romana. He and I trained around the same time. We started Evanston Athletic Club. We were both boxers, and we started training fighters at the same time that we were doing Pilates. We shared a common interest in the connection between what was necessary for boxing and what Pilates asked of the body.

I now work in a martial art called Aikido, which is very much based on the blending of energies when people are attacking. In martial arts you spend thousands and thousands of hours trying to get out of your own way to find that connection. It's like when you first learn to swing a baseball bat. First you try to swing it, and you can't hit the ball. You're swinging really hard, and you hit the ball really hard, but the ball doesn't really go anywhere. Then one day you swing the bat, and the ball goes flying. You think, "Wait a minute, I didn't feel like I did anything." That's when your coach looks at you and says, "Now you've got it." And that "you've got it" is the relaxation and the power of allowing your limbs to be an extension of the center of your body.

If you watch any sport, you'll see Pilates all the time. It's just there. Watch Roger Federer hitting a tennis ball. There's a tremendous relaxation and rotation through power. But in order to get that power on your serve, you have to release the tension that's in your neck; you have to release the tension that's in your arms, in your legs; you have to find that deep connection to the center of your body. As soon as you do that, you start hitting hard.

Every movement that Joseph Pilates constructed helps you to connect to your center. Whether your event is trying to walk up a flight of stairs or work as a Cirque du Soleil athlete, Pilates is hands down the simplest way to find the real connection to muscular strength, flexibility, power, and concentration. It's completely efficient in that way.

Currently, I am a Professor of Movement Theater in the Professional Actor Training Program at the University of Connecticut, where I've been teaching for the last six years. Pilates is an integral part of the work that I teach to my graduate M.F.A. students as well as my undergraduate B.F.A. students in preparing them for the profession as actors.

An actor has to be a balance of flexibility and power. And although the bulky muscles are necessary for the industry in terms of looks, they really don't have a practical application for the things that you have to do onstage. One of the things that I find really useful for the performer is that Pilates gives you the longevity that you need for long days of rehearsal and physical activity.

Acting is a physical process if it's done properly. It's physical theater, meaning that we're engaging our bodies in what we do. Because of Pilates, I know exactly what I need to do to mold my body to work on specific things and to do it efficiently. Acting is about being totally present in the moment. That may take 25 years to learn how to do, to put all the garbage aside so that you can really listen with your whole self and your whole body. Pilates work constantly asks me to do just that.

So, if I'm going to play an old man, it requires a certain kind of physicalization. Pilates gives you the background to be able to do that without injuring yourself. Even though I can do the exercises in the system with great skill, I don't even think that way anymore. Now I'm thinking about what I need to do to get through my day. How do I need to train my body to prepare for what I'm going to do?

In terms of performing, I can do things physically that 30-year-old actors can't do. I'm 42 years old. I can roll on the stage. I can flip over things. And that's all a result of the Pilates training. I also know when I can't do something. Pilates has given me that awareness, that sense of control and confidence, so that I know what I can do and also the limits of what I can't.

I'm in much better health than my colleagues who haven't done Pilates. They say, "Well, I can't do that anymore." But I'm thinking, I can do this probably for another 20 years. I can do that roll on the stage, and I can fall down backwards. I can do the Pratt fall. I can do the Buster Keaton/Charlie Chaplin bit that those men did only when they were young men. Pilates gives your body a vocabulary by which you can continue to do very athletic, gymnastic things late into your life. Thank God for that. That's the absolutely practical nature of Pilates.

Pilates builds muscular endurance and suppleness that I really haven't seen in any other form. I also teach Gyrotonic®, which is a wonderful system as well, and various other styles of movement. I've been a personal trainer for almost 15 years. But Pilates is simply the safest and most practical system that I know in the exercise world.

Part of Pilates' genius was initially putting people flat on their backs. In fact, the majority of our health problems are a result of our complete misunderstanding of our relationship to gravity. Joseph Pilates knew that people just didn't know how to hold themselves up. In his work and through its very careful progression, Joe reshapes and trains the body to be balanced in a sustainable way against the force of gravity.

We've all heard the wonderful stories that Romana would tell, about Joe's taking homeless guys off the street in New York, massaging their bodies for half an hour, working them—and suddenly they can walk again, or they start speaking. That kind of power is remarkable. What Joseph Pilates was able to do in 10 lessons is amazing. I've never been able to do that in 10 lessons to anyone, and I'm really good at this stuff. Sure, I can help them, but I haven't been able to totally change their legs and their backs and their entire bodies within 10 to 15 lessons. That's remarkable.

We're still chasing his genius. Every day that I work with clients and performers, I find out more and more about what Joseph was doing.

When I start getting bored with the work, it really means that I'm not paying attention. If you do too many sessions, you start feeling like a mechanic. You're not enjoying the creativity and the spirit of what Joe was doing. You aren't investing your full attention, and that's absolutely necessary with the authentic method. If you are fully present with your client, you will give them an impression of something that's really rich and powerful.

From the moment you start a lesson with Joe Pilates' work, you're sweating. You're doing the Hundred. It hurts, and it's not fun. But I can feel my breath working; I can feel my lungs working; I can do this movement. So people leave a lesson feeling like they've done something really powerful if you work them out right.

Pilates teaches people to listen to their bodies. If I have an injury or if something's hurt, I know exactly what I need to do in order to fix it. I still get hurt. I'm doing very dynamic and dangerous stuff onstage: rolls, fighting with swords, whatever. I get hurt. But I can say, "Okay, I know what that is, and I know how to fix it."

That seems like a small thing, but people have a complete misunderstanding of how their bodies relate to being alive. We need to get people to feel that again. Maybe they've never felt it before, or they only felt it when they were high school athletes. Back then, they had strength and power, but they really didn't know what they were doing physically. Their bodies let them get away with bad habits; then they got injured and couldn't perform anymore.

The restorative power of this work brings people to an understanding of what it is to be human, what it means to be alive. That's the real power of this work. When I have clients who say, "You've changed my life," I try to be very humble. I say, "I didn't do that. That's Joe Pilates' work." I'm a messenger, and I hope that he continues to teach me. But if we don't keep Pilates pure, we're not going to have that genius anymore. The well will become poisoned, and we won't really know what we're doing and why we're doing it.

If the work is done with any kind of integrity, you have to not put 15 people on Reformers and teach a class. It's impossible. I struggle with trios, and I'm an expert. You can't focus all the attention and the power that you need for individual bodies when there are too many.

Groups are just fun for people who already know how to move, and they have a good time.

Mat classes are simply an advertisement for individual lessons. That's how I've set up my business; the Mat class is a way to get the general public to feel something so they'll come in and take a lesson. Then they can enjoy the legacy of this incredibly precise and beautiful classical system.

There is only one method. There is The Method that Joe Pilates taught. I liken it to the Japanese tea ceremony. In ancient Japan, the tea ceremony was done meticulously. Every movement learned, choreographed, and precise. It is taught with ultimate precision, grace, and understanding. That same system of teaching is repeated through thousands of years; it has a lineage. So the Japanese tea ceremony can only be a Japanese tea ceremony. It can't be anything else.

Misrepresentations of Joseph Pilates' work are everywhere, which saddens and angers me. Pilates is a masterpiece. It is a very particular form. So you need to learn it if you want to understand it, instead of making half-hearted attempts at learning. If you learn the system, then you'll get all the benefit from it. If you don't put in the time to learn it, you won't.

The funny thing is, people who've taken a shortcut to learning always come back to us for the information. They literally come back, take a lesson, can't do a Teaser, then go off and teach. At one point, I couldn't teach them anymore because I was so upset by it. Now I've come back around, and I think that I might as well try to represent the work as it is. I try to bring back the joy of Pilates and not be so angry. No good can come of anger.

Now we need to invite people into the fold. Unfortunately, there has been a great deal of in-fighting among the classical teachers. People won't talk to each other and hate each other. All of that is useless, and not what Pilates intended. From everything that I can ascertain, I think Joseph Pilates was a wonderful, jovial guy who approached his work with incredible discipline and dedication and a great spirit.

Pilates and its construction are a masterpiece to me. I feel like every day that I teach or work with the equipment, Joe Pilates is teaching me. In a deep way, his spirit is in all of those pieces of equipment.

I was blessed with an excellent education through Juanita Lopez, Romana and Sari. Pilates has unquestionably improved my boxing, martial arts, and acting. Pilates has connected me to a body that will last a lifetime.

About Greg

Greg Webster joined the performance faculty at University of Connecticut in the fall of 2006. He is also the Movement coach and the resident fight choreographer for the Connecticut Repertory Theater. As a performer, choreographer, and teacher, he has worked from Broadway to the West End. Webster holds a M.F.A. degree in acting and directing from the University of Missouri in Kansas City, and he is a graduate of London International School of Performing. He is a certified teacher of the Authentic Pilates Method of Body Conditioning and the Gyrotonic Expansion System®. Webster holds a black belt in Aikido, and he has been a licensed personal trainer for more than ten years. In addition, Greg is a former Golden Gloves boxer.

Chapter II

On (Our) Teachers

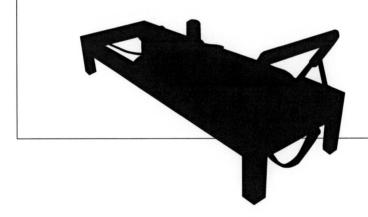

The Apprentice's Tale

By Amy Baria Bergesen

...from then on, every day was an adventure in discovering Pilates.

I spread my yoga mat on the gym floor, the cleanliness of both in question. The gym where I worked as a fitness instructor had officially gotten Pilates. This wasn't "The Method" or the "based-on" stuff that I'd seen around town. This was the real deal with a real instructor. All the gym employees, myself included, were clamoring to get into a class, and I had, at last, succeeded. As any instructor taking a fitness class knows, this is not a comfortable situation. The class participants and other instructors all know you. They expect you to be fit. You expect yourself to breeze effortlessly through any new challenges. It is a command performance with the spotlight on you. So I did my best, taking breathers disguised as clothing adjustments whenever it got to be too difficult. I wasn't about to pant in front of these people. The next day, it hurt to touch my abs. From outside my clothing. Wasn't I a super-fit aerobics goddess? Something had to be done.

Intrigued, I scheduled a private Pilates lesson. I'd never taken a private anything before, so this was a big deal. Private lessons were for rich people or people too uncoordinated to do things without assistance. I was neither—or so I thought. On the blistering afternoon of July 6, 2000, Pilates instructor Carrie Crestman Leal strapped me in for my first Frog on the Reformer. Ever the eager student, I straightened my legs into their extended position with enough force to break through the wall in front of me. Straps and hooks clanged as my legs veered wildly to the left and bobbled in the air. My unruly spine, as yet unassisted by any abdominals, bucked off the carriage. My chin lurched up, and my hands clutched the vinyl.

Even though she was holding my feet, Carrie was so surprised that she literally stepped back, her head quickly dodging my errant feet as she reined in her wide-eyed expression. She grabbed my legs more firmly, and a hasty "bend your knees" followed. With the care needed to instruct an infant, Carrie slowly helped me repeat the exercise: straighten, bend, straighten, bend. She held fast to my feet and the straps, all but arresting the force of my previous attempt. "Now do it with your stomach in," she instructed. The energy I had previously directed to my legs now contorted my face. I performed the Frog again. My legs still longed to stab the air; my interpretation of Frog was a literal one. Frogs jump, right? Shouldn't it be more like that, more froggy? Carrie didn't appear to share this interpretation. Nevertheless, I didn't want to injure Carrie, and she seemed bent on holding my feet and keeping her face dangerously close to them. My Frog was forced into submission.

Satisfied for the moment, Carrie eased the straps off my feet. The session had barely begun, and already I poured sweat. "That's the hardest thing I've ever done," I panted. I kept my literal interpretation of what a Frog should be like to myself. Perhaps, I imagined, Pilates Frogs weren't like real frogs at all. Thus began my Pilates experience.

I became a regular at Willow Pilates Studio in Nashville, Tennessee. Every afternoon I spent there, felt almost like being invited to join a club that was far too good for me. I breathed in the intoxicatingly clean scent of the tea tree oil used to clean the equipment; even the cleaning solution was too good for me. The afternoons when I took lessons were a slow time at the studio. Almost always, I was the lone client. I would walk into the cool, empty, clean-smelling aura of Willow to find Carrie (whose body was the most convincing advertisement for Pilates I've ever seen) in the studio with its owner, Pilates instructor Bambi Watt. They wore amazingly hip workout wear! They didn't wear shoes! They exuded height and confidence and blondeness! I felt squat and lumbering in the presence of The Cool Girls and their super-cool Pilates. On one such afternoon, I began a lesson, trying to squelch the groans of effort that involuntarily escaped my lips, so that the lovely Carrie and Bambi would invite me into their aromatic world. The noises I made were embarrassingly loud. I had walked in on my beefy thighs wearing spandex shorts (Shorts! In a Pilates studio!), my muscles puffy from my devotion to the gym where I worked. Now my body had the audacity to betray me with humiliating noises. I was certain The Cool Girls would not approve.

We began Elephant, which had heretofore been an exercise devoid of any purpose that I could discern. Push out? Pull in? I'm upside down. This is weird. You want my toes up? Utter nonsense. I didn't get it, but I wasn't about to let on. Carrie placed her hand on my ribcage and instructed me to lift. All at once, the three spectacularly large and greasy cheese enchiladas (not to mention the chips and salsa) I had had for lunch let their presence be known as my abdominals actually pulled in the carriage. I had found my powerhouse. I was just a hair shy of vomiting. I would never eat Mexican food before Pilates again. Ever.

Enchiladas aside, I was hooked on the feeling of doing new things with my body—things I hadn't been able to do before. So from then on, every day was an adventure in discovering Pilates. I crammed in lessons at every studio in town in order to learn enough to audition for the Pilates instructor program, then headed by Pilates, Inc. If not adept, I was, at least, dogged. I knew my order. I knew my springs. I knew my transitions. The purpose of the exercises was a bit fuzzy, but I was certain that enough repetition would remedy that problem. With this determination, I entered Springs Studio and began a session with Julie Kraft. I bludgeoned the exercises with my trademark determination, accepting calm, precise instruction from my dark-haired instructor. My brow furrowed with deep concentration. Repetition, repetition, repetition. I refused to be beaten by an exercise method. I already taught all manner of group exercise classes, in addition to being a personal trainer. I would conquer Pilates, as well. Under Julie's direction, I plowed through moves until I arrived at the Front Splits on the Reformer. I stood with one foot on the footbar, executing the second part of the splits. Julie stood, her head just level with my hips, spotting me. We both faced the mirror in front of us, silently taking it all in. I moved the carriage out, and my serious demeanor shattered as I delivered a fart that would make any teenage boy proud. My eyes met Julie's (hers being dangerously close to my behind) in sheer horror. I was so floored by my body and its foul behavior that I could scarcely think. All I could do was avoid further eye contact and continue the exercise, never saying a word out of sheer embarrassment. This same embarrassment kept me from ever entering Springs again. I would have to take lessons elsewhere and hope for a less gassy outcome. So, this is my apology for farting on you, Julie Kraft. Please forgive me.

My embarrassment at Springs coincided with a financial reality check. Private Pilates lessons, an absolute necessity if I wanted to pursue a Pilates career, were something I simply could not afford. I had hoped the gym where I worked could offer some assistance. I hoped to win the lottery. Neither happened. Demoralized, I entered Willow one afternoon and told Bambi and Carrie that this was my last lesson. I fought back tears. I didn't want to imagine my life without the challenge and satisfaction Pilates had brought to it. Then Bambi Watt changed my life forever. "Well, I need more instructors," she began. "Willow could pay for your certification, and you could work for me." My mouth hung open as Bambi's blonde hair glowed like what was, surely, a halo. "I will be the best instructor you've ever had," I stammered. Within 24 hours, we had worked out an agreement. Willow funded my lessons and tuition for the instructor training program, and I would repay the studio by working and teaching there. My Pilates career was officially back on track.

In the fall of 2000, I was accepted into the Pilates instructor training program in Atlanta, Georgia. I still felt like a large, overly-muscled interloper in a world of tall, flexible people with light footsteps. So far, I loved Pilates for the constant challenge it presented to both my mind and body. But my body, though stronger, remained as yet unchanged by the Pilates miracle of which I'd heard tell. I longed for words like lithe, willowy, or even lanky to be used in reference to me.

February 2001 brought my intermediate seminar with Juanita Lopez, and found me floundering in a sea of body image despair. I was a pear-shaped woman, from a long line of pear-shaped women, and a pear I would remain. With her laser gaze seemingly directed right at me, Juanita admonished our apprentice group for our "big bottoms." She stretched the word "bottoms" so that it seemed heavy and round coming out of her mouth. Continuing her tirade, Juanita pointed at the Reformer. "Do you know why it's called the Universal Reformer? Because it Universally Reforms." Eyeing the Circle, she commented, "It's called the Magic Circle because it is magic." Her tone left no room for dissent. I was cowed into silence, now believing not only that my big bottom was a destiny I couldn't escape, but also that Juanita just might be a bit looney tunes. I kept practicing, hoping that sweat would spark a little of that magic Juanita had talked about.

With March came the advanced seminar taught by Romana Kryzanowska. It was my first time to meet the woman, the legend. All of us apprentices had heard magical tales featuring Romana at the center of the action: "Romana knows bodies. She can take one look at you and know exactly what your body needs." Statements like this were common in the Pilates world, and universally believed. I wanted Romana to take one look at me and know how to make me not a pear. And for that transformation to happen instantly, with the touch of the magical Pilates wand she surely possessed. That weekend Romana worked us relentlessly, smiling all the while. After we'd muddled through the "businessman's luncheon," a series of 12 Teasers done in a circle like the numbers on a clock, Romana expounded on luncheons and the like. She told us we needed to do Leg Springs every day: "You don't need a snack. Leg Springs are your snack," she reasoned. Her metaphor echoed Juanita's "big bottoms" comment. I practiced harder. Then I began my apprentice hours in New York.

New York. Drago's Gym. Mecca for all Pilates devotees. Another chance for me to work with Romana and for her to change my body. I was still waiting for the magic wand. When Romana finally did look at me, she determined that what my body needed was not the touch of a magic wand, but a good butt-kicking. During my first lesson with Romana at Drago's, I prepared to get back on the Reformer after Balance Off, a movement resembling a Front Walkover. As my head tucked under, my shoulder slipped out from under me. I had fallen in a pool of my own sweat, landing like a belly-up turtle, legs waving wildly in the air. Romana chuckled. When I met the same fate the very next day, Romana, smiling, suggested I keep a towel handy. The third time I began to slide in the sweat pool, I was able to right myself just in time. Progress. Romana nodded approvingly. The effort and humiliation of it all were, at least, not making the pear that was me any worse.

Apprentices in New York spent afternoons learning our craft at 2121 Broadway under the tutelage of Michael Fritzke and Ton Voogt. They were the den mothers we apprentices all so desperately needed. Affirming and instructive, they brought thoughtful teaching and keen observation to life for me. Even better, they didn't make me feel stupid for asking questions—even stupid ones. They were the teachers I wanted to be.

Almost a year after my first lesson with Carrie, I had a private lesson with Michael. I was on my stomach, doing the beats to transition from one side to the other during the Side Kicks series. Michael stopped me. "Try using this part of your butt, rather than this part." I tried and failed. I tried again. By the end of the lesson, I had just begun to feel my muscles working differently, and I was intrigued. I practiced all afternoon, the next day, and the day after that. I had my hands on my bottom almost constantly, checking my muscles for cooperation. When at last my muscles reacted accordingly, I shared my breakthrough with the apprentices, especially the pear-shaped ones. Soon we were all touching our bottoms, compulsively tightening different muscles to see the effect. Three days after my lesson with Michael, I truly had a brand new butt. I checked myself out in every shop window, mirror, and reflective surface I passed, happy beyond belief at the disappearance of the pear.

My apprenticeship wore on, with one or two week intervals in New York, followed by a few weeks at home in Nashville. I spent more and more time at Willow, practicing teaching Pilates to any friend who was willing. Each time I made the trip to New York, I followed the flight plan as dictated by priceline.com: Nashville to St. Louis to New York. What the trip lacked in efficiency it made up for in price; there was no cheaper way to get to New York from Nashville. And by clicking the "fly anytime" button, I saved even more of my precious dollars for my Pilates travel expenses.

If not afraid of flying, I was at least respectful of it. I always flew wearing some kind of jeans or sweats with tennis shoes. I wanted to be able to leap, legs protected, from a burning fuselage and make a run for my life. I always tried to sit on an exit row, and if this proved impossible, I counted the seats between my own and the nearest exit. I was not about to trust my life with a row of little bitty lights to a distant doorway. Not me. I wore my hair up in a ponytail—less likely to catch fire or slow me down. And because of my intense germophobia, I never used a pillow or blanket supplied by the airline. But I digress.

The sheer number of flights I made that summer finally wore me down. I decided to quit acting like a scared baby and enjoy my frequent flying. So what if it wasn't vacation. I was going to New York. A lot. That in itself was cool. And I was training to teach Pilates. Cooler still. On the morning of August 9, 2001, I was scheduled to fly to New York again. I put on my favorite miniskirt, a floral wraparound that I'd gotten on sale. And my high-heeled black sandals. When I boarded TWA flight 1019, I sat on a non-exit row and didn't even bother counting seats. I wasn't Rain Man, after all. I was 32 years old, I was embarking on a glamorous new career path, and my ass looked great. I kept the ponytail. I liked my ponytail.

The plane took off from Nashville only to find there was inclement weather in St. Louis. We landed in Springfield to wait it out. There went making my connection to New York. I was in a dither. Each of my trips to New York was calculated down to the last hour: apprenticeship hours. I needed six hundred, and this delay would cost me at least eight. That meant another day off from my job in Nashville. More chagrin from my boss. More lost wages. I called my husband, Eric, while the plane was grounded in Springfield to vent about the situation. The next time I called him I would be in a field in Missouri.

At last we took off for St. Louis. We started our descent, and cruised by the airport without landing. That's odd. We flew by again, but more slowly. This time there were a group of men on the runway, pointing up at us. We were close enough to see their white, short-sleeved shirts and ties. Again, we arced back up into the air without landing. Passengers started pressing flight attendant call buttons all over the plane: "Ding. Ding. Ding." No flight attendants came. People leaned from their seats into the aisle, looking for someone to answer their questions. My heart beat faster.

After several minutes, the flight attendants emerged. The one nearest me had mascara streaks running down her face. She didn't say a word as the captain came over the intercom, explaining our situation. Someone in Springfield had failed to remove the wheel chocks from our front wheels before we took off for St. Louis. Now our front landing gear wouldn't come down. Our previous fly-bys had confirmed this. That explained the men on the ground. The cabin buzzed with instant conversation among the passengers. On a row alone, I sat dumbfounded. I struggled to breathe. I was nauseous with fear.

The pilot detailed our plan of action. We would dump our fuel while practicing crash position. We would move able-bodied and willing people to the exit rows and teach them how to open the doors. "I would say this is a very survivable situation," he concluded. Very survivable?!!? Very?! Survivable?!!? Surely the pilot had been schooled in soft-peddling the truth to distraught passengers. Was "very survivable" the best he could do? If that was his idea of a positive spin, I reasoned, we were all going to die.

Silenced by disbelief, I robotically followed along with the flight attendant as she instructed us in proper crash position. Big, young men were asked if they could handle opening the door of an exit row, and were seated there when they agreed. A tall, friendly-looking man of about my age in a navy blue baseball cap had been chosen for an exit row. He listened earnestly to everything the flight attendant said. He nodded as she explained the handle mechanism. His blue eyes were very wide, but not afraid. I wished I could be at his exit.

In this manner, an hour passed. We flew what seemed like miles away to dump fuel over a field. I extracted my wallet with my driver's license from my purse, and shoved it inside my bra. We wouldn't be allowed to carry anything off the plane (assuming we survived the very survivable landing), and I wanted someone to be able to identify my lifeless body. I tried to cram my phone into my underwear, but I couldn't make it fit with my seatbelt on in extra-tight crash mode, so I left it in my purse. The amethyst earrings that were a birthday present to my sister-in-law would also have to stay on board.

I longed to call my husband, but feared any illicit calls might crash the plane earlier than planned. I wished myself home. I wished myself at Drago's, falling in a pool of my own sweat while doing Reformer exercises. Or any exercises. I wanted to be anywhere but on this plane. Then began the bargaining: God, if you let me make it through this alive, I will show Eric how much I love him every single day. I will be a better person. A better daughter. I won't check out my ass in every shop window I pass. Then, with my arms tucked tightly under my legs and my eyes squeezed shut, the plane crash-landed. I managed not to pee myself.

Even with my head down and my eyes shut, everything went orange. Fire. We were sliding fast, not banging or jolting like a car wreck. The ground crew had prepped the runway of the MidAmerica Airport for our arrival with fire-extinguishing foam. By the time we stopped moving, smoke had filled the cabin. You couldn't see a single one of the tiny lights on the floor. Not one.

As I reached the bottom of the inflated slide, my wraparound skirt flew up around my neck. Fire-extinguishing foam shot straight up my thong underwear. My high-heeled sandals were barely on, but the ponytail was intact. A beautiful, young, blonde man in a flight suit—surely no more than eighteen years old—extended his hand down to me. I fought to push down my skirt. "Ma'am, may I help you up?" he said. The Air Force had been called to our aid (and from what I could tell, the Air Force was comprised of nothing but young hotties). I took his hand, and, minutes later, I borrowed his phone to call my husband from the field next to the runway. The passengers stood stunned while the Air Force hotties and the airline personnel took turns counting us. Over and over again. By the time they were convinced we were all present and accounted for, it was dusk. I shared a celebratory pack of menthol cigarettes with some of my fellow passengers. Around 2 a.m., we were at last bussed to an airport hotel. I had to catch my rebooked connecting flight in two hours. And I hadn't eaten since breakfast the day before in Nashville, a lifetime ago.

Sleep deprived and badly shaken, I arrived the next afternoon at Drago's. But now I was a changed person. Clearly, if I could survive a plane crash (emergency landing, the official term, just didn't seem to do justice to the whole experience), I could survive a Pilates certification program. I would no longer live my life in fear. I called Eric to share my new resolve: "I'm gonna go camping, and I'm gonna have kids, and I'm gonna spend as much money as I want!" Not only did I have a new backside, but a euphoric new lease on life, as well. Open Leg Rocker seemed a bit less daunting, to say the least.

For the first few days after the crash, I walked around the Pilates studios in New York in a daze. I was so happy to be alive! I was so sore from the landing it hurt to move! I interspersed my apprentice hours with a few visits to Larry, the resident massage therapist at the 2121 studio. He, and the introduction of bio-freeze, helped me get over the soreness and on with my life. I smelled like menthol almost constantly, but I was feeling better. I worked on the Arm Weights series, and Side-Kicked until I lost count. I bought some life-affirming glitter jeans at H&M. I couldn't wait to parade around Nashville in them. Because life is too short to not wear glitter anytime you want, even on your bottom. And nothing's better than a brand new booty—except a sparkling brand new booty. With no back pockets. That's some serious butt confidence. (And, regardless of all the myriad benefits Pilates truly offers, from a supple spine to pain-free joints, wouldn't any woman trade all those for the butt of her dreams? Seriously.) I slowly began to settle into my usual New York routine.

Mornings, as usual, were spent at Drago's. My hands had finally figured out how to best help the client. I could zero in on a ribcage with no problem at all. I never had to think about the order of the exercises; it just happened. I could move around the Reformer as a teacher, something that had seemed so awkward just months before. Afternoons and evenings were devoted to 2121 Broadway. I did Leg Springs for "a snack" almost every day. If we (the apprentices) forgot our socks, Elba, the receptionist, would offer her own. When she needed us to shake the love potion she'd made to send her wayward boyfriend running back, we were happy to oblige. We practiced teaching each other. We Rolled Like a Ball. Elba filled in the gaps by reading our tarot cards. The apprentices I'd been working with all along were close to completing their hours, and I was, too. We had regular clients, and we could help their bodies. My body needed help, too. The seatbelt had damaged my hip flexors during the crash landing, but Pilates was helping my recovery. For both myself and my clients, Pilates was really working.

A novice in my Pilates career, I nonetheless felt ready to teach. The crash landing had helped put Pilates into perspective for me. It was (and is) a life-affirming career choice, and I was thrilled to be changing people's lives, beginning with their bodies. I was also ready to fly home, convinced that lightning—in this case a plane crash—wouldn't strike twice. I felt ready, even, to start a family. Pilates felt like the puzzle piece my life had been missing in order to move forward. Now I was ready on all fronts.

My post-crash welcome home was glorious. I threw embarrassment to the wind and flung myself at my husband, who was waiting at the gate in Nashville. It was summertime, 2001, and it would be the last time he could meet me at the gate. I had to make one final trip to New York to complete my apprenticeship and final exam.

Sometime around 5:00 a.m. on September 11th, I quietly waited on the platform in Pelham, New York (where I stayed with my sister-in-law on my Pilates junkets. She did get her amethyst earrings.) to board the commuter train to Manhattan. Still dark outside, it was a cool morning. The man next to me, wearing braids and a hoodie, was there every morning, too. We exchanged glances. Then the train came, and I was off to Drago's.

It was my last day of practice before my final practical exam, scheduled for September 12th. The early hours were spent observing Romana and nibbling a pumpernickel bagel. Around midmorning, clients arrived at the studio buzzing about something happening at the Trade Center. Some clients didn't show up. Pilates studios are short on televisions and radios, to say the least, so I and my apprentice friends pulled out our cell phones and started calling. But none of our phones would work. Slowly news arrived, via incoming instructors and clients, of the plane crashes. If not hysterical, we were all puzzled, even spooked. We needed a full story, some explanation. Drago closed the gym.

With nothing to do but earn our hours, the apprentices left Drago's and began the walk to 2121, which we hoped was still open. The streets of the city were thronged with pedestrians, all of whom were strangely quiet. Every store was closed, save the street vendor who sold me cigarettes, my go-to in times of stress. Lines for banks and ATMs were hundreds of people long. My phone worked long enough for me to reach my husband, and he filled in the details of the attack on the Trade Center. We all spent a strange afternoon and evening at 2121 Broadway, stunned and questioning. At closing time, I couldn't go back to Pelham—the trains had all stopped. Fellow apprentice Zan Walker graciously led all of the Pilates homeless back to her nearby apartment for the night. The next morning was my final exam.

September 11th was no crash landing. September 11th was a plane crash. Now I understood the difference. No one had died in my crash, and I had emerged a little dazed and mildly injured. What the crash landing had done for my mental clarity, September 11th put into sharp relief. So although my final exam with Sari seemed a little surreal, it had none of the gut-wrenching anxiety I would have brought to it prior to August 9th or September 11th. We all had bigger issues to consider. The exam was fine. I was fine. It was done.

I got back to Pelham on September 12th, and returned to the city the next morning to complete my very last apprentice hours. The man with the braids and hoodie was on the train platform. Relief washed over me. Our faces registered mutual happiness to see each other alive. We smiled and introduced ourselves. He gave me a business card. He was a karate instructor. I told him about Pilates. So September 11th did that, too. Everyone was nicer for a little while.

I flew home to Nashville on September 17th, one of only two passengers on the airplane. With my new backside and newly minted certification, I was ready to go. Now, after nearly 12 years and 2 children, Pilates still delivers. My lingering hip flexor injury only flares up when my Pilates workouts flag. Even though all I'd hoped for was the end to my pear-shaped figure and thick thighs, I had emerged fully transformed. The injuries I sustained, literally on my way to my certification, brought me the means and understanding to handle chronic injuries. Pilates enabled me to help and teach my clients, whether they suffer from back pain or just want a perkier behind. I'm a teacher who teaches from personal experience, changing bodies and lives every day. I still work hard to make my muscles behave, gaining control with practice and hoping for a little of Juanita's magic. And I'm back to sitting on the exit row when I fly.

About Amy

A native of Houston, Texas, Amy Baria Bergesen holds a Ph.D. in English from Louisiana State University. She completed her Pilates certification at the Pilates Studio of New York under Romana Kryzanowska in 2001. The non-impact environment of Pilates, as well as its personalized care of injuries, has not only reshaped her body, but healed it as well. She lives and teaches Pilates in Nashville, Tennessee.

Pilates and Kathy Grant

By Blossom Leilani Crawford

...she was a force of nature.

The first time I heard the word Pilates, I was a dance student in Hawaii. Then I went to N.Y.U. in 1993, and I majored in dance in my freshman year. During my first or second week, I had a Mat class with Kathy Grant. That was my introduction to Pilates. I always think the way it was introduced to me was funny, because Kathy didn't start with the Hundred. I think she taught three exercises, and maybe we did one abdominal exercise. There was definitely nothing I recognized as Pilates, but I remember knowing that it was going to help me.

At the time, I had a back injury. I couldn't do any sort of backbend without pain, and for some reason I just knew that this woman was going to help me. I just knew that she was going to make me stronger. In the first week of class, I realized how weak I was. If I really wanted to be a professional dancer and keep up with the schedule, I should be able to do a sit up. But the way Kathy taught us to practice a sit up, I could barely do it.

So I took Kathy's class a lot, as many times as possible during my freshman year. In my second and third years of school it was no longer required, but I kept going because I saw and felt results. During those years I studied with Kathy privately in her studio at N.Y.U. She was the one who helped me regain my strength. I could do backbends again. I also became a better dancer. I actually felt the connection between my limbs and my torso. Just doing the work of Pilates improved my mental stamina. I remember Kathy saying, "This is just the alphabet. You have to put it together and use it to do something." I learned how to take care of myself because of The Method, not only because I knew which exercises to practice, but also because I learned how to listen to my body. I really learned to listen to it.

When I graduated in 1996, I had a crazy summer when I didn't get to dance much. I was out in the real world, and I was waiting tables, making a living. I was eating a lot, and gaining weight and not exercising as much. I was very unhappy with it all, because I didn't have the structure that school had given me. I remember one day very clearly. I was at a terrible bartending job, and I was thinking, "How can I convince Kathy to let me take her morning class again?" If I were able to take her morning Mat class, it would set me up for the rest of the day, even for the rest of the week. Just after I had that thought, I checked my voicemail during a break at the terrible bartending job. Kathy had left me a message, saying, "Blossom, I'm having a little procedure done. I could use someone to demonstrate for me for a few weeks." I leapt at the chance.

After the first couple of times I demonstrated for her, Kathy came up to me and said, "You know, why don't you just keep coming?" So I continued to demonstrate and started assisting Kathy for two or three years for free. The work eventually became a position at N.Y.U. I assisted Kathy for 10 years and continued to help her at workshops that she taught all around the country. Eventually my role developed into much more. I ended up being the person who assisted Kathy in the studio. Sometimes I was teaching, or maybe showing someone how to do an exercise, or even completing some type of administrative work. I continued all of those activities until she passed away.

Kathy was a woman unto herself. Each person brings his own point of view and life experience to Pilates. Kathy's life experience of the work came from a place of rehabilitation. She had had two knee surgeries in one year with no rehab, and when she chose to go back to dancing, she was in ridiculous amounts of pain. So, when Kathy went to study with Mr. Pilates, she didn't do the Hundred. Her approach to the Pilates work was different, and I think that really shaped her teaching. She was very independent: she was a black woman going to Mr. Pilates in the 1960s.

Kathy said that Mr. Pilates didn't verbally articulate many words when he was teaching. When Mr. Pilates said, "That was good," Kathy had to figure out what was good about it. She wasn't coddled. Kathy's teaching was very much like Mr. Pilates' teaching. She didn't use a lot of descriptions. She would never say, "Blossom, I really need you to not use your hip flexor so much. I want it to come from this place." Instead, she'd poke you or push you and say, "No." You would try again, and she would say, "No." Later on in life, when Kathy and I would talk, I said, "Kathy, sometimes you're really mean, and sometimes you don't explain. You could describe more of what you want." She would reply, "Well I don't want to explain because I need students to think. I want them to think about what they're doing, and how they can improve. They can't afford to have me around all the time." That was Kathy's experience with Mr. Pilates, and that is how he taught her.

Using your mind and being independent in the work; that's what is missing in Pilates today. I struggle with it myself. The way the work is taught now, people pay good money for a private session, so they expect a certain amount of attention from the teacher. Some students want their teacher to do the work for them. The Pilates Method, however, is best when both teacher and student are working equally. The client should be thinking and giving you feedback, just as much as you, the teacher, are thinking and giving feedback. The teacher can't do all the work, and the student can't do all the work. I understand my role as a teacher, but after a while, you've got to take the training wheels off. So I would like to have open studio time when people can exercise independently. The test of a good teacher is what your students are doing when you're not in the room. As much as I loved Kathy, she taught me how to not need her. But I still do.

It has been two years since Kathy passed away, and I still can't believe she's not around. It's so hard for me. After she died, I wrote that she was a force of nature. I still think this way because there's no one like her. She didn't lie. She didn't mince words. She would be either the first person or the last person I'd want to talk to, because she'd tell me the truth. There's a sense in which Kathy keeps teaching me today, which I find even more amazing. I still hear her words in my head. There are many things I didn't quite get while Kathy was alive, and now I'm beginning to finally understand them.

For example, the first time she taught me on the Reformer at N.Y.U., she gave me a one- or two-minute explanation of the apparatus. She said, "This is the footbar, and it goes up like this and it goes down like this. This is the head rest; it goes up like this and down like this. The handles, when they're not in use, they go here." At the time, I was thinking, "Lady, can I just get on the apparatus?" But now I get it. She'd had the Pilates studio equipment since the 1970s, and it had been with her. There was a history. She took really good care of the equipment, and she didn't want you to break it. Also, when she said, "Put your headrest down," she wanted you to know what that meant.

Now when I have people who push or bang on my machine, I cringe. I get it. I understand why Kathy taught us this way. So, in many ways, she still teaches me now.

Even when Kathy was alive—and could have rested on her laurels—she kept learning. She wanted to go and see and be involved. Once I told her that I was going to go check out a Chair workshop. She said, "Let's go together." She could have said, "Oh, that's not how I do it," but she was truly interested in what people were teaching, what they were practicing and why. Kathy also wanted to know how the work may have changed or evolved. She really saw things from a larger perspective.

One of the greatest lessons Kathy taught me was when she sent me to Romana's studio to get certified. In my mind, my loyalty was with Kathy. After a couple of weeks, I went back to Kathy, and she asked, "Well, how's it going?" I was in the process of getting certified. I started saying, "Oh, it's terrible. They just put you right on the Reformer, and they just make you do this stuff"—but Kathy stopped me. She yelled at me. I kept saying, "Kathy, you don't understand. They do this." She slammed her hand down on the Chair, and she said, "No, Blossom." Then I said, "Kathy, it's so different." She slammed her hand down again. "No. It's the same." I protested. Yet she said, "Blossom, it's the same. What is the point? The point is to get the food from the bowl into your mouth. I use the fork. They use chopsticks. The point is to get the food from the bowl to your mouth." Kathy made me realize the point was to move people. Once I looked at it from that point of view, as opposed to my judgmental point of view, I was able to learn and see and understand. I came to a point where I actually learned something, instead of just judging. That's one of the biggest lessons she ever taught me. I truly had one of the best teachers ever. Being in the room with her and listening to her talk was like a gift every time.

I was very fortunate to witness the boom of Pilates while I was assisting Kathy. So I started in 1993, as a student. Seventeen years later, it was a totally different Pilates world. Kathy's former students were teaching Pilates and opening studios. Kathy was deeply respectful of The Method, and she worried about people just going off and teaching it. What hurt Kathy the most was that she didn't hear about these things from her students. So, I learned that respect is something especially important in your Pilates business. You must be ethical. So, when I started thinking about opening my own studio, I spoke to Kathy right away. I told her, "This is what I'm thinking about doing." It's always best to be ethical and as respectful as possible. That's something that Kathy definitely taught me.

Kathy's view of ethics extended to individual exercises. When Kathy asked me to teach Eve Gentry's exercise called Threading the Needle at N.Y.U., she made me say, "Eve Gentry's Threading the Needle," every time. When I asked her why, she said, "These people will be forgotten if we don't say their names. And, this is not my exercise." Kathy wanted teaching done the right way, with the utmost integrity. So, when I teach a workshop, I actually call people from whom I've learned exercises and ask them if it's okay. I feel that's the right choice to make; it's something Kathy taught me. It's being respectful of the people in your community.

Kathy defined her work by the people who studied with her and by the individuals who teach with the same values. She believed it was a big democracy of different people who studied with her. Even though it's difficult to organize all of these individuals, Kathy's work lives on, the way she intended it, as a collection of different memories for each person. Each of us has our own collection.

About Blossom

Blossom has been practicing and teaching Pilates for over 15 years. Her introduction to the Pilates method was in 1993 through Master Teacher Kathleen Stanford Grant, while Crawford was a dance student at N.Y.U. Tisch School of the Arts. Using Pilates, she learned to heal and care for her back, easing her chronic back pain. From 1997 to 2007, she was teaching assistant to Mrs. Grant's Pilates Mat class at Tisch. Certified by Romana Kryzanowska, Blossom is owner and director of Bridge Pilates in Brooklyn, New York. She continues to teach Mat classes at the Mark Morris Dance Center in downtown Brooklyn.

The Spirit of Pilates
By Brett Howard

> *...for the work to hold its integrity, the spirit has to be passed along.*

As a student of Romana Kryzanowska, Lolita San Miguel, Mary Bowen, Kathy Grant and Jay Grimes, I feel I have a unique perspective on Pilates. I have spent the most time studying with Romana, and she has the greatest influence on my teaching of the Pilates method. Her perspective is the lens I see and teach through the most. I feel very fortunate to have been around such a passionate person and remarkable teacher and to have learned from her vast knowledge of the method. I am also grateful to all of my other wonderful and passionate teachers of Pilates. I am blessed to be able to gaze through their lenses and incorporate what I have learned from them into my teaching. I have learned much, not only from Romana's perspective, which I value, but from the perspectives of all my teachers and from that of Joseph Pilates and his method of Contrology.

I often ask myself how I should teach with these different stored experiences and perspectives, and at the same time retain the core values of the traditional method and my own voice as a teacher? How do I retain the plurality of perceptions and understandings, yet still find that core of teaching the Pilates method of body conditioning, of Contrology and Physical Culture? I have a definite intention of staying true to the work of Joseph Pilates. I try to honor his concepts, his exercises, his objectives and his beliefs. My goal is to stay true to Contrology. But what is Contrology? What is the Pilates Method? The Pilates method of body conditioning is an exercise system focused on improving flexibility, strength and balance for the total body. It is a series of controlled and systematic movements coupled with focused breathing patterns. But most important, I believe Pilates is a balance of Body, Mind and Spirit, all functioning perfectly as a coordinated whole. Joseph Pilates wrote, "The acquirement and enjoyment of physical well-being, mental calm and spiritual peace are priceless to their possessors if there be any such so fortunate living among us today. However, it is the ideal to strive for, and in our opinion, it is only through Contrology that this unique trinity of a balanced body, mind and spirit can be attained" (Pilates, Return to Life Through Contrology, 1945). Furthermore, "Perfect balance of Body and Mind is that quality in civilized man which not only gives him superiority over the savage and animal kingdom, but furnishes him with all the physical and mental powers that are indispensible for attaining the goal of Mankind—Health and Happiness" (Pilates, 1934).

While staying true to the work of Pilates I need to maintain my values and identity as an educator. I honor all of my past experiences, which define who I am and how I perceive things. My experiences give me a unique perspective that is unlike any other. This is the same formula that makes every teacher unique. Teachers pull from their own past experiences, which color who they are. On the flip side, the more I learn and the greater knowledge I acquire, the less I feel I know. This becomes a constant struggle. Am I accomplishing what I'm aiming for? Is there is a right way to do the work, and if so what is it? How, exactly, should I be teaching this? How can I best stay true to what Pilates created as well as to his vision and mission? The list of questions is endless.

This path of self-reflection and uncertainty is a path I believe I will continue to travel for the duration of my Pilates experience. I am very critical of myself. I have a great thirst for knowledge and understanding. Knowledge is never-ending. I want to be a sponge and soak up as much as I can. I reflect on the "Empty Your Cup" story my good friend Clare Dunphy told at a workshop we were coteaching that resonated with me. The story goes: A university professor went to visit a famous Zen master. While the master quietly served tea, the professor talked about Zen. The master poured the visitor's cup to the brim, and then kept pouring. The professor watched the overflowing cup until he could no longer restrain himself. "It's overfull! No more will go in!" the professor blurted. "You are like this cup," the master replied. "How can I show you Zen unless you first empty your cup?" I strive to be an empty cup that can always learn more.

I have had the special privilege to learn from the archival material that Joseph Pilates left behind. I consider these materials a valuable reference, similar to the first-generation teachers, whom I consider to be living references. Pilates is an oral history, passed down through the generations. I learned from Romana and many of the other first-generation teachers, they learned from Joseph Pilates and Clara, and my students learn from me. All of the first-generation teachers had their own unique and separate experiences with Joseph Pilates, and they all took from and contributed to the work in their own special ways.

When I look at how Romana Kryzanowska taught the work, I find some small differences between how she taught and how Joseph Pilates taught, according to the archival materials. And Romana's teaching differs from many of the other first-generation teachers. Was Romana wrong? I would say no. Her changes and additions to the exercises further substantiated the method while retaining its core values. Romana helped to systematize the method. Romana also simplified some of the movements to make them more manageable, so that difficult skills would be more attainable later in one's practice. This is not changing the work. Yes, influences of dance appeared in the work from Romana, but this was something that helped her understanding and teaching of the method. Romana's past experience was definitely a part of what makes her such an amazing teacher.

I studied the least with Kathy Grant, but I believe that she took the exercises in a different and valuable direction while staying true to the method. She developed ways to help students understand what skills are present in which exercises then strengthen those skills, so that later in their practice, when they were required to perform the skills in combination, they had success in the execution of the exercises. I believe this is what she called the "Before the Hundred Series," a concept very similar to what Eve Gentry did with Pre-Pilates: giving basic breakdowns or modifications to allow for success. I call this scaffolding, based on a theory in education that can be found in the work of Lev Vygotsky and Jerome Bruner (see, for example, Vygotsky's book Mind in Society, 1978). Scaffolding is the provision of sufficient support to promote learning when concepts and skills are first being introduced to students. Supports are gradually removed as students develop autonomous learning strategies, thus promoting their own cognitive, affective and psychomotor learning skills and knowledge. I apply the theory of scaffolding in my teaching, and I applaud Kathy Grant and Eve Gentry for fostering this in the method of Pilates.

I applaud all of the contributions from all of the first-generation teachers. They have all stayed true to the work but have made the work their own by pulling from their own experiences. They have their differences and similarities, but in the end they teach the exercises they learned from Joseph Pilates in more or less the same way. I remember attending a workshop with Lolita San Miguel during which she emphasized really pulling the leg in on the Single Leg Stretch. I remember her saying, "You don't just place the hands on the leg, you have to pull the leg in. Why is no one pulling the leg anymore?" A couple of months later I attended a workshop with Jay Grimes, and he lectured on the Single Leg Stretch as well, saying, "Why doesn't anyone pull the leg anymore? You don't lightly place the hands on the leg. You have to pull the leg in."

The first-generation teachers have their own plurality. They all have or had great admiration and respect for Joseph Pilates and the method he created. Studying with them, I came to realize that they all share a very special energy, which I believe is the Spirit of Pilates. Many times we emphasize an integration of body and mind, but we must remember that Pilates is a balance of body, mind and spirit. "Es ist der Geist, Der sich den Korperbaut" is a favorite quote of Joseph Pilates by Friedrich Schiller, which roughly translates as: "It is the spirit that builds the body." The word spirit comes from the Latin word spiritus, which means "breath." Spirit is a noncorporeal substance, in contrast to the material body, that in living things usually refers to or explains consciousness. It survives the body. This is something that is hard to explain or pinpoint, but this is the plurality of the first-generation teachers. This is the energy they all possess, the common thread that links them together. It was passed to them by Joseph Pilates, and they in turn have passed it on to my generation. I hope my contemporaries and I pass it on to the next generation.

I am a product of my teachers. Some are no longer with me, and some I continue to learn from, but they are all inside of me. Their passion and energy, as well as their voices, are still present within me. The words and corrections they gave me are still in my body. I remember that feeling I had at Drago's Gym; there was something special there. When I learn from and talk with Lolita San Miguel—a woman who is not just my teacher and mentor, but someone I consider a dear friend who has always been there for me—the same special feeling is present. It's a feeling you have deep in your body. You can't describe it, you just feel it.

Sometimes when I'm teaching, I'll say, "Arriba!" and it's just like Romana jumped out of my mouth. It's not intentional. Another memory I have is of Romana teaching the Hug on the reformer. She would make you push her away with your arm when you opened your arms. She'd say, "Push me. Push." Then she'd say, "You can't push me, can you, because I'm using my powerhouse." Sometimes at the end of the day, Romana would sit on a couch at the front of Drago's Gym, by Drago's desk right where the elevators opened, and have informal apprentice meetings. She often called me Young One. She'd say, "Young One, did you learn something today? What did you learn?" Then I would say to myself, oh God, think of something quick, even though I had gained a plethora of information. With my apprentices, I say the same thing: "Did you learn something today?" And I always say it with the Romana voice. I share my journey with them. I tell them my stories and experiences from working with my teachers, and I tell them the stories my teachers told me of their experiences with Joseph Pilates. These things can't be lost. It's about passing the torch. I love these stories. Sometimes Romana would imitate Joe. She'd say, "Strong like bull" in a German accent. Mary Bowen once told me, "I had had a really bad day one day, and that day Mr. Pilates was on me relentlessly. You could feel the tension. All of a sudden you hear 'Pow.' The spring just snapped in half and broke. I believe it's because my energy was so strong and his energy was so strong." Every time I hear Lolita talk about her experiences with Joseph Pilates and Carola Trier, I feel so happy to have been let into this place that I wasn't able to see with my own eyes. These stories are part of carrying the spirit. All of my teachers had and still have that spirit, even though each of them had a different experience with Joe.

All of my apprentices have a different experience with me. I try to provide them with the most quality experiences I can. As an educator, my role is to organize and facilitate direct experiences of phenomena under the assumption that this will lead to genuine, meaningful and long-lasting learning. This is experiential learning, a theory developed by John Dewey, an American philosopher, psychologist and educational reformer whose ideas have been influential in education and social reform. I base my teaching and learning on these very ideas.

Experiential learning is learning that develops through reflection on everyday experiences, with an emphasis on the quality and nature of participants' subjective experiences. There are two principles that explain the nature of experience: continuity and interaction. In continuity, all experiences are carried forward and influence other experiences. In interaction, present experiences arise out of the relationship between a situation and an individual's stored past.

It is my feeling that all of the first-generation teachers had their own, different experiences with Joseph Pilates. They were different individuals and came from different backgrounds. They studied with him at different times in his and their lives. They also had different challenges within their bodies. Romana first came to Joseph Pilates with an ankle injury. Lolita, Kathy and Carola had knee issues. He gave each of them different advice and instruction so that the method made the most sense for their own body. Each was a different kind of learner as well.

Everyone learns differently. When I teach my clients and apprentices I teach them in a way that helps them best understand the method. I make sure I don't teach everyone the same way. I have to teach to the intelligence of that learner to create the greatest success for them. I pull from a theory in education developed by Howard Gardner, called Multiple Levels of Intelligence. It's a model that differentiates intelligence into various specific (primarily sensory) modalities, rather than seeing it as dominated by a single general ability. Gardner differentiated nine different intelligences: Spatial, Linguistic, Logical-mathematical, Bodily-kinesthetic, Interpersonal, Intrapersonal, Naturalistic, Musical Rhythmic and Existential.

This can help explain how there can be different interpretations of the Pilates method. All of the first-generation teachers stressed and emphasized different things from the same body of work. They might have interpreted the work differently, but that has only enhanced the method. I can be teaching a group of apprentices the same material, but they will all walk away with a different interpretation of the material. One apprentice might focus on what type of verbal corrections I give, another might focus on what type of tactile feedback I give, and another might focus on where and how I'm spotting. Some might focus on why I'm giving particular modifications to the client in front of me, others on my rhythm and dynamics of the exercises, and others on the imagery I'm giving. The list is endless, but everything an apprentice might focus on is valuable. Different people will stress different things. That's why it's important to be able to look through multiple lenses, which I am fortunate to have acquired from my various teachers.

If I have a client, and a concept is not quite coming across how I want it to, I have to decide what is the best lens to use to help the client understand. For a client who comes in the next hour, I might need to use a different approach. I might have to use a different lens to make that client understand the same concept I was trying to get across to the previous client.

All of my teachers passed the Spirit of the Pilates Method to me, and they all made sure to pass down key concepts of the work. They might have had different ways of explaining those concepts, but in the end, I've found that they all were the same concepts.

As an example, in regard to engaging the powerhouse, Romana says, "Navel to the spine"; Lolita says, "Zipper up"; Kathy had her song: "Zipper up tight jeans, Push-pin to the lowest part of your spine, Fasten a tight belt around your waist, Put your vest on and wrap measuring tape around the ribs." They all had the same concepts Joseph Pilates had taught them, but they made it make sense in their own bodies and then taught it that way. Are the words identical to his? Probably not. Are the modifications—the way they break or broke the material down for the learner in front of them—the same as those Joseph Pilates would have made? Maybe not. Was everything they taught created by Joseph Pilates? That would be no. But if Joe saw them doing some of these things, he might think, "Hmm, that's a good idea. Maybe I'm going to do that." Sometimes I watch one of my apprentices teaching, or I'll have them teach me so I can give them feedback, and they'll cue something or spot slightly differently from how I normally do, and I'll think, "That's not exactly how I do it, but I kind of like it. I might just steal that one."

The more I teach, the more I see how valuable these different perspectives are. The more I teach, the more I learn. I learn from teaching my clients and I learn from teaching my apprentices. I learn what works and what might not work as well. Teaching many hours with many different bodies enriches my experience. It gives me a great appreciation for the Pilates method and how well it works. It truly is an amazing exercise program to live by. I think what Joseph Pilates created not only improves bodies but also changes peoples' lives.

I have made it a mission to bring the beauty of Pilates to the next generation, to the children. Joseph Pilates said, "First educate the child." I think that if he had lived longer, he would have gone further down that road. I've seen pictures and films of him working with children, and I know that it's something he wanted to do. Joseph Pilates said, "In childhood habits are easily formed-good and bad. Why not then concentrate on the formation of only good habits and thus avoid the necessity later on in life of attempting to correct bad habits and substituting for them good habits." I remember something Lolita told me once: "In schools, children learn how to read, write and perform arithmetic, but they never learn how to get in touch and live within their own bodies." She couldn't have been more correct. In this day and age, for children, it's all about computers. There is a large disconnect between the body and the mind. I think that if people learn to connect with their own bodies early on, it will help them to have a better sense of self-embodiment later on in life.

I have developed a special children's Pilates program that I hope Joseph Pilates would have been proud of were he still alive. It's Pilates directed to the child learner. The skills that an adult learner can execute are going to be different from those of a child. Educators Marliese Kimmerle and Paulette Cote-Laurence maintain, "Developmental limitations of children restrict both the choice of material selected and the method of teaching, which must be adapted to their growing body structure and a developing brain" (Kimmerle and Cote-Laurence, 2003, p. 87). A teacher of young children must be aware of the limitations of a child's growing body, lack of past motor learning experiences, immature perceptual and cognitive skills and allow a child to enjoy the experience of moving and exploration, while offering external guidance, instruction and evaluation (Kimmerle and Cote-Laurence, 2003, p. 111-112). I am happy to be following in the footsteps of Carola Trier, who wrote a children's book of exercise called Exercise: What It Is, What It Does. It's a wonderful book that teaches Pilates in a way that makes sense to a child.

It's important that people know who Joseph Pilates was. People need to know what his mission was, what he was trying to do, and pass it on. I think this is my mission, but not only mine. It's the mission of everyone of my generation. It's our mission to pass it along to the next generation. I don't want the method to be lost. I don't want that spirit to be lost.

You may write things down in a book, but they won't translate the same way to everyone. Pilates is in your body. If you're going to pass down something that's in your body, it has to be done physically. It is in my body that I remember the corrections I received from my teachers. I remember what I learned. I was taught differently by the same teacher at different times, depending on how my body was that day. It is all of these little things that I have to pass down. If people just do Pilates, it works. If they just follow the system, it works. Every once in a while, you may have to change the order a little bit, or break down the exercise, or emphasize something a little differently than you would normally, but you teach the body that's in front of you within the framework of Pilates.

That's how my teachers have taught it, and it's important that it remain that way. When I'm teaching, I always say, "This is the Pilates Method. This is how Romana taught it. This is how Lolita teaches it. This is how Jay teaches it." That way, my apprentices can see those different lineages, while I try to stay as true to the work as possible. I feel very fortunate to have trained with all of them, because I got not only many different experiences from them but also their spirit and their energy. Because that's what it's about. It's about passing on the work, and making people feel the spirit.

About Brett
Brett is Director of Education and Senior Teacher of Teachers of the United States Pilates Association™. Certified by the New York Pilates Studio®, he is an expert in the Joseph Pilates Archival Exercises. Howard created a Pilates curriculum for children, and worked on many projects to bring Pilates to the schools and youth programs. Featured in the book, *The Pilates Method of Body Conditioning*, Brett is "Distinguished Instructor" on Pilates Anytime and featured on Pilatesology. He owns the Pilates Haus and holds a M.A. in Dance Education from N.Y.U. and a B.F.A. in Dance from S.U.N.Y. Purchase College Conservatory of Dance.

WORKS CONSULTED

Howard Gardner, *Frames of Mind: The theory of multiple intelligences.* London, England: Fontana Press, 1993).

Muska (Moshe) Mosston & S. Ashworth, *The Spectrum of Teaching Styles. From command to discovery* (White Plains, NY: Longman, 1990).

Pilates, J. (1945). *Return to Life.* Incline Village, NV: Presentation Dynamics Inc.

Lev Vygotsky, *Mind and society: the development of higher psychological processes.* (Cambridge, MA: Harvard University Press, 1978).

Training in Authentic Pilates
By Daphne Peña-Higgs

...the sense of being a part of a family.

When I first moved to London in 2000, heavily pregnant and blindly keen to start my own business, I told a few friends that I had spent the last few years training to teach Pilates. They congratulated me on learning how to fly. I looked bemused and thought, seriously... an 8-month pregnant woman with a constant fetish for corn chips in the cockpit of a trainee aircraft? Was it such an unrecognized word over here? Things have certainly changed in the U.K. over the last 12 years.

As a performer touring in the U.S., U.K. and West End shows in the 1990s, I started experiencing more and more injuries to my neck and back. I soon became a permanent resident in the U.K. and decided to stay. In those days, "Pilates" in London was a word bounced at dancers and actors by osteopaths any time injuries occurred. I tried a few different studios and teachers and felt better for it. However, once my injuries healed I didn't notice my body changing as all my recently devoured books said it should. There was also this horrible little voice in the back of my brain saying that I must be an idiot because although I could learn an entire cast's choreography for a major musical, or 20 pages of dialog for a script, I could not get my head around any sort of sequence or "through line" of this Pilates stuff. It didn't make sense. Every studio did different things, used different equipment or none at all, called the same exercises different names and different exercises modifications of original ones. So frustrating! Where and what were these original exercises? It was like trying to find the Dead Pilates Scrolls.

Well, thankfully, they were not dead. In fact, they were alive and kicking, stretching, pushing, pulling...all supervised by an amazing woman, Romana Kryzanowska, a protégé of Joseph Pilates. However, I couldn't just breeze in to do a session with her without knowing what the hell I was doing. It would have been like asking Da Vinci for a lesson after only having done finger painting. Without the generosity, patience, complete love and intricate knowledge of the human body of

Master Teachers Jacqui and Bill Landrum, I would never have completed or even been able to enroll in what was then called authentic Pilates training. They started me on the road to Romana.

At that point I was one broke dancer, figuratively and literally. Work had dried up in the U.K. for Americans due to an Equity strike; after a bad break-up to boot, I had moved back to Los Angeles. I hadn't had enough money to keep up any sort of Pilates in London and was feeling the niggles of all those old injuries again. Jacqui and Bill gave me a few authentic Pilates sessions and my body started changing rapidly. This was powerful work, and we soon spoke about my learning how to teach this stuff. The pinnacle would be getting to work with Romana herself.

It took a lot of steps to get there. Besides my twice-weekly sessions with the Landrums, the invaluable help of Michael Levy and Zoë Studios in Los Angeles gave me enough hours to get to Chicago for the long-awaited Pilates Intensive Teacher Training Course.

It made me giggle every time I watched Michael Levy giving a seemingly ridiculous exercise to the intimidating head of the Jewish Women's League; he would look at me deadpan, saying, "Yes, it is a real exercise. Romana says this is great for the neck and shoulders." I thought he might have just been trying to clean the wall or stop the client from fainting!

I started Belly Dancing evenings and weekends to make enough money to stay in the Pilates pink. Leave it to a former showgirl to discover an old dance and add new tricks. This Pilates stuff was allowing me to dance sometimes eight shows a week and have no aches and pains. God, all this was certainly nerve racking, exhausting and thrilling!

Besides going over every bit of training that I could, Jacqui and Bill gave me more tips for my first big intensive course with Romana at the Evanston, Chicago studio: make sure you have good looking outfits as Romana really appreciates a sense of style; get your dynamics right as she hates boring-looking work; give her a bottle of champagne, not as a bribe, but more as a way of getting to spend the time with her in order to hear stories from her work with Uncle Joe. Once she went up to one of the girls in our group, a slight little thing with a very pale face, "Joe would have told you to go out and have a big steak and some red wine before you come back again, honey. You need the energy." Then she'd go off chanting, "Tight seat, loose feet," or "How long is your Achilles?" Without waiting for an answer, she'd say, "Nope, it goes from your heel right out the back of your neck, now show me." I still think of this line every time I do Tendon Stretch on the Reformer. At that time, around 1998, Romana's other favorite things to say were, "Use a freedom of movement, never stop the movement, this ain't yoga," and "Psoas be it," when we did the ending stretch of Front Splits. Apparently, authentic Pilates had just been publicly criticized by a magazine or newspaper article saying this method of Pilates did not stretch the psoas muscle.

So, twelve of us arrived at the Chicago intensive. The opportunity of working with Juanita, one of Romana's right-hand women, and Romana herself, was like being firmly rolled out and perfectly pieced together by a military cook and then having new life baked into you at the end. Juanita was scary in a Stockholm syndrome type of way; by the end of ten days, I couldn't imagine a day without her guidance. She set the scene, making sure that we knew every technical detail of every exercise we could fit in before Romana would see us four days later. She had such a clever way of working; I owe any technical expertise that I possess to her meticulous teaching. Once Romana arrived, the Diva hit the stage. We were so awed to watch Juanita's humbleness in the presence of Romana. She had gravitas and exuberance enough to get you to try any exercise, no matter the skill level, and internally dance the dynamics while doing it. She truly carried the spirit into the work, and it was contagious. I watched my colleagues around me performing sequences that five days earlier had looked like a good gym workout. Now they performed these same exercises as if Martha Graham and Balanchine possessed them. Romana said one of the tricks was not teaching your client any sort of anatomy: "Watch how the body moves and get it to move where it's not... and always starting from the powerhouse!"

Full of beans, I went back to L.A. to finish the pre-requisite hours that would finally get me to New York. I had all this information and now needed to see how it would work on real people's bodies instead of a load of apprentices like myself.

500 hours later…

I finally saved enough money and had enough hours to complete my last 100 hours in New York with Romana and Co. I walked into what was then called Drago's. The elevator door opened into a mildly frenzied reception area. People to the left were swinging on rings suspended from the ceiling. Small groups of confused apprentices were rifling through papers and arguing about spring settings on a Wunda Chair or following the trained teachers around like faithful pets. Drago came up to me and asked in a forceful Russian accent if I was a new apprentice. When I answered, "Yes," he told me to put my bag down and do a backbend. When he spoke, you didn't talk; you moved. I went backwards; he pulled my legs over my head into a back walkover and told me to roll up slowly. He paused, and then said quickly, "Ok, you stay." What a welcome!

Mornings started at 7:00 a.m. with the apprentices' Mat class. We usually started the first part of the day at Drago's with Sari, Romana's daughter, and different teachers whom she asked to show us certain apparatus. Later, we would watch Romana teach privates, duets—really just anything she did. The second day I was there, two teachers from Spain were in, Javier and Esperanza. Their work was so beautiful; they made the super-advanced workout look effortless. You could tell Romana was really enjoying this, lifting their toes to the ceiling, guiding their lower backs up and off their hips, positioning her finger on the front of the ribs fixing the whole body's alignment. She was conducting them with a master's touch. Her happiness was contagious; it was like the whole room was stoned with delight. That was it. I was hooked. It didn't matter that my Sagittarian nature had me out salsa dancing until 3 a.m. every night; I was in that studio each morning soaking up every bit of knowledge that my blurry eyes could handle.

Afternoons were spent on the Upper West Side studio with Bob Liekens. He was so organized and approachable. It was actually a welcome respite from the haphazard glory of Drago's. His precision and eagle eye would not only correct something you were doing wrong in an exercise, but would also fix how you were describing it to another student. Doing the exercises properly is one thing, but correcting a body's movement to attain the goal of an exercise is an entirely different talent. I remember feeling so down when I heard that Bob had left "the fold."

What struck me most then, and does still when in the presence of the "old school" Romana teachers, was the sense of being a part of a family. Everyone was struggling and suffering together because we all believed that this work was deeply important. We had to know it. We had worked extra shifts doing anything that paid, borrowed money, spent many hours away from loved ones to get here to New York, to saturate ourselves with the truest Pilates training available, to get that certification from Romana and soak up her spirit, her genius and sense of dynamics. Pilates was all we talked about day and night. Really, I suppose it's what it must feel like to join a cult. Here was the power to change your own body and very soon, other people's bodies. At that time, there was a really good balance of being mentored by the master teachers, combined with enough leeway and encouragement to find your own teaching voice. Regrettably, some teachers, myself included, emerged with a superiority complex. Always a sure sign of a newbie. It took a few good years to come to grips with the fact that it was not me changing people's bodies, but rather Joe's method. I was just a toddler channeling his work.

The final day of certification with Romana was thrilling. There was a hurricane outside. I felt as though I had manifested it with everything I had been going over in my head in order to pass the practical exam. The tales of older teachers passing through my thoughts made me buy a bottle of champagne to stick in my bag…just in case! The actual exam is now a blur, clouded by former nerves, but my 10-minute interview with Romana will always be with me. In a word she made it clear she could see I knew the format, but that it was just the beginning. She praised some of the wording I had used for the Rowing exercises, she emphasized more of the dynamics of my Mat teaching, then she looked me square in the eye and said, "Do you really know this work and really want to continue with it?" I was shocked. Had I not passed? Did I look like I didn't know what I was doing? Was I that BAD???? Then, I swear, her eyes seriously twinkled. There is no other fitting cliché. She patted my knee and said, "Keep learning. Don't ever stop moving. Smile. Breathe. Don't look so worried; you passed." She laughed as she signed my certificate and looked concerned as the windows shuddered again under the force of the wind.

During the last part of my training, I had decided to make things easy on myself and fall in love with an Australian. One of my clients in L.A. was the wonderful Susan Nash, wife of singing legend Graham Nash (Crosby, Stills and...). The man I was in love with lived in Sydney, and I was in L.A., apparently looking so lovesick that Susan said she couldn't stand to work with me anymore. She immediately demanded that he and I meet at her guesthouse in Hawaii to see if this was going anywhere. That was a dream week, not only cultivating a romance, but getting serenaded by Nash and Crosby to boot! After continually pinching ourselves over the course of the week, we went back to our respective cities, all pinched out and focused on finding a plan to be together.

Luckily for me, there was an authentic Pilates studio in Sydney, Australia. Once Romana had certified me, I pretty much booked the next flight over and prayed that customs would let me in (I'd been going back and forth with the owner of the Aussie studio regarding working documents that were far from totally clear). It took over an hour at customs to go through the documents, each of us holding our breath as the world moved in super slow-motion. Would they deport me? Was this too soon? Where the hell was the green form I filled out? Was I really meant to be here? My lungs and legs nearly collapsed as I was waved through. I took a deep inhalation of the humid, electrified air only to see my partner take the same breath as he finally caught sight of my relieved and emotional gaze.

It was a tumultuous adventure working in Sydney, one of the highlights being Romana's visit to the studio. It was the first time I could watch her work with the apprentices with a sense of ease, feeling proud and supportive, as I had already passed my grueling test. I marveled at Romana's stamina; she had just done the intensive in Brazil, then the U.S., down to Sydney and was leaving a few days after, on to another country. I mean, I know she had been "82" years old for quite a few years now, so how did she keep this pace up? It was still the norm for her to lithely lie on the Cadillac and show everyone how the Hundred was MEANT to be done and then flip herself around the bars like a gymnast. No wonder we would finish every day with champagne. She deserved it!

I was soon married, but with both of us missing Europe, we were a little discontent staying so far away from the rest of the world. My husband still had a flat in London, so we made the huge decision to move away from both of our cities and start a new life back in the

U.K. When Brits look at our Aussie and U.S. passports, they often ask what the hell we are doing here. We usually say we moved here for the weather.

We moved into a two-bedroom flat in Queen's Park, London. One bedroom was my husband's office and the other doubled as a mini Pilates studio and soon-to-be baby's bedroom. We slept in a little conservatory at the back of the house. I put out one ad and soon had a few clients. I would answer the door to new clients, heavily pregnant, and say, "This is what happens when you try Pilates. You too can look like this!"

Things started going so well that soon I had to find larger premises to work in. I didn't even put another ad out until three years later. Everything had been word of mouth. Many clients came to me saying that they had done some Pilates before, but never like this. It was exciting, dynamic and effective. Many of those original clients still attend the studio—they've never gone back to those old ways of just lifting your arm and breathing. What kind of a workout is that? I often tell my clients that Joe had developed Pilates as a challenging method of working out a healthy body, with specific exercises to fortify certain weaknesses that a body might have in order to attain symmetry. It wasn't developed as a therapy or to focus on breathing, but meant to incorporate movement and breath together in a way that should challenge a client to progress to a higher level of fitness than where they currently are, whatever that level may be.

Newspapers and magazines started calling, asking us for opinions on posture and weight loss and what celebrities were working with us. They wrote articles on all the different styles of Pilates now in the U.K., putting us at the London helm of what was now called classical Pilates.

Now, of course, with the recognition and success of the studio came criticism. I was soon able to find more teachers trained by Romana, most notably Greg Webster, without whom my studio would not be what it is today. And it just kept growing. I have to explain here what Pilates had come to be like in the U.K. by the time I started teaching in 2000.

Instead of clients understanding the Method for their own bodies, they were put in groups ranging between three to seven people and given different exercises to do at different times on different pieces of equipment with no sequence taught at all. Sometimes clients in these groups would start at different times, and the teacher was expected to guide them into a new exercise each time they finished a series, no matter what their level, and expected to remember if anyone had any injuries. This was quite a lot to ask of one person, and a task that only a very few can do well. This certainly brings in good revenue for the studio, but the integrity of the exercises suffers severely. After many years of doing this, teachers were training other teachers who'd never been taught the original exercises in the first place. Because the teachers weren't taught all the complexities within each exercise in The Method, they kept looking for new ideas for their clients. This led to a variety of problems: exercises were continually being watered down, or modified by physios and osteopaths for a specific client; exercises and equipment were borrowed from other systems such as Feldenkrais, then taken on as a widespread exercise in the Pilates world, ignoring the fact that the original exercise was meant to be part of a system and performed with a specific dynamic. I can't tell you how many times teachers trained in other styles of Pilates have come into the studio and said something like, "I don't do Swan on the Ladder Barrel because it hurts my back." I ask them to show me how they are doing it, and I will usually say, "No wonder! You're not starting from your powerhouse. You're relying on your back to perform the exercise and are not using the correct dynamic at all." Done the way Romana taught me, the exercise should actually be good for your back. (Every one of those teachers now does Swan on the Barrel with no back pain at all!)

So after many years of studios teaching Pilates in this slow, ongoing-group sort of way it became accepted in London as the norm. Other Pilates schools called us Pilates Nazis. Once I received a phone call from another studio posing as a client who shouted at me over the phone for calling myself London's first classical Pilates studio— even though upon questioning she could not name one master teacher by whom she had been trained. I was told to my face that my studio would not succeed because of the way that I was teaching; asking clients to start with privates before going on to any sort of group classes would never make me any sort of profit. Well, I will admit we are not the most profitable studio in London, but we are extremely success-ful and have a huge following of clients and teachers who attend our seminars.

I can't express how proud I am of our London studio and of the teachers who work there; sometimes they have even turned down trendy new studios and posh gyms so that they can continue to teach in a classical setting with original Gratz equipment (which, in my opinion, is still the best stuff around). Clients email me from L.A., Chicago, and New York wanting to pop in while they're in town. They're used to doing their twice weekly classical Pilates sessions and know that they can find the same quality sessions at our studio.

When interviewed in regards to the different styles of Pilates in London, I will often explain that I've seen some great teachers and really interesting modifications to exercises. My only criticism is that often teachers who've gone through training systems in the U.K. have not been taught a complete "Method," and have not been given the reasons for doing what they're doing. That is why when I started doing Pilates in London, nothing seemed to make any sense. The best way I can think to describe all the different styles of Pilates is it's as if they've become the French, Italian or Spanish strains of a method that was started from one root source. Joseph Pilates' method of Control-ogy, given to Romana Kryzanowska to maintain and uphold, and now most commonly called classical Pilates, is the Latin that started it all. There is an old saying, "Find yourself a teacher..." I couldn't have done better than finding Romana and all the master teachers who've dedicated themselves to continuing this work. Vivat Pilates!

About Daphne
Daphne was certified in The Pilates Method by Romana Kryza-nowska in 2000. She holds a B.A. from The University of Southern California and lives in London with her husband and daughter. Her studio, New York Pilates London, was the first classical Pilates studio to open in London and is devoted to keeping The Method alive and kicking in the United Kingdom. Coming from a long-standing career in the U.S. and West End Theatre world, she also writes and choreo-graphs her own one woman shows that have been sell-out successes in London and both the Edinburgh and Brighton festivals.

Kathy Grant and the Pilates Path to Bodymind

By Cara Reeser

Everything was meant to strike us in a very personal way...

Learning Pilates from Kathy Grant gave me the confidence and courage I needed to dance, live and play happily in my body after a serious injury. When I later became a Pilates teacher, Kathy taught me how to encourage my students in the same way. By telling her story, and mine, I hope to inspire those of you who practice and teach the work of Joseph Pilates. The possibilities are endless.

In the summer of 1989, after graduating from Sarah Lawrence College with an undergraduate degree in modern dance, I had an accident. While hiking on vacation in California, I accidentally stuck my hand in a ground wasps' nest on a cliff side and was immediately swarmed by wasps. Knowing I was allergic, I panicked, running off the edge of the cliff. For several months, the multiple fractures in my spine went undiagnosed, so by the time a diagnosis was finally made there was nothing to do but get caught in what I refer to now as the "wheel of healers." I was going to Dr. Bacharach, the famous New York back doctor for dancers, three days a week. I was going to acupuncture, going to massage, and my dance career completely stopped. I was medicated for fibromyalgia, put in a brace, and I began to feel depressed.

There was a moment when I decided I was over it. I had lost control of my relationship with my body and was constantly at the mercy of others. I was fed up. I was going to stop seeing all these practitioners and start dancing again. No longer in my brace, I went to New York University's Tisch School of the Arts, auditioned for and got into their Masters in Fine Arts dance program. I was elated.

On my first day of school, the very first class of the day was "Morning Barre," Kathy Grant's Pilates class. She started by asking us to sit up straight, to shut our eyes, to breathe and to find center. This was all fairly new to me. I remember thinking, what are we doing? We are not even moving! I had studied dance my whole life, and no one had ever begun a class like that. I was used to very traditional dance training.

We had been in that room for maybe five minutes. As we executed a simple spinal twist with cervical rotation, something Kathy called "Listening Heads," she came up behind me, inquiring, "What's wrong with your back?" I was shocked. We were hardly moving. What on earth could she be seeing? Of course, when you apply to Tisch, they ask you about your injury history, and I had not revealed any of my history. My eyes filled with tears. She said, "Come up at the end of the day and see me at 5M," which was her studio. I thought, "I'm going to get kicked out of this program." I didn't know who this lady was. Reluctantly, I went up to her studio that evening. It was a small room with very eerie looking tables with springs and chains hanging about. I was the only person there. She shut the door and sat down on the Cadillac, again asking, "What's wrong with your back?" I immediately burst out crying and told her that I had fractured my spine in three places, that I hadn't told the school, and if she told them, I would probably lose my scholarship and get kicked out of the program.

She looked at me and touched my spine a little, assuring me, "I'm not going to tell on you. But you can't come to my morning class because you're not ready. So what you're going to do is meet me here every morning at 8:00 a.m., and I'll set you up with your program. Then I'll go down and teach class and meet you up here afterwards." And that was what I did. She eventually allowed me to take class, too, but for two years I faithfully followed her instructions and she never revealed my injury history to the department.

In my sessions with Kathy, I learned simple exercises that built a foundation with which to strengthen my body. She had a big piece of foam that she wrapped around the Roll Down bar and tied with elastic bands. In the beginning, she had me lie down with my neck over the bar, performing very tiny motions, allowing the springs to assist me in cervical flexion. In my memory of these early lessons, she always had her hands on me, often directing me to breathe into just one area: into my upper ribs or into one side. She would tell a story and have me visualize the steam rising or feel the rain falling down on my chest. She stayed very close and told me to feel or listen to the springs.

In the studio, there was a recipe box with 3 x 5 cards. Each time I learned a new movement or exercise, I wrote it down on my card. Then I led myself through my program and she came around, using her hands to guide me, always working with imagery and using the props for which she became famous. It was a creative and sort of hypnotizing experience, and, in most cases, my lessons with Kathy lasted for two hours or more.

Eventually I was doing movements I never thought I would do again. She just set up an exercise and moved me through it. There were so many times during that period when I just screamed or burst out crying or completely collapsed. Whenever I freaked out, she just laughed, declaring, "You did it!" She always reminded me of what I had done, that I had just performed a backbend or a rotation that I had been told I would never be able to do again. Kathy never believed any of that. She never asked how I felt or if anything hurt; she just set up the exercise and asked me to do it.

But no one was allowed to move at all until her imagistic way of aligning had been established. If we were about to do a movement in poor alignment and with irrelevant tension, she stayed on us with her hands. She never let us proceed if we weren't relaxed and settled. So the first exercises were micro-gestures meant to teach us to move without strain: her "Ribcage Arms" exercise, for example, was often the first exercise she had me do. Lying supine with my hands knitted together, she guided me to visualize the oval shape that my arms were creating. Then she encouraged me to let the shape rise over my head and back down again, teaching me to use only the exertion necessary for this movement. This type of exercise was meant to get us to move inward and leave the experiences of our day behind us, so that our starting point was not a prepared position of the body, but rather an attitude of relaxation and receptivity. And then we went through our routines. There were numerous people in the room, but Kathy was always watching, calling out to each one or coming around as we moved about on the equipment from the Reformer to the Cadillac to the Chair.

There was no uniform protocol, and there was never a prescribed placement, or spring tension or breath. We each wrote down on our cards what springs we used and what side they should be on. Since I had torn one of my deep back muscles on the right side in my accident, all of my work was initially done with the spring on the right side. Using the springs in this way brought both my awareness and increased resistance to the weaker side. Kathy also had me hold a little ball in my right hand or armpit or even under my hip, enticing my right side to engage when it did not, or release when it was holding. It was all personally designed. I had no idea what anybody else in the room was doing. They might be doing things I had never seen before. There wasn't a sense of somebody supervising us all the time. We were often flailing, trying to figure something out, and Kathy would watch us flail for quite a while before she stepped in. The learning process was completely experiential. We had to give up any expectations. This sense of discovering the work is lost now that so many students have done Pilates before, certain that they know what they are supposed to do. Later in life, Kathy confessed that this was one of the things that spoiled her teaching experience. Students' expectations and ideas about the exercises thwarted the very type of experiential learning that she was guiding them towards. In the earlier days, we went in with no idea what to expect. I didn't know anything about Pilates, had never even heard of Mr. Pilates.

Whenever I asked Kathy if I did something correctly, she replied, "I don't know. I'm not you." There was never any answer unless I was out of alignment, using excess or not enough tension to support my body relative to gravity. Then she stopped me and said, "Cara, your head." When I had worked to center my head on my spine, she said, "Okay," or just made a gesture that meant I could proceed. If I were about to begin an exercise and inquired, "Where should I sit?" Kathy answered, "I don't know. I'm not you. Find your position." It's not about where you place yourself on the machine. It's about whether you can keep an awareness of your center.

Later on, when Kathy told me about how Mr. Pilates had taught her; it was very much like that. He just said, "No, no, no, no, yes, no." Then, on the subway ride home, she reflected on what she had been doing when he said, "Yes." She tried to feel yes again, and during her next session she worked to reproduce the sensation that was the yes. This was how she learned to find her way out of pain and back to dancing.

Kathy's experience of meeting Mr. Pilates was in many ways similar to my experience of meeting her. She was a professional dancer and she was injured while performing in a variety show. The act before her had left water on the stage, and she fell. I'm not sure what the diagnosis was, but she hurt her knees badly. At this time there were no physical therapists or dance medicine doctors, so she worked on her own to heal her injury. One day in ballet class, she began crying because her knees hurt so much that she couldn't do the plies. Pearl Lang, a great early modern dancer, told Kathy to see Mr. Pilates. He was known in the New York dance world as the miracle worker for injured dancers. Kathy said that in her first session with Mr. Pilates, he stood her up, put her feet in parallel and adjusted her feet, knees, hips, spine and shoulders. And then he walked away. After half an hour or so, he came back and asked, "Have you learned anything?" She replied, "But Mr. Pilates, I've only been standing here." And he responded, "Well, then today you learned to stand."

She said that she often wondered why she went back, but she could tell by the way he adjusted her that he was a healer and that he knew something that she didn't. She wanted to dance again and believed that he would help her reach that goal. And she did dance again, just as I did.

Kathy explained that Mr. Pilates taught the person in front of him. What he did with the other significant lineage holders (Romana Kryzanowska, Carola Trier, Ron Fletcher, and many others) was different from what he did with her. I was fortunate to spend time together with Kathy and Ron Fletcher, and it was always interesting to hear them reflect on their experiences learning from Joe and Clara. They sometimes agreed and other times they looked at each other with a bewildered gaze, as if to say, "That was not what it was like for me." Then they both laughed, realizing that although they had the same teachers, they had been taught the work differently. Later on, when there were arguments in the industry about the correct way to perform an exercise, Kathy remarked, "How do I know what Mr. Pilates taught Romana? Romana was Romana, and I was me." She never disagreed with anything anyone said Mr. Pilates had taught him or her. She had a deep respect and curiosity for the variety and diversity that had been passed down. Kathy's first job teaching Pilates was as Carola's assistant, and she always made a point of noting that certain exercises or interpretations that she gave us came to her from Carola.

Like her mentors, Kathy taught the body in front of her. Students often remarked, "I thought you were supposed to start with the Hundred." Kathy would say, "Mr. Pilates didn't start me with the Hundred. I went to him with a knee injury. Why would he have started me with the Hundred?" The idea was that you first learned exercises that worked to address the issues or patterns that were in your way and later, once you were more organized and pain-free, you learned the rest. In her class at Tisch, it took the whole semester to learn the repertory. There were lots of little "Kathy exercises" that we learned first. Then they came together in a brilliant way, and suddenly we were doing Teaser or doing the Hundred. We learned how to lift our heads, how to pump our arms, how to lift our legs off the floor, and then there was the Hundred, right in front of us. The way she taught Pilates was to teach the skills that allowed us to express the repertory fully, rather than using the repertory to find the skills. We went little by little into the vocabulary, and the last day of the class we had something like a performance, with Kathy giving the rhythm as we went through a sequence following the order from the Mat plates (pictures). The next semester we started at the beginning again. It was understood that we hadn't done our "Morning Barre" all summer, and we had to get into condition again.

If she thought we were being too serious or had become too uptight about doing everything right, Kathy introduced all sorts of other crazy things. Suddenly we were doing cartwheels, handstands and rolling exercises in a clown position. She understood that if we were trying too hard, holding too tight, we thwarted our ability to express ourselves freely in our movement. She was trying to help us move naturally, freely, understanding that our potential was already there. She sometimes gave us a simple task to remind us how easy it was. Once, when I struggled with the Roll-Up, she handed me a pencil and asked me to roll up and place the pencil at the end of the mat! When we made the exercises harder than they should be, she reminded us, "Don't give me all that choreography." What she meant was that we were performing the exercise, duplicating the way we thought it should look. By using ordinary, functional movement, she got us to realize that the thing she was asking for was something we already knew how to do. Her view was that our bodies knew how to do this. And if it wasn't happening, it was because we were somehow stopping it.

She also gave us cues that were specific to each person. Later when I became a teacher myself, she said to me, "How are you going to give a truck driver an image about playing a piano? How are you going to give the same image to someone who lives uptown and to someone who lives downtown?" Everything was meant to strike us in a very personal way, personal because it was relevant to us and our experience in the world. It gave us a reference point for the movement.

The thing I remember her saying the most was, "Move, but don't move." She meant, "I don't care if you move. I care that you're doing everything you can with your mind. I don't care if you can lift your leg or not. If you're going to disregard the whole setup to lift your leg, you're not doing the exercise." The exercise was much more internal. This supports the whole idea laid out by Mr. Pilates that we're not just entering into some mundane regimen of exercise. If we were to get back to the roots of the work, originally called Contrology, this idea of "move but don't move" is key. Control is about using the mind to direct us. It's not about getting into a position and holding it. In fact, the idea of getting to a position or a static hold in the body is completely counter to the goal. The goal is movement and the vehicle is the mind or, more concretely, the central nervous system. The question is, What stops us from moving as fully and expressively as possible?

In *Return to Life Through Contrology*, Mr. Pilates uses a phrase about moving with confidence, ease and awareness.[1] As I look back on the lineage to which I am connected, I see a commonality in the way that Mr. Pilates taught Kathy, the way she taught me and the way I now mentor and teach in my studio: the idea that we must engage our minds and commit to our goals, while finding a relaxed and alert relationship to ourselves. Mr. Pilates wrote that the goal of his work is the coordination of mind, body and spirit.[2]

There are three essential ingredients to regaining and maintaining mind, body and spirit as a coordinated whole: awareness, alignment or skeletal centering, and easeful movement of all the joints of the body. These key ingredients allow us to express ourselves fully in the world.

Another of my teachers at N.Y.U., Andre Bernard, defined movement as a "neuromusculosketetal event," meaning that in voluntary movement, the nervous system is the messenger, the muscles and tendons the workers, and the skeleton the support structure. If the nervous system is the messenger, where do the messages come from? From our sense perceptions and from our thoughts. We create movement responses through listening to cues, through mimicking what we see and by thinking. These thoughts are important to consider when engaging in a movement protocol such as Pilates. How we talk to ourselves about the movements we are performing dictates how the muscles, tendons, ligaments and skeleton will work to help us along.

The starting point becomes very important here. If the goal is to send clear messages from the periphery or thought process to the workforce (the soft tissue), then we have to begin from a place of relative relaxation or what is sometimes referred to as neutral. This use of the word neutral is not about a position or placement of the pelvis or trunk, but rather a quiet, simple state of body/mind that is not fixed or held. It was always the case in Kathy's studio that the first few exercises we practiced were designed to quiet our nervous systems and relax unnecessary holding patterns in our soft tissue.

These concepts are not new. Bernard states that this technique of using thought or imagery to create movement is "one of the oldest mind-body training techniques."[3] Developed by Mabel Todd in the early part of the 20th century, the term ideokinesis was later applied to this work by one of Todd's students, Lulu Sweigard, who borrowed the term from an American piano teacher named Bonpensiere. Ideokinesis comes from two Greek words, ideo, meaning idea or thought and kinesis, referring to movement. This technique is designed to direct, change, improve and discover movement patterns with "the image or thought as facilitator of the movement."[4]

Using ideokenesis is not as easy as it may sound. It is a complicated and subtle system that has been taught by a long line of students influenced by Todd and Sweigard. For the purpose of this conversation, what is important is engaging with our nervous systems to organize our muscle patterns by having clear movement goals, starting from a relaxed and receptive position of both body and mind. So when Kathy implored us to, "Move, but don't move," she was teaching us to see our intention clearly, starting with locating our sense of direction towards center, then developing into big, bold and glorious movements.

Today in my practice, I am blessed to work with Pilates teachers from around the country and abroad. We spend most of our time together learning to get out of our own way. If I notice a student holding himself tightly against his potential range as he moves through the Mat or apparatus workout, I ask, "What are you telling yourself right now?" The answer is almost always the same: "I am trying not to move my ___," or "I am trying to stabilize my ___." I respond, "If the goal is to move, why start with a cue in your mind of not moving?" It is much more effective to use an image of moving, even if at first it is only an image, rather than sending a message or image to the body that is based on holding or not moving at all.

Our bodies are filled to the brim with stories about how we should stand, sit, dress, behave and move. We have been receiving this information from the very start of our lives. Much of this internal dialogue occurs on a subconscious level. The idea is not to create more rules governing our movement; rather, the goal is to release ourselves from the story altogether.

Recently, I was teaching my dance technique class at Naropa University. While working with one student, I noticed that in all of the standing work she continued to hold her knees in a slightly bent position. I asked her to straighten her knees over and over throughout the class, using my hands to guide her. I said it in as many ways as I could. At the end of class I asked her why she kept her knees bent, even though I asked her to straighten them. Again I inquired, "What are you telling yourself?" She considered my question for a bit and then informed me that when she was about six years old, her first ballet teacher told her that if she straightened her knees all the way, her back would break (at least this is what she heard her teacher say). She wasn't aware that she was holding on to this notion; it had become a pattern she was completely committed to with little awareness. Suddenly, she realized she had been unconsciously keeping her knees bent because of a comment made to her over 12 years before, an instruction that was absolutely untrue and did not serve her dancing.

In Will Johnson's book, *The Posture of Meditation*, he reminds us that, "Acts of clinging or aversion, no matter how overt or subtle, are expressed through systematic tensing of the musculature of the body."[5] Coming to a place of neutral or a relatively relaxed relationship with gravity's support requires attention, concentration and willingness to change our minds and attitudes of body. This idea, well explored by many, reminds us that our posture or position of body that we hold and carry in the world is directly and unconsciously related to our idea of self. It is made up of a complex and historic multitude of attitudes, memories and experiences that are expressed through our bodies. In order to move towards a balanced sense of center, we have to let go of the patterns of body and mind that keep us in undesirable holding patterns. Changes of body attitude work to reshape the mind in the same way that changing the mind's rigid ideas work to reshape the body.

When I think of those first lessons with Kathy, as well as many of the later ones, she always took the time to help me calm myself, focusing on my breath, center and tension levels. In my case, Kathy was constantly working with me to let go of a post-injury holding pattern I had in my neck. She had me look at myself in the mirror, taking note of my head placement, which was always slightly tilted and forward —she called this position my "talking head," meaning the place where I held my head as part of my "attitude of body." She said we all had a "talking head," and that was fine when we talked with our friends; but when we did our Pilates with her, we had to take off our "talking heads" and find our centers without attitude, so that we could listen to the subtle guidance of her hands, the images and springs.

In Pilates we spend a fair amount of time practicing in a supine or prone position. These positions provide added support from gravity, allowing our bodies to let go of excess tension and exertion. The beauty of this is that we can more easily find neutral. We can feel the pull of gravity, but don't have to primarily organize our structure in the vertical plane as we do in everyday life. Giving our bodies a chance to release on the horizontal plane helps us re-set our tension levels. We then have more choices when we return to our usual, upright relationship to gravity.

The springs are then added to the body, working to support our movement through assistance and resistance. Kathy always emphasized our relationship to the spring tension with which we were engaged. She told us to listen to the springs as we worked to open and close the coils with just the right amount of tension and release. "Don't fight my springs," she would say. "Let the springs help you." If we yanked or pulled too hard on the springs, they often made a moaning sound. With her back turned to us, she warned, "I heard that. Go easy and listen to the springs." There was always a view of partnering with the springs, and it took a sensitive awareness, like moving across the stage with a dance partner. She always required us to tune in, pay attention and regulate our tension levels.

Years ago, I came across an article in *Movement Research Journal* written by the dancer, choreographer and educator Elaine Summers. It is titled "Bio-kinetic Tension: Loving tension, because without tension there is no movement; without movement there is no life." The title alone was so thrilling to me that I adopted the view right away. The idea that we learn to love our tension—what a concept! In this article, Summers offered a long list of different types of tension exertions used in the body, including irrelevant, compensatory, eccentric and conflicting, among others. She defined each type of tension, allowing me to see that tension alone wasn't necessarily the problem. The trick was what type of tension we use and what quantity, direction, duration, intensity and power we give our tension.[6]

Inspired by this article, today in my practice, I often ask my students to imagine that they have a dial deep inside their bodies. A tension dial. They can visualize the dial however they choose. The idea is that they can use this dial to increase or decrease the tension levels they use at any given moment in their moving bodies. The dial can regulate the tension in all areas of the body and can be tuned at any time. Knowing what levels of tension are necessary to achieve a balanced position towards center is the first step in knowing how much tension volume we need to perform the movements we desire.

I like to help my students visualize their center. We spend time at the beginning of the session imagining a vertical axis of support, regardless of the plane in which the body is placed. The vertical axis of support is the plumb line that is described by gravity's pull. We start by placing this imaginary line through our bodies.

Closing our eyes and noticing our breath, we visualize that the breath fills the entire cylinder of our bodies, including the volume of our head, trunk, and legs. We work to lengthen and expand the volume of our cylinder with each inhalation and each exhalation. Once we have established our cylinder, we then imagine dropping a line or cord directly down (and up) the center of the cylinder. I always imagine my cord being made of an elastic material in bright red.

Once the line is established inside the cylinder, in our mind's eye we begin to work towards visualizing our body (the cylinder) centering around this line. Like a strong elastic cord, we note how we can stretch and shorten this line, how we can change the orientation of our cylinder and cord and as we do, how our tension dial continually needs to be tuned to allow support to exist on all planes and in all our gestures.

Center is not a place to find and hold. The idea of ex-centering, which is a term originally coined by Mabel Todd, is just as relevant as centering. I love the explanation of this concept by Bernard. He states, "Ex-centering is not a bad word. It is not a villain. What I mean is centering is not a static condition. Ex-centering is not bad, because that is what you are doing in life: you are constantly ex-centering and centering, ex-centering and coming back to center. There can be no centering without ex-centering. So do not get the idea that you want to be in a constant state of being centered. You have to have a center to come back to, so please think about it in this way; otherwise you get a static concept of what center is."[7] When we are expressing our bodies using the Pilates techniques and equipment, we are constantly taking ourselves off center or "ex-centering the body." Our success depends on having a strong relationship with our direction towards center, just as we must have a relationship with gravity to understand how much effort it takes to move our bodies in balance with its force.

Finding the right formula for success during any given exercise or gesture is primary in my teaching. Each person will find his or her individual challenges based on his ability to organize the body with gravity, space, momentum and range. The further we take our bodies off center with fewer contact points and added weight or pull from the exterior or, in our case, the springs, the more difficult it becomes to balance our tension exertion. For each student, the formula is different. Some need to add tension as they begin to collapse to gravity's pull, while others need to release the holding in the soft tissue so that they can use gravity to support them. Giving my students time to locate their sense of center and then encouraging them to utilize the brilliant system that we today call Pilates allows them to center and ex-center. They use the springs to guide them to assist and resist without unnecessary struggle or rigidity. I use images more often than cues to guide the body towards center, away and back again.

When working with injured or physically compromised clients, I need to help them build strength and flexibility, as well as courage and confidence. There are many reasons we develop unhealthy movement patterns in our bodies. Our fear of pain is one of them. Summers referred to this type of tension as compensatory, a pattern of movement and or posture developed in the body with the goal of adjusting away from pain.[8] When these patterns are unexplored, they become fixed in the body long after the pain is gone. Recognizing and changing our compensatory tension is part of reestablishing healthy movement patterns.

Pain is a complicated response system that needs to be respected and understood. Like the other changes in movement and alignment noted previously, getting out of pain requires us to work to regulate our nervous systems, so that we are not reacting to input that is no longer there. As I work to help my clients change unhealthy holding patterns in their bodies with less pain and more confidence, it is primary for them to recognize the changes that they are making and the potential they have in their bodies to move with new range and direction without triggering pain. Since pain is regulated by our brains, helping our clients find new pain-free movement has to involve working with thought. Put simply, we have to see our potential in our mind's eye, let go of excess holding or guarding, and as we begin to move pain-free, our success must be confirmed.

I was always surprised when Kathy guided me without pain through a movement, particularly in extension, which I always feared would hurt me. It often took a while to get me ready and then suddenly I was there, shocked that I could move pain-free in this way again. "You did it!" she would declare. "And it didn't hurt, did it?" Little by little I gained courage and understanding in my body and mind, allowing me to recreate what I did in the studio in the dance classroom, on stage and in my life.

Using images that are relevant to one's life experience allows one to access the confidence needed to go a little deeper. This is what Kathy taught me. She said, "One size doesn't fit all." The exercises, the images, the spring tension, the position, the range and breath were chosen for each of us. This allowed each of us to locate our personal formula of tension and expression for our movement.

In many cases, students create their own images. I have a male client in his mid-fifties who has a farm. One day I was trying to help him find a way to use the strength in his arms without hiking his shoulder blades prior to lifting his limbs. As we worked to find the correct balance of tension for pushing and pulling with his arms, he discovered this image: when he opened the grain door on his barn, the movement felt the same. Now when we are working, all I have to do is remind him of his "grain door muscles," and he is able to find a correct pattern of exertion and relaxation for these gestures.

Kathy often told me Mr. Pilates said that Contrology was for the unexpected. She explained that the increased awareness, control and resilience that Contrology brought to the body and mind gave us the confidence and quick coordination we need to fall without injury, sprint for the bus with our kids in tow or get down a tricky mountain trail without injury or strain. For a dancer who had been severely injured, this meant that I had to learn to know my body and trust myself.

In his essay "Contrology Restores Physical Fitness," Mr. Pilates states, "In practically every instance the daily acts we perform are governed by what we think we see, hear, or touch, without stopping first to analyze or think of the possible results of our actions, good or bad…ideally, our muscles should obey our will. Reasonably, our will should not be dominated by the reflex actions of our muscles."[9] As I reflect on these words, I see that Mr. Pilates was guiding us with his thoughtful and sensitive movement practice to open our minds to our endless potential as movers, starting with a deep and direct relationship with our minds (our imagination), our bodies (our playground) and our spirit (our joy).

About Cara

Cara Reeser achieved a B.A. degree from Sara Lawrence College and M.F.A. from New York University. Cara is a dancer, choreographer and Pilates instructor. She received her initial training in Pilates from first generation master teacher Kathleen S. Grant. Cara is the owner of Pilates Aligned (www.pilatesaligned.com) in Denver, Colorado, and she teaches workshops around the U.S. as well as overseas.

REFERENCES

[1]Joseph H. Pilates and William John Miller, *Return to Life Through Contrology*. Edited, reformatted and reprinted (Incline Village, NV: Presentation Dynamics, 1998) 10. Originally published by J.J. Augustine, 1945.

[2]Pilates and Miller, 9.

[3]Andre Bernard; Wolfgang Steinmuller; Ursula Stricker. *Ideokinesis A Creative Approach to Human Movement & Body Alignment*. (Berkeley, CA: North Atlantic Books, 2006), 5.

[4]Bernard, Steinmuller, Stricker, 3.

[5]Will Johhnson, *The Posture of Meditation*. (Boston, MA: Shambhala Publications, 1996), 15.

[6]Elaine Summers, Tension: loving tension, because without tension there is no life bio-kinetic. (New York: NY: *Movement Research Journal*, 1999). 7-8.

[7] Bernard, Andre; Steinmuller, Wolfgang; Stricker, Ursula, 94.

[8]Elaine Summers, 7.

[9]Pilates and Miller, 10.

WORKS CONSULTED

Bernard, A., Steinmuller, W. & Stricker, U. (2006). *Ideokenesis A Creative Approach to Human Movement & Body Alignment*. Berkeley, CA: North Atlantic Books.

Johnson, W. (1996). *The Posture of Meditation*. Boston & London: Shambhala Publications.

Pilates, J. (1945). *Return to Life*. NV: Presentation Dynamics Inc.

Summers, E. "Bio-Kinetic Tension: Loving tension, because without tension there is no movement; without movement there is no life." (1999). *Movement Research Journal*. pp. 7-8.

Todd, M. (1937). *The Thinking Body*. NJ: Princeton Book Company Publishers.

Lessons Taught, Lessons Learned: My Days with Romana

By Cary Regan

...how to support yourself so gravity doesn't take you down...

I was a dancer when I started studying Pilates. Since then the world has changed. I was in a world of dancers using Pilates as a tool for their profession. And now I'm in a marketplace where very affluent people study Pilates for general health, often not to enhance their skills in an athletic profession. Joe Pilates' exercises definitely work for the specific needs of the dancer. His exercises enhance our strengths, save us from injuries, and help us recover from injuries. And now in this age of technology, you have more people getting further and further removed from their bodies, so thank God they have enough money to come in to learn Pilates, so they can get back to finding out what their bodies do for them.

Over the decades, there have been different ways to use Pilates and different environments to use it in, but the one thing that never changes is you can never escape your body. If you don't know your body, and you need to be "introduced" to your body, Pilates is a fabulous way to get to know yourself.

When I worked with Romana, we were very familiar with teaching dancers, disciplined actors, or other individuals who practiced a complex athletic skill. Then there were people who studied directly with Joe Pilates who had a physical discipline such as boxing. These individuals had an appreciation for the work he was giving to them. When a wealthier clientele started coming to the studio, that kind of appreciation for the work was absent because many of these individuals did not devote themselves to a complex physical discipline, sport or athletic art form; it could be frustrating for both teachers and students.

You wouldn't believe how people have grown so uncoordinated. They don't know where they are in space, don't know where their muscles are, and don't know that they're not breathing. So, in some ways, teaching now means teaching people who need Pilates forever. Especially, if individuals keep getting and relying upon more technology, they'll keep multitasking, and they'll keep getting away from their bodies. Pilates isn't multitasking. It's a mind; it's a body; and it's an intention that all activate at once. Today people live much of their lives through BlackBerrys and computers and other screen-dependent activities. As a result, it seems that that Pilates is changing; it's changing to a different market.

Originally, when I worked with Romana, Pilates happened in a studio where you taught five hours per day. This is the rule that Joe Pilates established. At the end of five hours, you did your workout. In Joe Pilates' time students learned their exercises and practiced them. They were observed by teachers who would correct a few things; but teachers didn't need to prod students to do their exercises. Students just worked out. Now, studio culture is different. There's a one-on-one lesson or a class with instructor involvement, meaning we're always there as your personal cheerleader to bring you to the next level of exercise.

There are multiple ways of working with the Pilates method. Even though it's been changed in every decade, in every different environment, the bottom line is that Pilates works. The exercises work. Pilates eventually brings people back to their bodies if they've been away, that is, if they have not consistently stayed in relatively good physical condition. Pilates gives more strength, more control. I can see in the way students hold themselves that they feel good.

So I love the work. I love to teach it. I adore working with the person who needs it for a high-end skill, for that athlete who wants to tweak his performance: the Cirque du Soleil artist, the ballet dancer. But when you get someone who's an investment banker who is super stressed out and working 13-hour days, he often disregards his body's need to move and sustain a relatively good body conditioning.

Romana trained us all to see the full spectrum of clientele that would walk in the door. It's just amazing to see how the exercises bring healthiness that's not just for physical fitness, but also for well-being, energy, and self-confidence. When I attended the State University College at Purchase, New York, I was working on a B.F.A. in dance. The program required each member of the dance program to have Pilates in their curriculum in order to earn the degree. Having never heard of Pilates, we all attended the class. In walked Romana and her assistant for our first session.

She took us first through exercises on Mats, on the floor. I thought it was strange, and I wondered why I knew at least three-quarters of these exercises already. I thought, "Why do I know this?" I had no idea, but I'd been doing them since I was nine and didn't know they were called Pilates. Then Romana showed us the equipment and started teaching us the system. That was all new to me. She was like a magician of physical feats. She approached an apparatus called the High Chair. We didn't know what it was. She stepped up to it, pressed the pedal down, placed her other foot on top and floated up. After finishing the exercise, Romana asked one of us to try it. We figured well, she looks like a middle-aged woman; there's no reason why we won't float up on this thing. Suddenly we didn't move. The pedal was down. It didn't go anywhere, and we hadn't a clue. And here we were, 18 years old. Young dancers. We were strong, but we didn't understand the Pilates system or apparatus at all. That was how I began in Pilates.

That first semester of 1975 was amazing. It was amazing to realize there could be a specific set of exercises geared to enhance everything we needed in dance: the lift, the center, the standing leg, the muscular "wrap" of a turnout. The Pilates system was so skillfully taught; it was wonderful to reduce the effects of gravity by starting in the supine position. This way, we could encounter and strengthen core stabilizing muscles and strengthen them with more focus and attention. Back in 1975 this was something only done by a few people.

Pilates started from the Mat, but it moved, it evolved, it rolled. It didn't just lie flat on the floor. It used the floor as a surface, as a reference for the front of the body or the core of the body working to the back of the body as a support.

So, in one sense, Pilates was something very new to me. But the reason it was so familiar is that I had taken some version of Pilates Mat at the Alwin Nikolais/Murray Louis School in the '60s. It was probably around 1967. I attended school at Henry Street Settlement House, where Alwin Nikolais and Murray Louis were the resident choreographers at the dance school.

It wasn't until years later that I found out it was really Hanya Holm who set up the warm-up for Nikolais and his company. What he had wanted was something that had no affectations. He just wanted something that would totally warm up the whole body. And Hanya Holm studied with Joe Pilates, so she extrapolated exercises from the Pilates method and put them together as a Nikolais warm-up. Consequently, I'd been doing the Nikolais warm-up since I was nine years old, which would have been about 1966. So at S.U.N.Y. Purchase I realized how important the teaching aspect of Pilates is. The exercises I learned in 1966 were done totally for flow. But if you don't concentrate on the breath, and use the abdominal wall, or pull the navel towards the spine to get speed and fluidity when you stand up, you will not have the same strength. It's impossible to use the floor without really understanding how to teach. The floor is not a surface to fall into, relax into, but to work from and away from.

The funny thing was that a lot of the Nikolais dancers did not have enough strength when they stood up. So, instead of doing their Pilates, they would run to Zena Rommett to take ballet floor barre. This watered down the Pilates work. It's like that old game when someone tells you something, and then you tell the next person, and the next person, and by the 100th person, you have a whole different conversation from what you started with.

That's what can happen with the Pilates work as it gets changed and changed and changed. I take liberties and do variations, but I always try to come back to the original exercise, because the original method works, and it's great. The changes I make with Pilates work are for an individual's needs; then I bring them back to the original. You might teach somebody who has a rod in their back from a scoliosis surgery. You're not going to get spinal articulation. It doesn't mean they can't do Pilates work. You're just going to have to let that kind of roundness go from what you want. But that doesn't mean they're not going to be able to do the work. Those same principles of working with balance of stretch equal to flexibility, with breath, with awareness, with focus, with concentration, and working against resistance, all apply.

In many ways, there are so many exercises within the Pilates method that you're always going to find something a student can do. They're redundant in a sense, but not in a bad sense. You may not be doing exactly the same exercise, but it's engaging the same muscles in the core, in the trunk of the body. So if you can't do it lying down, you can do it sitting down. If you can't do it sitting down, you can do it kneeling or standing up. If you can't kneel or stand up, you can lie down. There's always a way we can get muscle groups to work advantageously. Also, it changes it up for you, so your mind doesn't get bored. Then your mind doesn't leave your body because it got bored after you did it 27 million times, and now your mind couldn't care less. Otherwise your mind's like, "Forget about it, I'm bored."

If your mind leaves you while you're driving a car, you'll tend to crash. If your mind leaves you while you are walking, you'll tend to hit things. So your mind should be present when you're doing physical activity, when you're involved in movement. Pilates always emphasized the mind being with the body, working with the body. Never take this for granted.

When I meet someone to begin working with them, I remember Romana. The first thing you noticed in the studio environment was that Romana was a host. She would walk in a studio, and you were in her studio. It was her home. It was her environment. It was hers. And we were the hostesses there, too. But as any good host—sometimes I would use the term "body bartender"—you see what's coming at you. You kind of know what's coming your way. I'm not known as the nicest teacher. And some people have said I'm pretty mean. But a funny thing they say in the studio is, "The harder they come, the more they like you." Because hard meets hard, and it just kind of balances out.

If you're a fragile person, I can be nice any time, but I work really well with people who are frustrated or pissed off; there's energy in anger. I'm not saying it's good energy, but it's something. I grew up with three brothers, really tough, and we'd fight. There were seven of us kids so, you know, I knew how to deal; and I'm the bottom, the last one. And I like that. I'd rather have that than a weepy sadness. Emotion has energy. When it's coming at me, I can redirect it or change it. I can manipulate it and switch it.

As a teacher, you're going to have all kinds of things come at you. Whoever comes to you has a personality. Usually the personality in that body is doing something to that body. You'll see the tension, the fear, the insecurity. For instance, with insecurity the head might tip to one side, or the shoulder might go down.

With fear, the arms might be crossed and the shoulders rolled in. You know, the "I'm so wonderful," the chest is popped so far forward that the back is arched. You're going to see that. I'm always going to go with the opposite of what I have coming at me.

With the person who is weak, or looking insecure, I'm going to give him a frame: put him in the High Chair. I'm going to put his back right up against that chair, get him Pumping. You've got to give them something. You can't give them everything, but you try within The Method; Romana would always see that.

I worked with one woman who had attempted suicide. Luckily, she didn't succeed. But at the end of working with me she started doing more lessons. By the end of six months, she was so amazed. She stopped working with her psychiatrist, but continued doing Pilates.

People start to see how important Pilates is in their lives. And Pilates becomes part of their budget. It's their life force. It's part of their life. It is part of their food. That's it. I always try to tell people if they really learn it, it's very cheap; you can do it at home on your own. Practice your Mat work every single day. Joe Pilates was out there in the sunshine getting a tan—you have your workout at the same time. So you can work it out! There is a sense in which Romana always was in her own studio, wherever she was, wherever her studio was. She worked every day. So whether it was a six-hour shift or a four-hour shift or whatever she needed to do, Romana physically worked with people and she physically enjoyed it. There was an enjoyment there that you could see from the beginning of a session to the end of the session. She had some cranky clients, and I have some, too. Not everyone of course, but, over the years, every teacher gets one; and you'll see how they change when they're at the end of the session. Their bodies feel better, and the work changes their personality.

Though it's not been realized yet, something that Joseph Pilates wanted to see was Pilates for children. The sooner people can get Pilates in their lives and keep it in their lives, the better their lives will be. I know Pilates is quite an expense. But, in relationship to the times, it has always cost money to do Pilates. But as I've always said to clients, "You give yourself a year of this, and, really, you have it for the rest of your life. If you really learn it, it's yours." It's Joseph Pilates' gift. Because it's a system of exercises that you can follow, and it works. Whether they worked in 1923 or 1993, they work. It's a constant. It doesn't need to be upgraded like a phone every six months. You don't need a new thing. That's another reason I love Pilates. You don't need any brand new toy for it and it is effective.

You can go to a fancy new gym and they can give you an anti-gravity running treadmill. La-dee-da! Then when they take you off your antigravity treadmill and put you back in the real world, what are you going to run on? You're going to have to walk on the real world with real gravity. So Pilates teaches you how to support yourself so gravity doesn't take you down, take you under.

No matter what exercises they have out there, the idea of the functioning core, what we call in Pilates the powerhouse, uses your abdominal muscles to lift you up and out of your limbs. It makes your limbs and your joints last longer. It always has made them last longer, and it always will make them last longer. There's no sneaker, there's no shoe, there's no special treadmill. You have to do the work, and you'll get the results.

I had a traumatic knee injury in college, tearing my anterior cruciate ligament on my left knee. I didn't just tear it, I severed it; it was gone. So, back then, 1976, that pretty much cut your ability to dance down to zero. I was told to give up dance. Romana looked at me and said, "Oh, they don't know what they're talking about. You don't have to do that." So Romana worked with me. I had an excellent knee doctor, but still not as fabulous as Romana. She said, "They haven't caught up to Joe Pilates yet. They don't know what we do." And that was in 1976.

And so I thought, "I love dancing." Romana said I didn't have to stop. So I said to myself, "Okay, I'm not stopping." And I did it, and there were other people doing it, too. One person was from the original Chorus Line, not the remake. Another woman was from American Ballet Theater, and there was a guy in the Joffrey Ballet. All of us, in 1976, had no ACL. But we were all working professionals. I worked without an ACL for 13 years before I actually got a knee reconstruction in 1989. If it hadn't been for Romana, I wouldn't have been able to believe that was really possible. But she had a way about her; when she said something, it was "the word." You believed it. That was it. And I guess I really needed that at the time.

Within a year and a half of studying with Romana, I was doing Graham knee crawls and everything with no ACL. Romana didn't seem to be surprised by it. I might have had a little set back here and there, but that was the dance world.

Romana would go to the person who seemed to need the most help. She could look in a room—and I don't know how she had that skill—but she would know. Romana would give that person three exercises to help pump up their spirit or to release tension in the muscles. She had a keen ability; she had magic about her. She carried herself with a kind of silk pajama magic. She was the gypsy, with the magical crystal ball. She read tea leaves. She always had that exotic quality in her, and she was physically exuberant. Romana had an amazing amount of energy. She loved people and life and happiness and the ballet and the world—she loved them all. Romana loved energy; she thrived on it and she would give it as well as she received it. She was that way, and she liked her studio to be that way. She liked her teachers to be that way, and she didn't like worrying. She didn't like fretting. She didn't like being down. Everything was up. Romana had that kind of spark. In my day, you were invited into her party, and she taught you. She taught you because either you could pick it up, or she saw that you had a spark. Then she could work with that. She never felt, in those days, that she could write a manual and then teach somebody. It had to be in you. It was like taking on the work of teaching a racehorse. Not everyone is a racehorse. Not everyone is a Pilates teacher.

Romana would just see it. You could watch her, and you absorbed her knowledge or you didn't. Once there was one woman, I forget her name now, but I know she had cancer. She would come every day for 20 minutes. Romana didn't charge her. Romana was like that. You just don't bill someone in that condition. That's who Romana was, you know. She worked with a woman who had multiple sclerosis. And you would think there was a party going on there. Romana would be giggling. I can't even imitate her giggle, but you would know it when Romana laughed. She had the woman on the Cadillac, holding on and pulling up. They were exercises, but they were not Pilates exercises. Romana was sharing the spirit of life. That client was on the Cadillac. She's doing something. She's doing whatever she can do, and she's out there every day doing it. She would rather be with Romana than in a physical therapist's office. There are some nice physical therapy offices, but I've been in them. With Pilates you feel like you're doing something; you're making progress, you're moving with your entire body and mind. In physical therapy, the focus is upon injury, the negative part of the body and rehabilitation. Naturally, a lot of times you feel injured, you're down, and the physical therapists are just going to bill insurance, then it's done.

Pilates is energy. You're around a lot of people who are all different ages, who are all doing different things, and who are all at different skill levels. This spirit, this energy that I'm talking about—Anthony Rabara saw it. He lived it. We worked on the same shift at the studio. Phoebe Higgins lived it. She worked on that same shift with Romana and Sari. At that time, those of us who worked with Romana, the studio was our space. That was 1981 through 1989. That was the spirit in the studio; it was alive: let's have fun, and oh, laugh. Yet there was serious energy given to exercises; it wasn't strictness, though, as much as it was to "live the movement," to have fun, to attempt new goals and keep aiming for excellence. In Romana's space, it was the spirit that I felt. She felt the most important way to grow is to have happiness, to have joy. You have to want something, desire something in order to change the body, for it to move.

I think Romana was the eternal optimist when it came to life. Romana believed the Pilates system helped sustain health and well-being; she was right. Years later, when I finally had knee surgery, the doctors asked, "How could you do so well for so long?" It turns out the body and the mind are well-connected; and eventually, within about a three-year period, the mind will retrain other muscles to replace what an injured ligament previously accomplished in the knee area. After about two and a half years, my knee dislocated fewer and fewer times. Pilates really targeted everything I needed. I don't know how many Standing Side Splits I had to do, and Cross-over Pumping at the Chair, and Magic Circle for inner thighs, pliés; everything to get the abductors, hamstrings and core working. It was amazing, you know.

Physical therapy never came close to what Pilates accomplished for knee rehab, at least back in the 1970s. I'm not saying they don't have more things, but Pilates was far ahead of physical therapy in the 1970s, and I'm talking about exercises developed in the U.S. since the 1920s. Of course Joe Pilates began creating his work many years before in Germany.

I guess what's sad for me now is that people think Pilates is just a female workout. Joe Pilates did not design his exercise system for women. This is not something they should simply do after lunch or before lunch. Pilates is not a new and humorous trend to appear on *Sex and the City*. This work is something that the male population used. I wish Pilates would get more respect for the physical work it is. The Pilates system can enhance so much in your entire body; it's not just for big hips and your loose tummy. It's for a much deeper skill level. Pilates is for balance, control and multitasking for fine-tuned athletes. I think Pilates is for the dancer, for the artist, and for the "everyday" person.

When I first started working with Romana, the studio was at 29 West 56th Street. So it's right between Fifth and Sixth Avenue. It was a long rectangular room. It was a one-room studio. It went from the front to the back of the building. So there were six Reformers, a desk, and then about four Mats, then two Cadillacs, a half-Cadillac, and a Guillotine. But everything could be seen from this one big rectangle. There were two shifts, and there were four to five teachers per shift. And we were all in the same room. There was someone working out on every Reformer and on every Mat. At that time, we did not have the approach of one student being taught by one teacher. So every student had the eyes of other teachers, and instructors could interject. A student could be working out with Phoebe. Well, Phoebe might go to answer the phone, and I would say, "Drop those shoulders" to the student. And that's it. And then I would go away. But if I'm across the room and you see me in the mirror, you already know I'm checking you. I'd say, "Oh, you're going to miss my correction twice?" So that was the kind of playfulness that was there.

As a student, there could be multiple people telling you what to do. So there was an energy. Between the teachers, too. There was the feeling that you had freedom of movement. I liked it; we all loved it. This kind of playfulness taught the client to be self-correcting, which is what the goal was, and is.

Pilates is a method for you to learn, and then as you learned it, Romana and Joe would expect that you're going to know your order. Romana tells the story of Joe saying, "What's the next exercise?" And the client said, "This." Then Joe said, "What is this?" And the client said, "Running." Joe said, "Good, have a nice shower." Because if you didn't know what came next, you did Running. If Running was an incorrect answer or choice, then goodbye; you're done for the day.

So Joe was tough that way. In the studio, there was the rolling cart with photos of Joe doing all his exercises. Students would roll it in front of their Reformers if they didn't know their workout order. If they had to ask which exercise came next, we would say, "You know you need another private." So, to save money, clients learned their workouts for themselves. I was just beginning as a teacher—a baby teacher—so clients might know more than I did. Sometimes Romana questioned my teaching. For instance, sometimes I would refer to a more precise anatomical phrase such as "pubic bone." Romana would call me aside. She did not like me to use that word. I said, "Well, what am I supposed to say, Romana?" She said, "Nothing. Don't refer to it at all." Then an old client said to me, "Oh, don't listen to Romana. Clara used to put her fist right down on your pubic bone and nail you right to the Reformer." So that's what I mean. You had clients who were there with Joe and Clara. So I even had clients telling me, "Oh, you teach like Clara."

Our clientele in the early 1980s was high-end Pilates in the sense that 75% to 80% of the studio was advanced. That's high. There was a high level of advanced practitioners. And, I mean, really advanced. After the first year, I worked afternoons. At the time, John Winters was teaching in the studio. John Winters was probably in his late 60s when I started working there. He wore white shorts, white pants, white ankle socks and white sneakers. He was dressed in all white with a little belt.

When I worked with John Winters, he would make variations. John taught me all the exercises that were considered men's exercises. John said that Joe made women do these things. And when you see archival footage, you see women in bathing suits, doing the High Chair, doing the Dips and everything. I would play sometimes with the Magic Circle or a piece of equipment and I'd ask, "Oh, John, what about this?" And he'd say, "Ooh, Joe would have liked that variation. Joe would have liked that. Oh, keep that, keep that."

So John was one who believed if the principles were all there, good, keep it. He did, unfortunately, push just like Joe. He could kill you when you did the Rowing. Don't ask him for a push because he was like, boom, boom, boom. When you saw Joe push people like that, it made you wonder a little bit. That's why you had to be really strong, bounce back.

Working with John was very, very positive. He liked working more on strength moves. And he worked very specifically. Romana emphasized tempo, while John was really all about form. He went for a strong form, and he didn't go for speed. I've never seen anybody quite like that.

John taught resistance with the Reformer. The way he taught it wasn't about speed, but suspension. And Romana did that sometimes, too. She would say, "I could snap a photo at any time," meaning, "I could stop you and you'd be right where you are." You could be in the Long Stretch and hold. And she's going to take a picture, meaning that you could stop at any point during the exercise because you were in control. So, therefore, you could support it at any angle.

We had a male population that was huge. And we had almost all male teachers. Doug Figachelli, Danny Burke, Rodney, Patrick Strong, John, Lori, and then came me, the baby teacher. Patrick Strong taught the divas. He had every star on the planet. He had Makarova, Candice Bergen, Louie Malle, Bill Hurt. I mean, everybody was there. It was unreal. Michael Romano, a star chef, was working with him. We had the conductor for the New York City Ballet orchestra and the New York Opera. James Lipton. It was unreal. So you just had this high level energy of people and male, all male teachers except for Royce Gandora, who was like Ms. Broadway. But she was a good teacher. She was a really good teacher. She really knew what she was doing.

Patrick Strong was caffeine city, espresso city. Out in 45 minutes; he kept to the Joe Pilates 45-minute mark. You had five minutes to tell Patrick what you were feeling in your body. After that, not another word. Forty-five minutes, bam. He would punch you in the stomach while you did the 100. And they all loved him. Loved him.

Romana made him the star teacher because he was so intense. He was five feet tall, my height. I danced with him, so I knew him. He had left college about a year early, and I guess he started working at Romana's. He was aggressive, intense. And any time there was any-body with a slight muscle tweak or an injury, he'd say, "Cary, this is for you." So that's how I worked with all the injuries. And watching

Romana, who taught me how to work with so many injuries.

One man I learned to work with had half a leg, and he was missing most of his left arm. He used a crutch. Anyway, we worked with him. And that man, about six months later, was fitted with a prosthetic for his leg. Then his physical therapist came in with him the next week because he wanted to see what kind of service we provided. He had never seen anybody get a leg and adjust in 10 minutes to all the balance, without using a crutch.

So far, I've seen some good physical therapists, but not as many as really good Pilates instructors. And I've seen what a really good Pilates session can do for someone. When Romana referred to bad Pilates, she meant taking something of a Pilates exercise and manipulating it until it no longer had the principles. For example, where is your powerhouse? Why are you calling it Pilates? If you're not using the principles, just call the system something else. Don't call it Pilates. We all know how to open our legs and close them together but that doesn't make the action Pilates. So, bad Pilates does not use the principles. Where's your core? Where's your powerhouse? Where's your breath? Are you focused? These kinds of things.

Romana would stop you at the top of Open Leg Rocker and make you hold it. She loved to do that. She loved rolling. She was like a little acrobat, a little gymnast. She could do anything. She could do plenty of tricks. Somersault, and Roll Back off the Mat. And roll onto the Mat. Romana loved Forward Walkovers and the Candle Walkover. These are strength moves that I don't practice now, although I did them every day when I was with everyone in the studio. Every day we would hang off the Cadillac and do the Beats. Then we would practice the Corkscrew off the Cadillac. You name it, we did it. My shoulders were the strongest things in the world. And all the guys were ripped.

You truly had an appreciation for Joe Pilates; his clients loved him so much, and they loved his method even more. Students would not stop coming to his studio to do the work. They were all there in their bathing suits and no shirts on.

The big new megagyms are like Starbucks now. They're on every corner. And they put Pilates in there, too. But I don't think there is enough independent marketing by traditional teachers for the public to understand that Pilates works best outside of that setting. The male population, 54, 55, 56 years of age, they could definitely benefit from Pilates. I don't know where they are. I don't think they're in the mega-gyms. They're our generation. Maybe these men think they're too old and they're giving up, but we as teachers should not give up communicating the benefits of Pilates for men. Remember, The Method was made for men. We could target these individuals with advertising and networking. Their health and well-being are at stake.

I think younger men don't find Pilates until they have injuries. Before then, younger men just don't come to the studios. They've got egos, man! In the past, I've attended conferences for male college athletics. These conferences were for the coaches, the colleges and the men. There were booths setup for sales and marketing different products and services. There was a guy next to me selling a type of shoulder girdle apparatus to improve tennis. And I thought, "What the hell is this? What are you selling?" So, there I was trying to promote Pilates in the midst of coaches and colleges, and they're all selling all this stuff. I was the only woman there. I finally said to one man, "Give me five minutes, and I'll give you a workout." Afterwards, I said, "Now do you see my point?" The guy said, "I can't believe it." Then other guys came over.

Finally, I think Pilates will survive and thrive. In this world of technology, Pilates can never die because we need it to balance our physical relationship to technology. Through the mind-body connection and Pilates system, humanity stays connected to itself so we can find and keep good relationships with each other. As instructors, it would be very beneficial to incorporate Pilates into public school systems, colleges and the corporate world.

Romana always said, "There are plenty of clients who want and need this work." In the spirit of Joe, he would say we have endless work ahead. There's not enough time to do everything that Joe would have done, and to improve what Joe would have wanted. The concepts he left us are still the ones that work beautifully. And the idea of reaching more people with Pilates is one that everybody would love to see happen.

About Cary

Cary Regan began her training in the Pilates method at S.U.N.Y. Purchase in 1975 under the direction of Romana Kryzanowska. She received her B.F.A. in dance from The State University of New York at Purchase and continued her Pilates training at the original Pilates Studio in New York. Cary has been teaching the authentic Pilates method since 1981. Over the years she has worked in collaboration with physical therapists, chiropractors, orthopedists, and dance companies to integrate the work of Joseph Pilates with the sports/dance medicine world. With more than 30 years of Pilates teaching experience, Cary is considered a Master Teacher. She is the director of teacher training at re:AB Pilates in New York.

The Joy of Pilates

By Mari Winsor

Inspiration comes deep from within.

I was trained and certified by Romana Kryzanowska in 1993. Anyone can teach a technique. But can they inspire you to really want it, and want more? Romana inspired me. She was joyful, she was commanding, and she made me want to be the best that I could be.

When I first started my business, I knew some movements on the Reformer. I won't call it Pilates because it wasn't. I realized very quickly I was a little short when it came to proper Pilates movement. I didn't know where to go or what to do to get this valuable information. Then a very dear friend who knew how I liked to gather information and study, said, "This is the person that you need to study with." So I said, "Done."

I booked an appointment with Romana. I took my lesson with her, and everything fell into place. The work we did made sense. I knew at that moment that I had to learn as much as I could from her because she had the flow. She had the information. She studied with Joseph Pilates, and this was what I was missing.

I have the capacity to teach. I can teach anything that I feel in my heart. I have the talent to do that. Romana saw that. She put her trust in me, and that was empowering.

Romana made me laugh, and we had some great times together. While I was studying with her, I couldn't wait to get on the Reformer. Anybody can buy a book or a video and learn the exercises. There is no heart behind that. Romana taught you the logic. It was something that oozed out of her pores: powerhouse, joy and feeling better. Empowered.

Inspiration comes deep from within. That element of inspiration is missing in some teachers today. The ability to look at the body in front of you and focus completely on how one can make that body feel better is becoming lost. Being positive and kind are necessary ingredients for being a good communicator. Also being joyful in what you do plays an important role for your clients. More teachers need to find that joy for themselves rather than having the work be just a list of exercises.

We can't forget that this is movement. As teachers, we already have a mindset of movement. That's our life; that's what we do. Most clients don't have that mindset unless they're athletes. Normal people take their kids to school, meet their husbands for lunch, or they work; their lives have not revolved around movement like ours have. We as teachers have a responsibility to be patient with our clients.

When clients come to you, you want them to get the most out of what they're doing. You want them to feel joy. You want their bodies to feel better than they did when they walked in. This has not as much to do with technique or alignment, and everything to do with moving and feeling joyful about it.

Once you get them hooked on that feeling, then you backtrack. Then you can say, "Well, if you did this on your Footwork, and squeezed here," it will work because they'll want it. They'll make that connection, and realize how much better they will feel if they do it really correctly.

The desire to work correctly has to come from them; you can't force that on people. Clients don't really want to hear about what's wrong. Especially if they've been doing Pilates someplace where they do it incorrectly, or, they've been doing something else but it's been called Pilates. Don't criticize. Embrace that. As a teacher, you embrace those differences. You want to help your client.

The client is putting their body into your hands, so you want to embrace them in every way. You don't want to be negative, and say, "Jeez! Who taught you that? Where did you learn that? Oh, that's wrong!" You don't want people to feel that they've wasted their time somewhere. You want people to feel empowered. Instead, the best thing to say is, "I'm really glad you have done Pilates somewhere else because it makes my job easier. Try it this way, and see if this works better for you. See if you feel this more. If you do, that's great. Then we can go deeper into the work that you already know, and we'll have a good working relationship."

It's so important to stay positive and to stay joyful about what you do. For instance, I love to move. I hate to exercise. When somebody says "exercise" to me, I think, Ugh. But I love to move; I love to feel my body in space. I like to be in control of my body in space and know where I'm going every second. That comes from my dance training, but I've found joy in movement my whole life.

So, when I quit my dance career and was going into exercise, I didn't really get the same sense of joy. When I met Romana, she rekindled that joy of movement in me; it brought me back to my early dance days. With that, I became committed to her and the work of Jospeh Pilates.

If you can instill joy in your clients, they will be committed to you; you will have clients forever, and the work will spread. If you make it drudgery, if you talk down to people and tell them what they're doing is wrong, you're never going to have clients. You have to really focus on the body that's in front of you and instill your knowledge, creativity, imagination, and intelligence into that body. Then, that body will respond to you in a positive way. That's all you want.

The joy of teaching is to have that joy reciprocated to you. What better words are there from a client to a teacher than, "Oh my God, I feel better! Oh my God, my spine feels longer! Oh my God, I feel taller!" It's as if they'd never felt anything like that before. The client will gush, "Oh my God, you're responsible for this." But I'm not. I just provide the tools; you chose to use the tools. You chose to do that, so you are empowered because you listened. You did it, and you're committed. Now you have joy.

There's nothing worse than a cranky teacher. Think back to when you were in grade school. Can you remember any of your cranky teachers? I only remember the ones who gave me joy. I remember the ones who inspired me to move forward and to go into my education in a different new way. Discovery.

It's the same in every profession. There are people who know this is a responsibility, and this is what they have to do. I love this work. Whether you're a salesperson or an executive or a Pilates teacher, you have to take responsibility and do what's best for the client. Because the work is not about you; it's about the client. If you make it about the client, then your needs will be fulfilled. End of story.

One way to make it about the client is to give them something that they can be successful at. Jay Grimes always says, "At the end of class, give them an exercise they'll be successful at, so that they'll leave your studio feeling that they can do something." Because the work can be daunting; as a teacher, it's up to you to make it accessible.

If you're with a client who has trouble connecting, and you just get them to move, it'll be better than trying to go into detail fixing them. As teachers, we're not here to fix people. The work fixes people. In order for people to do the work, you have to be patient; clients are not like teachers.

I come from a family of teachers. I am a direct descendent of William Brewster, who came over on *The Mayflower*. He was one of the religious leaders on *The Mayflower*. He was an organizer, leader, teacher, and orator. I have that in my bloodline. Cotton Mather, one of the first presidents of Yale, was one of the first people to write essays against burning witches. I am one of his direct descendants, as well. I have many judges and ministers in my family line. It's something that burns inside me, that explodes, and I can't explain it. When I'm teaching, I'm not even thinking about what comes next. It just comes next. I appreciate that talent, and honor that talent, but, most of all, I feel grateful that I've been able to find a place where I can use that talent. That, to me, is joy and responsibility. Clients are putting their bodies in your hands. You can be grateful, and joyful, and patient and kind, or you can be cranky, and suck your teeth and roll your eyes. You have a choice. I choose joy.

About Mari

In 1990, Mari, a former professional dancer, opened her first Pilates studio in Los Angeles, introducing her innovative signature workout to her celebrity clients. Certified by Romana Kryzanowska, with whom she continues to study, Winsor has brought Pilates to a national audience. She sold more than 29 million DVDs, co-wrote three books on Pilates, and her fitness expertise has been featured in countless magazines. Her Los Angeles studios attract some of the biggest names in show business. Committed to sharing her knowledge and experience with the public, Mari has created an Online Winsor Pilates Fitness Club.

Chapter III

Methodology

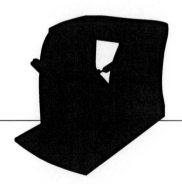

On Good Teaching

By Anthony Rabara

*Give them one pearl at a time, not
the entire string of beads.*

I first met Romana Kryzanowska in 1979 after a dance injury. Romana saw something in my work and asked me to teach with her at the studio on West 56th Street. The studio always seemed to have plenty of dancers and artists, and Pilates (Contrology) had not yet hit the mainstream population. Romana ran the studio, paid our salaries, taught mornings and afternoons, and trained us to teach Joe's work. My story is not unlike that of many early teachers. I learned the fundamentals of Contrology through Romana's understanding of movement and exercise. She taught me the benefits of each apparatus. I also learned the fundamentals of teaching by her example. Romana would say, "Just get the body to move, then work on the issues." It sounds simple, but what a regimen of bodywork!

Certainly, we all know that Pilates is physical and mental conditioning. I am sure that I learned Pilates as a physical entity first. I needed to heal my body so that I could continue dancing without pain. Most dancers possess the discipline to learn the work. It's engrained in our psyche. The beauty of the work came with balancing and challenging the body. Romana was a keen teacher. A single finger-tap was all she needed to get someone to understand what she wanted. Her musicality, her eye for movement and understanding of the body, was wonderful to witness and experience. I, like many, studied and performed music as well as danced professionally. Romana told me that she always felt that when she taught me that we were dancing together. I cherish that comment and have shared that with very few because it is so precious to me. Romana shared the best of herself—with everyone. Having the good fortune to train with such a gifted person and teacher helped to instill in me a passion for the work. I also easily developed a healthy vocabulary with which to teach others because I'd had Romana as my mentor and teacher.

The ability to see the body and "touch" are two important aspects of teaching. I am a hands-on teacher. We all emulate our mentors to some degree and develop our own styles of teaching. Gesture and touch have always been a part of my teaching; Romana was a genius at this. If your gestures are simple and instructive, you can often help a client/student through a lesson where words and images fail.

One focus of my teaching is working with people who have extreme muscular issues. My first such experience was working with a nine-year-old boy who had a form of muscular laxity. Weak and hypermobile joints meant that his joints could easily dislocate. He was unable to walk or sit up for extended periods of time. As a baby, he was carried in a scooped out sponge, so as to not damage his limbs and joints. Weight bearing was risky. His form of locomotion was a wheelchair. For nine years, we worked on developing his muscular system so that he could sit upright. Next, our goal was to get him out of a wheelchair and onto his legs with the help of braces. He is in college now and can walk with the aid of leg braces and a walker. He is a classical Indian singer, and he can sit upright through his performances without pain or assistance. In 2002, I presented him and his family to a Romana's Pilates conference in Las Vegas, where he demonstrated the Mat work and the Cadillac exercises that helped bring him to the current level of strength and mobility. And, for the second time only, he walked across the room with leg supports. That 25 feet was a dramatic moment for everyone attending. There were few dry eyes.

I am currently working with a boy who has muscular dystrophy (MD). Muscular dystrophy challenges certain muscles, and the person with MD may need the use of a wheelchair. Our job is to keep him mobile for as long as possible and out of a wheelchair. Working with children presents particular challenges. Teaching becomes a creative adventure utilizing the full scope of Pilates apparatus and tools. Often a playful gesture on a piece of equipment can be turned into an exercise that mimics a traditional exercise taught to a healthy body. Head pillows become Magic Circles, and breathing exercises can help build abdominal strength and balance the back muscles. Eventually, we transitioned these tools to the appropriate Pilates equipment. At the outset, I was not sure that I could help either boy, but through my years of experience and training and trusting Joe's work, I knew that I could make some difference. This young boy, now 13, and I are now Skyping lessons with a teacher and her student, who also has a form of MD. So now we are extending our work beyond my studio to another studio several miles away. Contrology is both a science and an art. The artist shares and passes on information. In this case, science helps us do just that. The science in Pilates helps teachers figure out and understand body function. Joe gave us that in his work. Romana passed this on to me and others. My intent is to do the same.

In my early years, perhaps around 1982, Romana asked me to work with a client who had Multiple Sclerosis. As her disease progressed, I worked with her at her home in New York City. Romana somehow sensed that I could handle more complex clients, and I think that trust was the spark that led me to working with those who are physically challenged. Lori Coleman-Brown, a physical therapist and Pilates teacher, brings her skill and science to the same group of people. There are many who find the same kind of joy in helping in this way. Both of the boys I mentioned were written about in *Pilates Style*. Articles like these help to educate the public on the benefits of Pilates. We pass it on. So in the spirit of Romana and Sari, we do as much as we can for the client.

Each of us has teaching strengths. The concerned teacher knows when he has taught a good class, though the criteria may be different from teacher to teacher. If after a lesson you feel good about what your client has learned, you've taught a good class. You work with the body in front of you and give it what it needs. That was always Romana's premise. You give them one thing to work on. She said, "Give them one pearl at a time, not the entire string of beads." All of us early teachers remember this mantra. She would say, "If they have learned one thing about their body when they walk out of the door, you have accomplished your goal."

Over years of teaching, one develops sensitivity to the body. It's a kind of kinesthetic sympathy that allows you to relate to what a client might be feeling as they progress through a lesson. My range of movement experience, for example, serves as a vehicle to sense what the body in front of me is sensing. I become sensitive to the person and better able to know how much to push a client and when to ease up. There is a lot to accomplish in one hour. We have to bring all of our sensibilities to that hour of teaching. The more skills you develop, the more you can bring to a lesson. Some skills are learned; some are innate. How many times has a teacher watched a lesson and said, "I feel what you are doing with your body! I feel you working!" I have heard many good teachers say that. It is a sense you develop or understand. Choosing the correct exercise for a client is also an element in teaching a good class. Identifying a client's movement habits is another element, and defining those elements might just become the theme of your lesson.

First, I should say that there are many good Pilates teachers out there who may come from other training backgrounds. I am just happy to have the years with Romana that I have had. Teaching is much different from instructing. Teaching comes from the inside, and not from a list of exercises. Teachers give of themselves. Romana and Sari are evidence of that. We have all studied Joe's videotapes. He seemed to teach with a kind of force that we do not use these days. Earlier teachers who worked in the original studio will attest to that. However, I think that Romana included her great sense of movement in this discipline. Sari said to me one day that there were many other dancers who contributed elements of movement also. But again, it was Romana who was asked to carry Pilates forward in Joe's studio. Romana has tremendous musicality. She brought movement and music to her teaching. I try to bring that to my teaching, as well. This is one way I carry on Romana's spirit. We all have our own specialness; Romana, Sari and Daria have theirs. You have your own specialness. Then your experience in teaching allows you to foster and improve that specialness and pass it on to those you teach. Romana continuously gave of herself. That was one of her greatest contributions to all of us.

In teaching those with complex physical issues, I had to trust in my teaching experience to know that I could help these individuals in some capacity. As you know, I help teach apprentices and newer teachers at our home studio in New York City, True Pilates. It was in one of those sessions that a new apprentice wanted to know why we do not have a book that shows pictures of all the exercises, an explanation of how to teach each one, and Joe's purpose in developing those exercises. Part of my answer to her was that she will need to trust that all of our combined experience will guide her to understanding this work and hopefully to be able to teach it. She wanted a shortcut to teaching. As I mentioned earlier, we are not about turning out people who read from lists, but developing those who have a passion for teaching

Pilates. I will never forget that back around 1988, Romana said, "We need to document our teaching." In our studio on East 56th Street, Romana made a video of seven of us performing most of the exercises in the repertoire. This was before workbooks and a syllabus existed. That tape became the first "certification" (with stamp and seal) of the Pilates method. Soon to follow were seminars, workshops and more certifications. In that same manner, I give as much as I have learned to others, in the hope and trust that they will follow suit.

It is our tradition. There is also another part of trust that comes from teaching experiences. If you are honest about what you do and how you teach, your students are more than likely to teach with the enthusiasm and quality that so many of our teachers possess. With that honesty and trust you do not have to feel threatened by others' teaching or the need to promote yourself. Trust is inherent in your person. That can be contagious. And, part of our Pilates "food" as a teacher is to watch other good instructors teach—experience their skills and not be threatened by them. I tell teachers that you never stop learning about your craft. You might be employed and have a certification, but your learning does not ever end. Romana has said many times that she never stops learning about what she does.

I know what the work feels like in my body. The continued work and lessons of my own help me to be a better teacher than I was 10 years ago. Also, through my former injury and the aches of getting older, I can identify with those who may have similar problems. I can get to the source of those problems more quickly and move to the next stage of Pilates development. All of your prior experience becomes part of your vocabulary from which to draw when teaching.

I am a better teacher than manager. Many who are in the same shoes will probably say the same. Pilates is global now and certainly has business needs. As a studio owner, I have always felt that the business should support the teaching, not the other way around. Surely we all need to pay our bills. Romana would say that, too. But I think that the business aspect needs to support the teachers and their teaching schedules. Your business grows because you and your teachers have good teaching skills. That brings in more clients, and then we develop business strategies to support the growing business. When I first started the studio, I did everything. Even now, when the telephone rings, I want to pick it up. Fortunately, the desk staff (who are also integral in supporting the studio) let me do what I do best: teach. Managing my studio is supported by the philosophy of what I do. If I teach well and realize each client's interests, I believe the business falls into place more naturally.

Like everyone else, I get up and have great days and not-so-great days. But here is one thing that I pass on to my teachers. If the first person of the day is Sally, I take a few minutes to think about her. I think about her last lesson and what it was like, her possible needs that day, etc. From the first words I speak, she knows that I am mindful of her. From there I develop my lesson as we work together. It sets me up for that particular hour. The anthropologist Margaret Mead said, "Never doubt that a small group of thoughtful, committed citizens can change the world; indeed, it's the only thing that ever has." That is our mission: to positively change the world through Pilates.

About Anthony

Anthony Rabara is a Master Teacher with Romana's Pilates. He was introduced to the Pilates studio in 1979 because of a dance-related injury, rehabilitated, and asked by Romana Kryzanowska to teach. Anthony left the New York studio in 1987 and opened his studio in Princeton, NJ. Articles have been published about his work with clients who have severe injury including muscular laxity, muscular dystrophy, MS and fibromyalgia. Anthony helps train apprentices who are enrolled in the Teacher Certification Program through Romana's Pilates. Anthony holds a M.A. degree in and Dance, a B.A. in Music and has danced professionally in the United States and Europe.

The Red Thread

By Kathryn Ross-Nash

> *...the connections between all movements in the traditional Pilates method.*

The Red Thread is my way of describing the connections between all movements in the traditional Pilates method. When you stay within the framework of the classical system, you can be creative. Yet there must always be a clear connection—Red Thread—that takes you back to original exercises.

At first glance, the Red Thread is a very simple concept. Yet it is an important key to the subtlety and deep complexity of traditional Pilates technique. First, the Red Thread provides a way to help teachers understand how to utilize The Method; it also demystifies the work for students. Say you asked a student to do Spine Stretch Forward, and she has practiced it ever since the first lesson. Then you ask her to practice Horseback on the Barrel. If you teach Horseback as a totally different exercise, it's scary. You're up on top of something. But if you say, "This is Spine Stretch Forward," the person thinks, "Oh, I know this exercise." And it takes some fear out of it.

There are many components to The Red Thread. I chose red because blood is red, and that is what Pilates is all about. Pilates is getting circulation through the body, and that's what makes The Method work. It gets circulation in areas of the body that don't get circulation, and that's why it's so powerful. We use the circulation, the blood, the pumping of the blood through the body to purify and to cleanse it. The Pilates system is designed to move blood through the body. For example, the Footwork stimulates various organs in the body through pressure points. Then pumping motions of the Hundred exercise intensify circulation even more. There are so many exercises where we're squeezing our thighs inward, reaching long in extension with the legs, and pulling up with abdominals that we're actually using the body like an accordion to squeeze the blood in and out to clean out toxins in our organs. So that's why I chose red.

Joe Pilates understood how human beings learn. One way we edu-cate ourselves in the Pilates system is to practice the same exercise in many different positions on different pieces of apparatus. Joseph Pilates took the same exercise and moved it spatially. For example, think of the Double Leg Stretch. You're on your back doing it, right? Then you can practice the same muscular actions in Knee Stretches. When you are practicing Going Up Front, you're doing the Single Leg Stretch because you bring one leg in and stretch one leg out; but it is the same exercise in all different planes, in all different body positions. The different positions change the effect on the body and prepare you to engage your stomach doing that exercise in all different positions.

Everything in Pilates is to prepare you for functional movement. It's not to prepare you to do cartwheels. We do cartwheels so that our balance gets off, and we have to catch it; we then experience that topsy-turvyness. Remember, Joseph Pilates was a martial artist. You get thrown as a martial artist. You roll. You have to get yourself right back up and be on your feet and have your center. And the only way that you can do that is to have experienced it. Pilates teaches us to move with a strong center no matter what is thrown at us. That's the beauty of it. It prepares us for the unexpected.

The other thread that I find running through the work is how bril-liant Joseph was with using planes of action. So in the very begin-ning, you're just using your frontal plane. It's very simple. Then we will teach an exercise with side flexion. As a teacher, you may notice asymmetries as one side might have more range of motion; the other side might exhibit more rotation. In yet another example, regarding the axis of our skull, one side naturally has more range of motion; the other side naturally rotates a little more. It's related to survival. If I have to look quickly, I want to be able to utilize that ability; but if they're equal then you don't know which way to go, you don't know which way to check first. Things that are innate to humans sometimes create imbalances.

In the Pilates system, you can learn about your own alignment. You may discover that you turn more easily to the right than to the left. It's important to be aware of that difference and practice exercise that helps both sides work equally. Twisting is the same thing. Then you go into rotation. As a teacher we might ask, How can we help someone achieve better alignment? How can we teach a student to learn and correct themselves after they utilize different planes of action within the Red Thread?

Joseph Pilates breaks down body movements to simple planes of action to retrain the body. Then he moves to two planes of action. For example, you have the Twist and the Reach. So you're using the frontal plane with rotation. Then he adds dynamic movement. You have the Snake and the Twist, which is actually the exact same as Twist and Reach, you just flip it upside down. Another example is the Tree. Everybody gets all complicated with the Tree, but it's so simple. It's the Roll Up. The leg is there. You bring your head to the knee, you take it up. It's your Roll Up. And then you go back, and then you come back up with the crown of the head to the knee. It's also your Control Balance.

The connections between every Reformer exercise and Mat exercise are to strengthen muscles that are weak and challenge what is biomechanically ineffective. Every exercise that we do is connected to the other. Every single exercise. If I look at Going Up Front, I know that it's the Single Leg Stretch. If I look at Standing Pumping, I know that's Going Up Front. If I look at Pumping on the Foot Corrector, I know that that's Going Up Front, which is my Single Leg Stretch. If I notice there is misalignment between knee, hip and ankle of a student, I can say, "Okay. Let me see Going Up Front." I may find the student is not quite ready or able. Their instability could be in the ankle. So I ask the person to practice Pumping Standing, so that they can strengthen the position of the ankle. If you see somebody whose foot is collapsing inward, utilize the Foot Corrector, or try Standing Pumping, or the Ankle Press. Every single exercise is interwoven, and that has always been how I have differentiated my work from other people's work. If it's not connected, then it is not within the traditional work. Everyone I've trained under who studied directly with Joe Pilates also had this line of thinking.

Joe's traditional work is a complete method of exercise, and method is the key. First of all, the Mat work that we do is complete. Each exercise supports another exercise, which helps you create a balanced body. If you want to prevent injuries to keep optimum health, you want to have stretch, strength, and control equally. That is, if you're too strong, you can tear a muscle. If you're too flexible, you can injure a joint. If you don't have the control, then you can't really accomplish anything because you don't have control over your own body. Pilates allows you to use the exercises that are all connected to create balance in the body.

Pilates is systemic work; physical therapy is reductionistic work. I'm not saying Pilates exercises aren't great for PTs to use in their work, but Pilates addresses the whole body. The knee might be injured, but the rest of the body is dealing with that injury. We're not made of parts. Our bodies and minds are interconnected as a system and Pilates works because it is an integrated system. Pilates was created for our entire body-brain system, not simply to be used for different body parts. Different exercise modalities address parts. For example, someone might say, "Oh, your inner thighs are weak. Let's go work the inner thighs." Well that's useful, but this action, in itself, doesn't connect us to the integrated system of Pilates or to ourselves.

Look at the Foot Corrector. Say you go to a podiatrist and he gives you foot exercises. You do the foot exercises, but they don't connect to anything else in your body. They don't connect to movement. They don't become functional. So you build a big muscle in your foot, but it doesn't connect to your alignment; it doesn't help you walk better. The reason why you're having problems in the first place is probably not because the arch was collapsed, but because there was some misalignment in your body that caused the arch to collapse that way.

From the time my son was little, his left foot dropped down. Well, it wasn't just because that left foot dropped down; it was because one of his legs is slightly longer than the other, so it was compensating, trying to make space. So it was best for him to fix the alignment and make space inside of his body for the misalignment, as opposed to correcting the foot collapse. You create space; you don't take away space. So he practiced Footwork on the Foot Corrector. The exercise lifted his arch, and it taught him how to stand. This action connected him up into his buttocks and abdominal muscles. He was getting taller, so his body found the space that was missing. So, when he would get off the Foot Corrector, there would be this buoyancy because he had opened space in the body. Then we would take that buoyancy and move it to the Reformer.

Next, we solidified in his Reformer what we had just created, without the gravity now, lying down, assessing the alignment, creating more space. Then we moved to the Mat. After that I would take him to the Electric Chair, where he then solidified it even more with Going Up Front. That's the same push-off action that he would need to walk, which was the same action that he did on the Foot Corrector. So these corrective exercises integrated into his alignment. They didn't just strengthen the foot muscles, but they trained the foot muscles to be in the correct alignment as they were strengthened. The Pilates method does not consist of a one-point approach. That's the genius of The Method; it's about integration, it prepares you for life, and addresses everything in your life.

Pilates addresses daily mental and physical challenges we use to have a very high quality of life. When we're missing one of those components—which Pilates challenges in every exercise—that's where trouble happens. As we age, we gradually lose balance and fluidity in our body. It is also possible to lose even more natural physical abilities due to various societal demands. When we're developing and growing at younger ages, we should be rolling, we should be jumping and we should be twisting. But if you're gifted with hand-eye coordination, all of a sudden you stop doing all those other components, and you focus in on one specific talent that you might have. But when you stop doing all those other activities, you will never reach your full potential. If you had kept up with those physical challenges, your abilities in developing strength, stability, stamina, and stretch would improve because your development would be more functionally advantageous.

In Pilates you challenge your balance from the very beginning with rolling. To be able to get back up, you roll and sit. You're not doing cartwheels yet, but you've already prepared for that. It's all in there—balance, alignment and jumping. Many times we leave jumping out, but jumping is something that is critical to keeping the nervous system alive and responsive. Think about how every time you land, the whole body has to respond. Then think about how many people twist their ankles stepping off of a curb. Well, if your body had been trained to land through that foot in response to that drop, you wouldn't twist your ankle stepping off the curb. But if you fall, and you've worked through your Footwork and the Jumping Board, then you've learned that you're not jumping with your feet. Instead, you're connecting to that lift and lengthening out of your head. As you're going down, you work on the feeling and physical action of going up. You have a secure center. As a result, you're not going to break your ankle when you step off that curb unexpectedly because your body will have been trained to respond to that.

It's like puppies playing. When puppies play, they are developing skills that they need for their lives. We as humans don't play much anymore. So, to me, what we do in Pilates is more important now than ever.

One reason why I wanted my kids to train in martial arts first was that it incorporates all the benefits of Pilates. Martial arts incorporates all the rolling, alignment, jumping, and equally using both sides of the body. You work on balance. You work on control: where you're putting a punch, where you're placing a kick. That is also the essence of what we do in Pilates. Joseph Pilates was a martial artist. There is so much of martial arts integrated into Pilates. For example, with the Side Splits, everybody thinks, "Oh, it looks like ballet." To me it's not. To me it's Horse stance. Horse stance comes from being in two boats. Martial artists would be boating along, and they'd come across other fighters, they would place one foot in each boat and fight. And they had to have that balance. And they had the balance in the inner thigh and the buttocks to be able to control the boats.

So when we do Gondola or Side Splits, I see the martial arts aspect of it. I see the balance that is needed and the strength that is needed to be able to hold two boats together while somebody's swinging at you and you're swinging at them. But look at that simple exercise. Look at how many exercises are incorporated in that. Your very first Side Sit-Up is the beginning of that, because that connects you to the stability of the lower part of your body. All the lateral movement—Leg Circles, Frogs—your very first Footwork is the beginning of that action. The Pelvic Lift is the beginning of that action. It just blows my mind. And you know what? It never stops; it never stops. One day I was working with my son, and we were doing the Mermaid. And he looked at me and he said, "Mom, this is the same as, you know, when you're kneeling on your side, and we do Swakate and we pull the arm." I was sitting there, thinking, "Yes, he gets it."

It's so complicated, yet so simple. As teachers, if we can expose that simplicity to other teachers, it will help them understand The Method. If you understand how to use The Method, you don't need anything else. The traditional work is so complete if you understand it. If you can find the thread between all apparatus exercises, then you understand The Method, and you will understand how to strengthen as well as how to challenge. Pilates has influenced my life as a mother, as a martial artist, as a trainer and breeder of champion dogs, and as a teacher of the traditional method. First off, both my children are physical. I think that their having spent a lifetime being exposed to the work has helped them become balanced human beings. You know, we are not separate. People often say the phrase "mind-body" but even this description denotes separation; mind-body describes different aspects of a singular process.

If your body is balanced, you are balanced. I think that the traditional method has positively enabled me as a mother. The more that I became balanced with myself by doing the work, the more balanced I became as a mother, and the more balanced I became as a person. The traditional work offers that.

Another aspect of the traditional work, which I think often gets lost, is practicing Pilates without music (as some other methods do today). When I was a martial artist, I had to meditate for my black belt test for three hours. I had to sit in one position for three hours and not move. When you are without music and you are paying attention to your own rhythms, and how your body moves and how you breathe and how you feel the exercises in your body, it connects you in a deeper way to yourself and gives you a better understanding of who you are. So often we do not access or utilize this deeper connection within ourselves. We live in a society that is constantly taking us out of being connected to who we are. We walk around with cell phones, constantly texting; we're on computers, constantly communicating. Look at the television. When you're watching the news there are captions underneath; there's a sidebar happening; there's a guy speaking. And many people have their phones on at the same time. We are so far removed from being inside of ourselves that when we have music, it takes our concentration out of the work. It takes away awareness of who you are, where you are, and presence within the Pilates system.

Every individual has different rhythms. Your heart beats in a different way than my heart beats. Your respiratory patterns are different from mine. If you have music, yes, it's driving; yes, you might get a great workout. But you're missing a component. You're missing the awareness and the concentration on yourself, which is imperative for change.

Now with my dogs, the work has put me on the fast track as a breeder because I really understand form and function. When you work enough with people who do not have correct structure to be doing the tasks that they're supposed to be doing, you learn how that lack of balance and movement quality affects them. When you are breeding or judging dogs, you learn to quickly identify those imbalances in the animal's body, just like in the human body. So my knowledge of Pilates really helped facilitate my ability to take what I knew as a teacher and as a Pilates practitioner and apply it to the structure and movement of the animals.

I've been fortunate. I have had great teachers my whole life. Regarding martial arts and boxing, Pilates gave me a whole different insight into actually fighting. I'm not sure that people who have never fought ever understand who Joe really was, because when you fight, you have to be so attuned to yourself. You can't waste a punch. If I don't have control of my punch, if I don't have control of my body, if I don't have my balance, if I don't have my breath, I'm done. I must have full concentration. You've heard about "the zone." You should be in "the zone" when you're doing Pilates. You should be so attuned to yourself, so present. It's the same when you fight. The second you lose your focus when you fight, you're on your butt.

Again, it's the same thing with the dogs. If you're not 100% present or aware, you lose your dogs; they go all over the place. It's a mess. This ties back to listening to music during a workout and not being focused on where you are, or, possibly who you are. I feel that is probably one of the biggest components that people have let go in Pilates. Listening to music has probably been used in an effort to motivate people.

I don't teach Mat classes. I understand that group classes motivate people, but I think that they cause us to disassociate. I think what teachers really need to concentrate on in Pilates classes is to help somebody come back into themselves because that's what the work is. It's creating a greater understanding of yourself.

Pilates can be a difficult mirror because you have to accept what is weak to make it strong first. You don't disregard what's strong and what's fabulous, but you have to understand all the components of yourself. For example, I've had clients who are in pivotal points of their lives, and they'll start training. Then all of a sudden they'll disappear, and two years later they'll call me and say, "I need to come back to training. I have to tell you what happened." Because they were starting to understand themselves, they ended up either getting a divorce or changing careers. They had huge life changes because the work made them look into themselves. The training was more than physical; they had to look into themselves.

In another example, I have a client, and when she first started training, every time she went back over the Barrel, she discussed her mother. Something about her mother would come out of her mouth, because we hold things in our bodies. I know of many times that a movement has recalled something from the past. It's like a car accident I had. I dislocated my jaw and my hip and my shoulder, my knee, that whole right side. There are times when I'm in the car and a car will swerve towards us, and my whole right side will freeze because my body recalls what happened, the habitual pattern, from the accident. Well, we have all that held in our bodies. We hold memories in ourselves because, like I mentioned earlier, we're not separate. So as someone is changing their body, they are unable to hold those traumatic experiences, or they have to address them because they're released. So, back to my client who talked about her mother. She must have been going through a lot when her mother died, bringing her to that forward mourning position. And as she opened up, she was forced to let go of what she held. And that is where the balance, the emotional balance, is connected to the physical, which makes us change.

I remember after my father died. I would drive home from being with Romana. And, you know, we'd have our lesson, and then we'd go out to lunch. As I would drive home, I cried the entire way. And I never really let it out. I had to be strong for my kids because they adored their grandfather. It was a hard thing, but the physicality and the Pilates opened me up. I had to address what had been exposed, and so I cried all the way home. It was part of the healing process. Although I may not understand everything you've been through, and you may not understand what I've been through, we can meet inside the movement, inside the Pilates system and know one another without talking. When you see a body moving, it exposes that part of it. So you try to balance that, and release that tension, and release where we're holding these emotions, where we're holding things in our bodies. Whether you suffer from a physical injury or an emotional injury, Pilates balances you out, and then that injury gets released. And, to me, The Red Thread does that.

The Red Thread is the traditional work. It's just the traditional work. And if you do the traditional work, it's complete. You need nothing else. If you truly understand connections between exercises, integration between exercises, and how to utilize that, it's the most complete, brilliant method that has ever been created.

About Kathryn
Kathryn began her study of The Method in the 1980s. She worked with five first generation teachers and strives to carry on their work by teaching and training instructors throughout the world. After years of studying side by side with Romana Kryzanowska, Kathi was the only woman asked to be in the Romana's Pilates Workout DVDs and she is featured in *Romana On Pilates: The Legacy Edition* demonstrating the various Pilates apparatus. Kathi developed the Red Thread™ workshop and the Add On Mat™ Class and she authored *Fix Your Feet Using the Pilates Method*™ and the Fix Your Feet - Using the Pilates Method™ workshop.

Pilates Archetypes

By Dana Santi

> *...all teachers have something*
> *amazing to offer.*

I will be the first to say, my studio and my teaching style are an acquired taste. There is nothing fancy about my studio; and I find myself to be a very straightforward, unedited, and fair person. I don't believe in competitive offerings from a business perspective; I believe in offering pure, undiluted Pilates—the kind of Pilates I think Joe would practice if he were still with us. I will never claim to know it all; no one can claim that, but I have made it my mission to practice and study Pilates with some of the best instructors in the nation. Through those relationships I've learned a thing or two about Pilates and the people who work so hard at the receiving end of our Pilates offerings: our clients.

I've been lucky enough in my career to have managed a training center in Chicago; I currently own my own studio and have hosted various seminars and workshops. These unique positions have allowed me to observe different types of instructors and to see those instructors instructing clients. In the end, I believe all teachers have something amazing to offer. Some I personally align with, some I don't, but none of that indifference makes for a bad instructor; it's all relative to one's training and goals. I believe every instructor needs to recognize what type of teacher they are, what type of educator they want to be, and in what ways they can adapt to different clientele, and vice versa, there is a perfect client for every instructor.

Back when I was a child, both of my parents owned their own businesses. Now, out of five grown children, two of my siblings and I currently own and operate our own businesses. Growing up in a self-employed ecosystem, I learned business in a way they don't always teach you in school.

I learned a very strong work ethic; I learned to look at situations very realistically, and I've developed reliable instincts to foresee and navigate problems. Multitasking has become a way of life for me, along with the ability to listen and learn from people. In the process I've become a good judge of character. From a very young age I emulated those around me, and I believe all of those traits have endured and helped me evolve into who I am as a teacher and business owner.

The Pilates Studio, Inc. in Evanston, IL, certified me in 1998. Much of my training back then was under Juanita Lopez. Juanita is simply one of the best teacher trainers who have ever existed, and a tremendous judge of character. She knew quickly who was right for the training program and who was going to struggle with it. Some took her advice and succeeded, and some did not. It was empowering to survey and learn so much from someone whose skills I so admired.

Juanita not only worked with apprentices and teachers, she had a regular clientele and became a constant set of eyes on all the clients who flowed in and out of the studio. She gracefully moved businessmen, mothers, traders, doctors, lawyers, the injured and many more through exercises, as if they were all coordinated, fluid and healthy individuals. Lessons with her clients were beautiful to watch. She would always advise an apprentice or newbie instructor in the most tactful way to move their clients through a lesson, without concentrating on, or more importantly, being aware any issues they had at all. I think that is a key take-away from my time with her.

Let's face it; every client has issues, some big, some small. If the instructor doesn't dwell on these issues, but instead focuses on the goals, the client will likely progress without ever knowing any hurdles existed. I was lucky enough to be an active onlooker within an amazing training center environment for five years. My tenure there also positively impacted both my teaching style and the way I choose to run my business.

Perhaps this statement seems a stretch, but I think Pilates takes at least a lifetime to learn, and I also believe that it takes a lifetime to learn how to teach correctly. There are a couple of different reasons for this. First, Pilates evolves in you. No one understood Pilates or "got it" after the first ten lessons. And trust me, no one understood how to teach after his or her first ten clients. Additionally, what you learned in your training was but a thumbnail sketch of the big picture. It was an early focus on how to keep your client safe and what words would help you better explain the exercises to them.

This picture then continues to expand, culminating in a progressive adaptation to one's own teaching style. After a few years, instructors begin to understand their Pilates universe more clearly; after a few more years, they understand even more, and so on.

I have never aligned with any instructor who proclaimed, "This is the way that it is." From my perspective, it can't possibly be that way for every client. This is where things can get a bit confusing. I can't speak for all training programs because I only know of the one I went through. What Juanita taught me was what Romana thought was best for her training program. I learned the exercises, how to spot and how to keep the client safe. Juanita explained when to leave exercises out and which exercises were good for your client's issues. I also learned the breakdown of specific exercises and how to transition from exercise to exercise.

Looking back, I start to appreciate that in the setting of a training program, rules had to be a bit more finite in nature because of who was learning them. There was no guarantee apprentices were going to stick around after their initial training. Some would leave immediately after they flew through their six-month program. So, of course, decisions were made on the safest way to perform and teach each particular exercise.

Staying so many years after my certification within that training environment, I learned that the more people I saw complete the program and become instructors, the more I understood that Pilates is the farthest thing from anything exact or definite. For new instructors it had to be, but once they embarked on their own, what they learned had to adapt and grow through their teaching, training and continuing education. But some still only saw Pilates instruction through a "training center" lens.

In 2004, after a move from Chicago to Los Angeles, I first met and studied with Jay Grimes. I came home from my first lesson with Jay and my husband asked, "Well, how was it?" I looked at him and said, "I think I've finally found what I was looking for." The best part of that revelation was—I'm not sure I was looking for a revelation. But after that lesson I knew I hadn't just found another teacher, I'd found someone who could help me take that next, necessary step in becoming a different and better instructor.

Jay doesn't teach for or affiliate himself with any single training program, he just teaches to others what Joe taught to him. I learned from Jay that Pilates is not black and white; as a matter of fact, it is very…gray. What you practice yourself may not be what you practice with your clients. What you do with client A, you may have to change up a bit with client B. Jay challenged in me the fundamental concept that nothing could ever be "exact."

Now, had I not gone through such a regimented program, I'm not sure I'd have been able to execute what Jay had taught me and what he currently teaches me as well as I do. At that time I was pretty confident in my teaching and I knew I had a good eye. I knew I had common sense and perhaps I was even teaching more "gray" than I was aware of. Maybe I just needed someone to point it out. Perhaps Jay wasn't the first one to tell me how much leverage you had within an exercise, but he is absolutely the one who brought it to light for me.

In 2002, I opened up a small studio called The Pilates Core in the suburbs of Chicago. I started getting busy, so I drafted a dear teacher friend to help me out. The space was very small, so small our butts would bump if we were both teaching at the same time. Within that first year, the studio grew bigger, our space grew exponentially, and today I have eight instructors working daily with people in 2,000 square feet of studio space.

Over the years, there have been many clients who have come through the door. Some come back every once in a while, and others have left to never return, but there are so many interesting people who have stayed with us for the long haul. My studio is basic and simple, a bunch of different rooms peppered with Gratz equipment and a minimalist décor consisting of mirrors, more equipment and pictures of Joe, Clara and Romana. I have decided that my studio is this way for a reason. The studio is filled with such strong personalities that between my instructors and my clients, that might be all the decorating it can handle. I am confident that amazing Pilates is taking place there, and the clients who have stuck it out know that, feel that, and see that.

As with all Pilates studios, clients are the reason for its success. There would not be clients without good teachers, and, if one attains the status of a good teacher, they will always have good clients. Like I said, the clientele at my studio, for the most part, have strong, loud, and confident personalities. They, like my studio, are an acquired taste. Dynamics exist between my instructors and their clients. This is the intangible magic that makes two (sometimes very different) ingredients blend. If you are in this business for the long haul, I can't tell you how important that combination is.

Every instructor is a different personality; this fact alone makes the presentation of each exercise as unique as a fingerprint. I can't tell you how many times a client has told me, "For all of you having the same training, you sure are different!" I always smile and reply, "Yes, we are." We ARE all different. Indeed, we are trying to reach similar goals with each client, but in every case, each instructor's methodology is particular and diverse—because different eyes see different things. One example is that we all develop distinctive terms and patterns of words that click with each client individually. It's part of how we personalize each interaction with our clients.

Through all of this time training, teaching, observing, and connecting I have noticed polarizing patterns in teaching styles and behaviors. I have watched so many instructors try to reach clients who are at different levels, some with great success, others without. I have also seen one phenomenon that I find most interesting—watching a client move between different teaching styles at different need states in their development. Let me explain.

The Archetypes

These ideas may seem a bit stereotypical, but I like that; it means they might actually be a little bit true. Whether true, false, or plainly subjective on my part, it makes it easier for me to know what "type" of person has just entered into a relationship with both my studio and with me. I have divided some clients I have seen into these categories:

THE PERFECT CLIENT—This client is always on time, works hard, has no issues, doesn't talk much, pays on time, cancels 24 hours in advance, gets his or her workout done and says goodbye. Does this person really exist?

THE PERFECTIONIST—This client makes every effort to make sure he is performing each exercise to its most "perfect" potential.

THE INQUIRER—The client who seeks information about the physical exercise. He asks many questions and wants to know the intentions behind each exercise he is performing.

THE MAINTENANCE MAN—This client has figured out the long haul recipe that's right for him. He knows how many Pilates sessions he needs per week in order to achieve Nirvana, be it keeping him pain-free, fit, stress-free or whatever he is looking for.

THE IN-CHARGE MARGE—This client is very direct in telling you what she would like to do today, and possibly how it should be done.

THE "LIKE THE TOUCH? NOT SO MUCH"—This client is not responsive to the direction of physical touch and needs to verbally understand what you are asking him to do. You will find the depth of your vocabularies helping these folks.

THE "LIKE THE TOUCH? VERY MUCH"—Need I say more?

THE "I'M IN PAIN!!! LET ME EXPLAIN"—This client has come to Pilates in legitimate pain, whether it be chronic pain or an acute injury or accident.

Just so you know I am an equal opportunity evaluator, I have also divided teachers into several categories as well:

THE SWISS ARMY KNIFE—This instructor is multifunctional. He can teach anyone, on any day, changes in his schedule don't fluster him, and he'll take the garbage out, if need be.

THE PERFECTIONIST—Just like the client, this instructor makes every effort to make sure he is teaching each exercise to its optimum potential.

THE NEWCOMER—A new instructor, not necessarily to your studio, but new to Pilates.

THE AUCTIONEER—This instructor can move a client through more exercises than the client will realize, in the allotted 50 minutes. The word "rest" to this instructor is simply a word.

THE CONVINCER—This instructor could sell you a goat, even if you already bought one last week. He has a style and confidence and whether he's been teaching for weeks or years—he is gifted in the art of selling Pilates.

THE EXPLAINANATOR—This instructor has been sent from the past to the present with extreme passion and a voice, and that voice is all about Pilates.

THE DIAGNOSER—This instructor always has the client's best interest at heart, but may need to remember we teach exercise.

THE CONTENDER—This instructor is strong, consistent, and can go the distance to better any client and his situation.

As I stated earlier, for every type of client out there, there is a fairly paired instructor, an instructor who can work within a particular personality to get the most out of each person during each session. Every person at the root of these archetypes, whether he is the client or the instructor, is, or has been, a little bit of all of these. Don't forget, all this is based on theory that is part armchair psychology and part practicing Pilates instructor.

One may think that THE PERFECTIONIST client needs to be with THE PERFECTIONIST instructor. There are times I believe this would be a good match, but sometimes not. It's almost like being in a good relationship—opposites tend to attract. I would like to see THE PERFECTIONIST client eventually move on to THE AUCTIONEER because it may speed that client up a little. These two might not gel right away, but soon they will move forward and progress together. THE CONTENDER may be a good in-between instructor because he will spar with that client for a while and, without him knowing, slip in more exercises and forward his progress that way.

You might find yourself telling THE INQUIRER client, in your best German accent, "It's good for za body," just like Joe said, but that answer won't be enough. One's instincts may be to put this client with THE EXPLAINANATOR because he would preemptively be answering all of his questions. That will work for a bit, but I think he will get wrapped up in too much explanation and detail and may only find their lessons getting to the Tree by the 50 minute mark. Soon the INQUIRER client won't understand why he isn't getting the results his friend is, but he can detail the specifics of why he's doing what he's doing. So, more balance needs to be achieved. A different direction for THE INQUIRER may be THE CONVINCER. Perhaps this client has a lot of questions because he is feeling insecure, and why wouldn't he—his feet go into straps during the third exercise and his pants fall down during the fourth. Let's face it, this can get downright intimidating. THE CONVINCER gains THE INQUIRER's confidence and makes him a believer in Pilates. Before you know it, THE INQUIRER'S questions will lessen and he will have no problem working with THE AUCTIONEER.

THE MAINTENANCE MAN (or woman) has been coming to the studio for years. He isn't looking for superstardom; chances are he probably isn't totally motivated to come in at all, but he knows what he needs from his Pilates. I'm not going to put this client with THE EXPLAINANATOR. If THE MAINTENANCE MAN is on an autopilot preservation program, I'm guessing he doesn't want to know which of his organs is being worked during Footwork. He knows Pilates works, and that's just enough explaining for him. The teaching style of the NEWCOMER would fare well with this client. It would give the NEWCOMER a set routine, and he'd be able to deliver the workout the client was used to, all the while getting to watch someone who is familiar with his body and workout go through the motions fairly consistently. THE CONTENDER would be a good instructor match, as well. He'd be able to hit the client with a new exercise without him knowing, thereby advancing him but not breaking up the workout.

The IN-CHARGE MARGE comes in and tells you what she would like to do today. Rightfully so, it's her lesson, and chances are she is more open to suggestion than we think. THE SWISS ARMY KNIFE would adapt teaching styles very well; his multifunctional approach will go with the flow. THE PERFECTIONIST instructor is also a good match. If this client is going to tell you what she wants to do, THE PERFECTIONIST can make sure she is doing it well, precisely, and with very good technique. I may keep THE NEWCOMER at a safe distance for a while, in case this client throws out some exercise that he may not be comfortable teaching.

Who's kidding who? It's tough to teach Pilates without touching your client. But yes, some clients just simply LIKE THE TOUCH? NOT SO MUCH. In reality, the NEWCOMER might be the best option here. During training he had to teach using his voice, learn the right words, etc., so words are fresh to him. THE EXPLAINANATOR has good use of words, as well, and if THE AUCTIONEER can move her voice as much as she can move the client, that's another good match. And lastly, the old standby, the SWISS ARMY KNIFE. So for not liking to be touched so much, this client has many options and can progress well.

Some clients seek comfort in the guidance of a touch from their Pilates instructor and LIKE THE TOUCH, VERY MUCH. Others need to be pushed, stretched, and manipulated into different positions because they are so tight; and the only way they will loosen is through constant poking and prodding. Some clients get lost in verbal instruction and can't imagine what in their bodies you are possibly talking about. They have to LIKE THE TOUCH, VERY MUCH and will have to depend on it. Most of the time these clients are men, and often they can be tough assignments; but because of the way men are built, results happen rather quickly. Whatever the case, any instructor who needs to touch, needs to be confident in his stretching techniques. I've already stated THE CONVINCER is a very confident teacher, but he needs to make sure he has a plan for what he's doing. THE CONTENDER can also handle this client, as he is tough and can last the whole fight. And just like in the previous examples, the SWISS ARMY KNIFE can always manage the job.

THE I'M IN PAIN!!! LET ME EXPLAIN client has come in to your world in legitimate pain or discomfort. A doctor, a physical therapist, or a friend who had similar issues has most likely recommended this person to seek your skill set. Many of these clients are so scared they are going to reinjure themselves that they go through life physically guarded and often stress other parts of their bodies in the process. Depending on each case, their pain can be managed, and they can maintain what health and vitality they currently walk in with. Perhaps, if they reinjure that bad back of theirs, the duration of the pain is shortened. So, as this client may ask for opinions, it's important to keep him from THE DIAGNOSER. Pilates instructors are not doctors, and I know this isn't the first time that's been said. Chances are this client not only needs Pilates, but he needs to be sold on it a bit, because nothing else has worked for him. THE CONVINCER may be helpful during this time. The day the pain begins to retreat, even slightly, is the day he becomes a believer. THE PERFECTIONIST may be a comforting teaching style to this achy client and progress him slowly at a calming pace, easing his expectations and focusing him on exercise instead of pain. In due time, THE CONTENDER may be good at drawing attention away from the injury by skillfully challenging the client to come out of his comfort zone, without him knowing his "safe" routine is changing all that much.

In truth, I think many things happen over the course of time in a client/instructor relationship. Both parties should be aware they have the potential to become a type. Because it's so easy to rely on previous patterns, we have to remember to constantly reassess and challenge both our clients and ourselves.

So back to that PERFECT CLIENT I spoke of before. I asked, "Does this person exist?" Yes, he actually does, and in so many ways. Perhaps not all wrapped up in one consistent individual, but THE PERFECT CLIENT is someone who is on the journey to discover Pilates and how it can enhance his life.

Each client, no matter what his or her type on this list, seeks out my studio or yours for fundamentally the same reason: wellness. Wellness is an intangible mind-body connection that each person can only truly define for him or herself. So, in many ways that PERFECT CLIENT is, at one time or another, an INQUIRER, a PERFECTONIST, and an IN CHARGE MARGE, perhaps even within the same session. Each individual is on his own path, and that path is to be illuminated if not defined by his instructor or instructors.

I have never told one of my instructors how to teach. Lord knows I don't need eight more of myself in my studio, because I know my weaknesses, and I work hard to correct them. My instructors have the leeway to find their own style and their own voice; that is the reason they are there. I am available to give the instructors advice or direction on a client, but the way each of us feels Pilates within our own bodies is special and exclusive. That automatically makes the words that originate from our mouths unique and memorable. We each get to define our individual "brand"; and, therefore, each lesson that gets taught is special and diverse because of the pairing of instructor and client.

I am lucky to have so many different teaching "flavors" available for my studio's client base. We are a tightly knit group of people and continuing education is very important to all of us. We always share what we learn, exchange ideas about exercises and how they work on different people, and we've figured out what is most important to us. We are also lucky enough to work with each other's clients to get ourselves closer to becoming SWISS ARMY KNIVES.

Because we are Pilates professionals, life doesn't hinge on what our present teaching style is or where exactly our clients are in their individual journeys. What matters is that every lesson we teach is one lesson closer to perfecting our craft through the molding and forging of our next PERFECT CLIENT.

About Dana

Dana began studying the Pilates method in 1996, under the direction of Juanita Lopez and was certified by Romana Kryzanowska in 1998. She instructed at and managed The Pilates Studio of The Midwest in Chicago. In 2002, she opened The Pilates Core, Inc. in LaGrange, IL. Two years later, Dana met and studied with Jay Grimes. That meeting changed Dana's life, and she is honored to borrow every ounce of inspiration and wisdom that he provides. Co-Chair and founding member of the Authentic Pilates Union, Dana organizes conferences with Gratz Pilates, bringing authentic Pilates nationwide.

Teaching Pilates

By Dorothee VandeWalle

> *...Pilates brings out a very strong inner*
> *beauty and inner strength that radiates*
> *through the body.*

I don't know if I can say I ever studied Pilates in the formal sense. I first did Pilates after an ankle injury in the early '80s, but there was no explicit method that I had to learn. It was more of a "just do this and then do that" approach rather than a comprehensive program. But it worked for me, and I loved it.

Then, for various reasons, I ended up in New York visiting a friend. I got up one morning, and my neck was stiff. My friend said, "I want you to meet somebody." So I went to watch Romana teach and absolutely loved the work. Watching her, I understood exactly what I wanted to do and what this was all about. I loved that she had worked with Joseph Pilates directly and all the stories she shared about "Joe." I loved the individual attention that she gave to people while she was teaching. It was a very organic way of teaching. It was not a critical approach, and it was really natural. There was nothing false about it. There was nothing egocentric, nothing academic, and it wasn't like anything else. It was artistic and organic, and everything that I felt I could relate to.

So that's how I decided to become a teacher. I was lucky that Romana let me become a student of hers without belonging to any program, since there was no formal program at that time. I learned through observing and by being part of the work. Romana would just say a few things here and there: "This is good for that. This is good for this other thing, too." There was never any formal instruction, but the education was based on observing, doing, and feeling what Pilates could do. Romana is not an academic person. She's a natural teacher. She teaches from her heart and from her understanding of the body. She is not about words and explaining, but more about doing, feeling, observing and just being simple about it. Proper technique is always fundamentally simple. That's what I felt, and Romana's spirited insistence on this point and the fact that anyone could master it was very contagious!

What Romana gave us was like a very basic geometry class. The shoulders, the hips, the ankles, and the knees all have to be in the right place. If they aren't, then eventually you will have problems. Your body will wear out. Learning that helped me with my scoliosis, my knees, my back and my ankle. I always tell my students, "I can tell you what works—because I've had that injury!" I think the body has to go through painful moments in order to learn. Maybe I don't learn any other way. I had to go through my own experience. I actually had to live the pain, and it has given me a lot of compassion. I have compassion for my students and my clients because of the injuries I've gone through, and I know Pilates works.

As a child I used to cross my legs Indian-style, then walk on my knees with my legs crossed. Imagine the damage I did! When I met Romana, she helped me with my knees. I've had knee problems for a long time, and a partial knee replacement three months ago. Pilates helped me delay that operation for almost 10 years, and it has also sped my rehabilitation. Growing up, I knew that my upper body was not very strong, but didn't know it was actually scoliosis. I wasn't well-connected to my body, even though I danced. My body worked in parts, but not as a whole, and Pilates helped connect my upper body with my head, my limbs, and my torso. Since learning that connection, I've gone back to it to help me relieve injuries I've had over the years. Every day, I try to think of the back. I always pull my stomach in and up. I try to be light on my feet, and lifting forward. Those things help me a lot, but it wasn't until I started practicing Pilates that I could hear what my body was saying to me.

So, when teaching Pilates, and when teaching teachers of Pilates, I emphasize that you need to learn with your body. The body first has to speak to you. It's not the words that speak to the body. This is probably the most important thing I learned from Romana. To me, it is the organic and spiritual core of Pilates that transcends all the technique and any program out there.

However, people sometimes need a more intellectual connection to the work in addition to the practicum, and I understand that. The

Pilates community has grown very large and is spread across the globe. People want to know they are taking Pilates from instructors who have learned their craft from authentic practitioners of Joseph Pilates' method. They want the valuable instruction that only a well-trained and well-practiced instructor can give them. So today, we have many teacher-training centers and conferences around the world, and I've been lucky to be able to contribute to that. When training teachers in my seminars, I think of it as a kind of base, a grounding start. It is the dirt, and you have to put the seeds in. To become a teacher, you have to be on the floor practicing the skills without being observed constantly. You do the exercises, and you feel it. You have to have a chance to be yourself and respect the work, but also have a chance to explore. So, I give my apprentices a lot of time for that, and I also tailor their instruction to the individual. Some apprentices cannot observe for two hours straight in the studio because they have a hard time focusing, so I won't make them do that. I will give them another mission. I observe the apprentices with their work, and I see what they need. One may need to speak more loudly, or stand farther away and absorb the big picture and stop looking at just parts of the body. So, I give them all something to work on. But I try to keep an eye on the apprentices from a distance, so that they have the chance to be themselves, and find their own voices with the work that they've learned. That way, they stay passionate, and this passion is so important to Pilates!

I believe Pilates brings out a very strong inner beauty and inner strength that radiates through the body. It permeates the spirit and affects your mood. People from all kinds of various backgrounds come to study with me. I am very welcoming, even if they seem, at first glance, to have little connection to their bodies. They start Pilates because of the passion it makes them feel and because they're passionate about it. I support that and welcome them.

What causes this passion? From the get-go, Pilates transforms us not only physically, but emotionally. That brings passion into people. Most people who study with me have done all kinds of other work before coming to Pilates. They're usually not 18-year-olds right out of high school. They're people who have been in the workforce, and they've contended with that lifestyle for years. Pilates grounds them, and creates a physical and mental connection that they crave.

Upon starting Pilates, most people feel better right away, even though it takes them a while to realize it. They don't always recognize the benefits right away, because they are disconnected from the body. But soon, they say things like, "Oh, I was driving, and my neck wasn't hurting. I was much more at ease with my body." Or, "Just standing, I felt lighter." Or my favorite, "I look like a truck driver, but walk like a ballerina!" People tell me things like that. Recently I had a student who felt the difference in her first session. She was a young woman, and she felt her whole upper body coming alive. She was putting her hands all over her torso, lower back, and stomach, and she was sort of talking to herself. Right away, she felt good, like she had a belt holding her in a strong position, and I think that's what a lot of people feel. They feel more secure: in their stance, in how they walk, and even in the way they approach things.

I have another client, a woman in her 60s, who needs a hip replacement. She's afraid to have surgery. She's been doing Pilates for about a year and a half, and she's keeping it a secret from her family. I think she wants to have something that's hers that she doesn't have to share with anybody. I asked her if people had noticed any difference in her. She said, "Yes, they've noticed that I'm not walking with a big limp anymore." She definitely has less pain. It's very nice to hear that, even in a severe case like that, she has relieved her pain, and her walking is so much better. She gets compliments on her health from her family, and feels stronger because she did something on her own that helps her family worry less about her. I think that's wonderful.

The people who are training to be teachers in my studio are passionate about these kinds of experiences, and this is what drives them to want to become teachers. They're not going to be the same teacher I am, but I hope they will share the same passion for the work and the legacy. They've got to find their voices as teachers, who they need to be. That is something that I respect. I try to teach by example. But our studio is also full of senior teachers who have worked with me for years, even decades, and our teachers-in-training also watch these other instructors and learn from them, too, absorbing their examples. They don't just follow me, but they have a group of people to look to who are working with the same philosophy of respecting the individual body and who are driven by the same passion for results.

When training teachers, I think that being in the studio with my own clients on a daily basis is really important. I'm a teacher, too, just like who they are becoming. We're peers in many ways. I look at it like that. We become a kind of family. I teach them that their career with Pilates will happen little by little, one thing after another just like mine did. First I was taking Pilates; then I was teaching it. Then apprentices came. Then came the bigger studio, and the business. With that comes the teaching of seminars.

I try to limit how often I teach abroad because it takes me away from the place where I should be spending most of my time, my studio. However, I do think it's important to be part of a broader community because you learn a lot by going to different places and then reflecting on what you are doing. You see if what you are doing is good in the big picture, and contributing to the broader picture of what Pilates is to the world is important to me. But for me, this can be accomplished most effectively by choosing quality events over quantity, and choosing partners wisely. And you cannot forget that your first priority as a teacher of teachers is to your studio, so that they can also be productive.

As for fitting everything in, I don't think too much about balancing it all. After all, I do Pilates! Balance comes naturally to my life! I teach clients and work out in my studio every day, and I teach my students. I don't think, okay, today I need to teach my clients, and I have to teach my apprentices, and I have to run the business, and I have to travel. Instead, I let things come organically. I teach my clients, and as I'm teaching my clients, I'm aware that my apprentices are in the studio and absorbing, and they are part of it. While that's going on, I have teachers in the studio with their own clients, as well as the whole business part. If you are centered, no one part of these can knock you off balance and make you lose focus.

I think as a teacher, you have to give what you receive. You received passion from the practice. You received knowledge from your teachers. Hopefully, I am passing on the work the way Romana taught it to me, and the way Joe taught it to her. I hope to pass on this idea of purity. Pilates is simple and true. If you are true to the work, then you will be true to yourself, too. My students respect the work because I tell them how important it is to keep it simple. You do not need to make the work more complicated or bring outside work to Pilates. If you stick to the authentic way, you will have the foundation that you need to adapt to your clients and the student teachers you may teach in the next generation. That is the tradition I try to pass on.

In the end, one of the most gratifying parts of being a trainer of teachers is seeing how Pilates teaches people who they are. To me, that's really amazing. The work transforms people not just physically but also emotionally. It gives them maturity, and helps them be more of what they want to be. They didn't know they had this voice, this power of being, this something else that they weren't before. That's a great transformation. Maybe they were insecure, unhappy, and unhealthy, and they're not anymore. Maybe they couldn't express themselves, but through this work, now they can. Pilates opens up so many doors: doors of opportunity, doors of friendship. I think that's fantastic. That's worth every penny and every hour that you invest in Pilates. And that's why I love teaching.

About Dorothee

Dorothee VandeWalle is a master Pilates teacher and is recognized as one of the leading teacher trainers in the world. She started teaching Pilates in New York with Romana Kryzanowska and was a teacher trainer for The Pilates Studio and Romana's Pilates for over a decade before starting her own training program, M.A.T. Pilates (Metropolitan Authentic Training). Originally from Belgium, Dorothee started dancing at the age of seven and was trained on scholarship at the Institute für Buhnentanz. She danced professionally for over ten years in Europe and the United States. She's been teaching in Seattle since 1993 and has had her own studio since 1999.

Chapter IV

Athletic Applications for Pilates

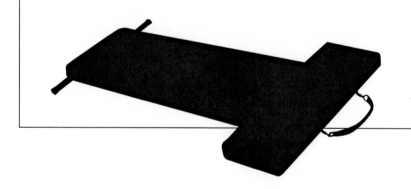

My Journey in Pilates

By Fatima Bruhns

...the answer to both my physical and professional transitions.

I have been a practitioner and teacher of the Pilates method for over 20 years. During my career, I have had the privilege and honor to train with renowned Pilates Master Teacher and mentor, Romana Kryzanowska, along with other talented teachers like Sari Mejia-Santo and Juanita Lopez.

What I would like to convey is not necessarily about myself, but about the invaluable knowledge and the experiences that I have gained as both a teacher and practitioner of the Pilates method. In either case, I have observed how Pilates has successfully enhanced healthy bodies, improved high fitness levels in athletes and non-athletes alike, benefited muscle function and shape, as well as proven to aid quicker recovery from injuries and surgeries.

As a classical, character, and ballroom dancer, I suffered from many common dancers' injuries, including a knee strain that resulted in several surgeries to repair a damaged meniscus. The medical treatment available at the time for this kind of injury was not capable of providing me with a full recovery, and consequently this ended my professional career as a dancer. As I transitioned into other potential career options, I discovered the fitness industry in the early 1980s. I began with high impact aerobics and circuit training, and continued with the newest and latest crazes of the time, like step aerobics, slide aerobics, water exercise classes, low impact aerobics, and, of course, jogging and weight training. I covered the entire range of exercises that were popular at a time when the general population was becoming more aware of their health, their fitness level and, more importantly, their physical looks. As time passed, however, I discovered that the intensity of high-level aerobics further aggravated my former injuries. For the first time, I noticed how my age began to play a role in my recovery process, thus adding a new factor into how I needed to care for and respond to my body's limits and needs. So I was blessed to meet Juanita Lopez and the wonderful work of Joseph Pilates. Shortly after this initial introduction to the practice, I decided that Pilates was the answer to both my physical and professional transitions. It was at this point in the 1980s that my journey and love affair with the Pilates method began.

Throughout my initial training, I studied with Romana, her daughter Sari, and other wonderful teachers like Roxanne Murata in New York City at Drago's Gym; it was a kind of mecca for the Pilates method of body conditioning, where people trained to be in better physical health and, ultimately, for the few of us who were interested, to become future Pilates instructors. Drago's is where for many years Romana began her workday promptly at 7:00 a.m., rain or shine. Her magnificent work ethic, as well as that of her daughter Sari, was something that was important to her to transmit to us new apprentices as part of our formation into instructors. This facility is where apprentices and the general public alike still find learning opportunities today.

Inspired by how Pilates changed my life, I subsequently opened one of the first training centers for the Pilates method outside of New York City, in 1994, in Evanston, Illinois. This was at a time when there were only two other training centers in the country in association with Romana's teaching method: one in Los Angeles, California, and the other in Seattle, Washington.

In 2000, six years into the success of my Chicago-based business, I expanded and opened two more studios; one in the center of Chicago, known as the downtown area, and the other in Highland Park, a northern suburb. Encouraged by this success, I organized the first ever International Pilates Convention. Attending and participating instructors included Romana herself, Sari Mejia-Santo, Juanita Lopez, Roxanne Murata, Lauren Stephen, Lori Coleman, Dorothee Vande-Walle, Brooke Siler, Kathryn Ross-Nash, and many other great Pilates instructors from across the globe, who brought their own wealth of knowledge and experiences to the discussions, lessons, and seminars provided throughout the weekend. We were also fortunate to have the presence of Basil Blecher at the conference. Basil, who at the time was a representative of Gratz Industries Pilates division, provided us with both equipment and support.

The convention was a great risk, being the first of its kind, and there were many skeptics who doubted the probability of the event's success. Some of the questions I faced included whether the seminars would be provided lecture-style in more of a traditional classroom environment, or if there would be physical demonstrations accompanying each seminar. Additional questions included whether there would be related mini-seminars addressing topics on specific physical conditions, whether physical therapy had a role in Pilates training, and which equipment was the best and why.

Since then, these "Convention Workshops" have grown and evolved as a great tool to expand the continuing education of professionals and non-professionals, as well as a path to promote the Pilates method beyond the fitness industry, and make it available to the general population. Of course various mistakes were made during that first convention, but overall it was a great success, and the highpoint of the convention was hosting a dinner to honor Romana for her lifelong dedication to preserve the original Pilates method of body conditioning as well as the education and formation of new students and teachers. There were surprise guests and gifts featured as well as acknowledgment of other great teachers who have worked so hard throughout the years to maintain the integrity of The Method.

During my years as a business owner and a supervisor of new teachers, I personally witnessed many different kinds of changes in both healthy and non-healthy bodies alike that Pilates could bring about in its followers. I saw the execution of The Method by some of the greatest Pilates practitioners. I also observed the emotional and physical changes that stimulate a positive growth of body and mind in many Pilates professionals and practitioners.

In this period I also witnessed the rapid evolution of the fitness industry and how it has sometimes affected the original Pilates method both positively and negatively. It was hard, and even painful, to watch private interests distorting the values of such a comprehensive fitness system. The disintegration of the Pilates method as trademark created confusion and misunderstanding throughout the industry and allowed private interests to take advantage of a situation for financial gain. I believe that this had nothing to do with the teaching and practice of the original method.

For personal reasons related to the growth and prosperity of my family, I left Chicago in 2002; and my personal and professional life took a turn once again when I sold the Chicago businesses and moved to New Jersey, where I still reside today. For a time, I became an independent teacher and worked freelance at several Pilates studios in Manhattan and New Jersey. The needs of my family, however, led me to the decision to open my own private practice out of my home. The flexibility this option offered me provided me with a balance in which I could harmoniously attend to my clients and my family.

My necessity to have a flexible schedule came from the commitments I made to my family, especially to my children. One of my concerns as a parent and a professional has been finding the appropriate balance between my family's goals and my own pursuits. Following this line of thinking led my husband and me to make the decision to home-school both of my daughters in order to give them the best opportunity to work towards their personal aspirations.

Both of my daughters, as athletes, were introduced to the Pilates system at a very early age, and both girls subsequently worked with Romana. My oldest daughter pursued the possibility of a classical dance career, but unfortunately at age 16 suffered a back injury that resulted in the insertion of a titanium rod in her lower back. Pilates helped her throughout her recovery, and today I am the proud mother of an aspiring Ph.D. candidate in philosophy and aesthetics. She is still involved with the arts, but this time from a different perspective.

My youngest daughter is a figure skater, and her commitment to the sport has developed her into a world competitor. As a high level athlete, she trains and competes all over the world, frequently training between six and eight hours a day both on and off the ice. She began competing internationally at the age of 12, traveling to cities like Seoul, South Korea; Merano, Italy; Dortmund, Germany; and Nice, France among others, which led me to make my decision to teach privately from home. Her extensive off-ice training has included Pilates work designed by Romana, who helped me develop a program for young high-level athletes like my daughter. Since then, I have continued to work with my daughter during the competitive season as well as the off-season, and through her sport, I was introduced to the world of figure skating at all levels.

Figure skating, like many other sports, creates an unbalanced strength and flexibility that is aggravated by the frequency and intensity level of their training. Common injuries to the ankles, lower back and hips are caused by daily pounding of joints while figure skaters practice their spins and high-intensity jumps.

In the last few years, I have had the privilege to train some of these top athletes in the Pilates method, some of whom include Roman and Sasha Zaretsky, National champions of Israel, two-time Olympians and world competitors. The extraordinary ice skater, Johnny Weir, who was a three-time United States National Champion, two-time Olympian, and Bronze Medalist at the World Championship of 2008, had this to say:

> Pilates changed my life as an Olympian and figure skater. I use Pilates to strengthen my body, while remaining "body beautiful," both of which are necessary for the art of figure skating. I was injury-prone as a young athlete, but as soon as I began training in the Pilates method, I was able to train harder and jump higher with no consequence, other than achieving my goals and attaining my best performance. I will do Pilates for the rest of my life because I couldn't be the athlete I am, or the person I am without it. – Johnny Weir, August 22, 2011

Another powerful affirmation of the remarkable benefits of Pilates comes from Natasha Popova, the National Champion of Ukraine and a World Championship competitor:

> Since I began doing Pilates, I have noticed and felt a big, positive change both physically and mentally. Pilates involves doing exercises that involve total body conditioning; this includes building the core muscles of the stomach, back, and pelvis. Pilates focuses on the quality of movement, rather than numerous repetitions. It elongates the spine and makes the muscles more elastic, reducing the risk of injury. Being a professional figure skater, I can feel the results during my on-ice training and performances. I feel much stronger, in control of myself, and aware. My endurance level has also improved. My muscles have become toned and lean. I have developed good core strength, since the majority of exercises involve engaging the core. In addition, I have learned about breath

awareness, and how to breathe properly while executing the exercises. During a Pilates workout every muscle is engaged, and you can feel it elongating and strengthening. The core exercises have definitely improved my balance on the ice. Another benefit from doing Pilates is that the pain I used to experience in my right knee due to overcompensation has diminished, because the muscles around it have strengthened, and the alignment of my feet has improved. I am very grateful for my great Pilates instructor, Fatima Bruhns, who motivates me and brings joy to working out. Her instructions are easy and fun to follow, making the workout seem to go by in an instant! In conclusion, the numerous benefits of Pilates include improved balance, strength, flexibility, and posture, as well as better circulation, a longer leaner physique, injury prevention, and rehabilitation. - Natasha Popova, September 9, 2011

During the last several years I have expanded beyond the teaching and practice of the Pilates method, and ventured into the field of translating Pilates-related books from English into Spanish. I was given this opportunity through my dear friend, Peter Fiasca. As far as my future is concerned, I see the Pilates method continuing to play a role, one way or another, in the rest of my life. Teaching will always be part of me because it is something that I truly enjoy, along with practicing The Method as much as I can to maintain my health. In this way, I hope to share Pilates and transmit its lessons to others the way Romana once taught it to me.

About Fatima

Fatima studied dance in Mexico City, where she was a member of Ballet Folklòrico de Mexico. Recurring knee problems brought her to Pilates and the watchful eye of Juanita Lopez. Bruhns received her teaching certification in 1993 from Romana Kryzanowska. Two years later, she co-founded The Pilates Studio of the Midwest, a training center for the Pilates Method, in Evanston, Illinois. She organized the first international Pilates Convention and now has a studio in New Jersey, where she trains Olympic athlete Johnny Weir and other skaters. She collaborated with Peter Fiasca in the Spanish version of his *Classical Pilates Technique* DVD series and first translation of their companion book, *Discovering Pure Classical Pilates*.

Dance Until You Drop

By Carl Corry

> *...it was the complete cross-training answer for any serious dancer or athlete.*

When I was very young, I used to watch my parents teaching kids to dance while I sprawled on a tumbling mat near what seemed to be the biggest piano in the world. It was my fort and a safe place for me to play while my folks kept an eye on me as they worked. I wasn't interested in dance then; I was too young. But as I got older, I paid more and more attention to what the other kids were doing. I even knew some of the songs they sang as they performed their routines. By the time I was seven, I became curious enough to begin imitating what I saw. Although imitation is how we learn most things, especially things of a physical nature, I was not aware at the time that I had already begun to experience exercise. There was not much so-called technique involved at that point, and it certainly never occurred to me to what level the art of dance could be taken.

By the time I was 11, things became more regimented. I had to wear tights! My parents began explaining how important it is to have good posture and line in the body, rotating from the hips and stretching the legs and feet from very specific positions. Holding the arms in defined positions became more and more complicated. I started to understand exercise in a much more formal way, again by imitation. Little did I know that ballet had been handed down from one generation to the next, just like this, for over 300 years. All of this became clearer as I grew older.

Ballet is one of the most unnatural things for the body to try to achieve. It demands things of the body that only a young lifetime of work can produce. And it takes years to build the kind of strength needed to sustain a full day and night of dancing flat out, without holding back.

Obviously, dancers are fit; they're always taking ballet class, and that's their main training method. But injuries in athletics, and in ballet especially, come from the multitude and variety of demands made on the body that are far from natural.

A professional male dancer is required to jump, turn, and beat (quick execution of the legs and feet) all day long. When partnering a female in a series of lifts, turns, and balances, he may try one lift 15 different ways to determine how to get out of or into position with his partner. This can be extremely demanding on the back and upper body. How many muscles could that work in just one day? The answer: too many not to be cross-training.

As I began my professional career as a dancer, I was completely unprepared for the toll it would take on my body. The intense variety of styles in the Joffrey Ballet's repertoire, moving this way one hour and that way another, injured many dancers. My path was to push my body until some hitherto undetected weakness broke it down, resulting in an injury severe enough to require rehabilitation. This pattern of building strength, breaking down, and being rebuilt became the ever-present process by which I withstood the high energy work demanded of me. It took lots of physical therapy to keep shoring up the weaknesses that were created by a completely inconsistent set of demands on my body.

It wasn't until I stopped dancing that I learned the Pilates method. Once I fully understood what it did for the body, I could see how much easier my path to total body strength would have been and how many injuries could have been prevented.

The Pilates method of body conditioning was purposely made to build strength and flexibility in the body in a completely consistent way, so there are no weak links. As I trained in The Method, I knew it was the complete cross-training answer for any serious dancer or athlete. In fact, it is the most comprehensive body conditioning system for any fitness level. What Pilates did for my aging and battered body after I stopped dancing was proof enough for me. It not only keeps me strong and flexible, but it keeps scar tissue and arthritis in check and the pain in my spine, hips, knees, ankles, and toes at bay. Without it, I would be a fossil right now. And despite the fact that I no longer jump, I am quite fit overall.

Pilates creates an environment for the body that is very consistent. Even when being challenged, you can never do more than progress at a pace that is conducive to growth rather than destruction. That is because it is your own body in Pilates that challenges you, not a technique like ballet, gymnastics, or tennis or an adjustable set of restraints like weights or machines that can be programmed to a level that the human ego thinks is correct for the human body. This is where most people get into trouble. Only when the mind is in complete concert with the body does a really powerful connection take place. I'm not talking about the ability to block out distractions, as the phrase is commonly used: "Whoever has the best mind-body focus in a 5th set tie break at Wimbledon is the winner…period." It is more a matter of the mind and body working together. Consider the fact that walking on the treadmill for 45 minutes while watching TV won't result in as much weight loss as one ballroom dance class. That's because in the latter, the mind is focused on recruiting multiple muscle groups to perform fairly simple tasks all at the same time with the proper amount of energy and coordination.

I have heard many times, "Pilates is not rocket science," but it is much more challenging than people think for a simple reason: it takes time. I have never seen anyone get Pilates overnight. I danced professionally for 22 years, and I am still working on Pilates a decade after being certified. This is a fast-paced world, and everyone wants everything yesterday. It is just not possible to build someone up in Pilates quickly. I've never seen it done well at all. Some people do make neuromuscular connections faster than others, but Pilates is much more information than people think. For me personally, the connection came one day after a hard advanced Reformer. Through rivers of sweat, I thought, "Wow, that felt like a really good ballet class." That's how many connections I had to make to actually be able to feel the mind working with the body.

Similarities in ballet and Pilates are numerous, but let me make one distinction right away. Pilates is pure exercise. Ballet is a 300-year-old art form. That being said, physically they go hand in hand. Both require and generate two essential qualities: strength and flexibility. You cannot have graceful athleticism without a very high concentration and balance between both of these components. Putting the artistry in ballet aside is difficult. The reason that I'm not uncomfortable making the comparison to Pilates is that you can't even think about artistry until you've mastered technique. Then we can compare. Pilates uses a number of movements many different ways to achieve a deeply conditioned muscle. Ballet requires the body to move hundreds of ways for which it is not always prepared. So there is a definite gap that needs to be filled in order for the body to be able to successfully navigate its many avenues of expression. Pilates fills the gap beautifully. It is comprehensive and leaves no stone unturned, provided the student has proper guidance.

But one must start with a solid foundation. An individual studying Pilates or ballet needs to have instruction that leads to the ultimate goal. The caliber of that instruction cannot be understated. It is quite literally the difference between the student being adequate or exceptional, no matter what his given abilities are. There will always be people greater and lesser than others, but a good teacher can make even the most limited person better. The great classical guitarist, Andrés Segovia, was able to pick up a guitar in the worst condition and still make it sound beautiful. A dancer is considered a living instrument. Robert Joffrey always wanted to know why we settled for being pretty on stage when we could be beautiful. A good teacher of ballet can refine the smallest movement to give meaning and clear intention to a single step. Similarly, a good teacher of Pilates can take a person with severe rheumatoid arthritis and enable him, over time, to advance remarkably on a Reformer. I've seen it.

It all comes back to basics. Are they lined up right? Are they in a good position? Are they using the muscles that need to be working? Are they working properly and together in coordination? Only now can we start to address good movement. In ballet it would be called adagio. In Pilates it is called flow. This is a physical state that is hard-won. It requires total control of the movement. Grace is a good word to describe it. When someone achieves this kind of movement, the body receives its ultimate benefit.

However, Romana taught us that as teachers, we have to be aware of much more than the body in front of us. In what kind of mood is the client? Has he had a bad day? Does he have underlying issues that are holding him back? Is some part of his body bothering him that he is not even aware of? People are complicated, and as Romana said, "You have to treat more than their body, dear."

A good teacher recognizes what each body needs both physically and psychologically. While some people are training for high level events and must be worked accordingly, others just need to lift up out of their hips a little more so that their legs can move better. Then, they can begin to deepen their performance in a more appropriate way.

At the end of the day the teacher must ask, "Did I really pay attention or was I striving to be mediocre?" If it is the latter, that is what the student will look like.

People are there with you for a reason. None of this is cheap, and they could be at Starbucks, right? In both Pilates and ballet, you have to give them the truth of what you know and believe. No one will follow a teacher just because he is passionate. They follow a teacher because they know that he is speaking truth to them. People are not so jaded that they can't figure out if you really don't have a clue or if you aren't certain about the truth of what you are teaching. It is always best to use the truth to get to the heart of the matter, especially in teaching. If someone has it all figured out, he doesn't need you. There is no need to be mean. Just show him the truth.

When I first started teaching Pilates, I had an older gentleman tell me repeatedly, "You can't pull your ribs in. It is not possible." I had to show him the truth of what I was saying. Telling him did not work, so I asked him to lie on his back, put his hands on top of his lower rib cage and cough! It hit him hard that I had, indeed, been telling him the truth and that it was possible. If a dancer draws the upper abdominals in, like Pilates clients, he can get many more turns in a pirouette simply because that action alone helps to line up the spine in a straighter stack, keeping the centrifugal force of the turn in alignment. Voila! He just went from 3 to 5 turns with an adjustment most people think isn't even possible.

Pilates concentrates on an inner movement which is uniquely yours, so it is quite personal. In ballet, a composer complements the dancer. This is a whole new animal, and it is what separates physical exercise (Pilates) from a physical exercise art form (ballet). Phrasing a section of music is so exciting that it is hard to describe, particularly if you are really moved by that passage. All of a sudden you have a partner, someone who can make you look great or someone who can make you look awkward.

There are other distinctions between dance and Pilates. Costumes and lighting designs are both obstacles to be overcome after dancers achieve movement quality in ballet. This is not something typically dealt with in a Pilates workout. A strangely weighted costume or intense side lighting on a stage can be a real movement killer. All of a sudden it is like being partially blind with odd motor skills. That turn and that balance in the normality of the studio are gone and must be recaptured, usually that very night.

Despite these differences, there are numerous similarities in the movement patterns of both methods. The Footwork on the Reformer, typically how a Reformer workout starts, is amazingly similar to demi and grand plié in ballet, typically how a ballet class begins. Coordination on the Reformer requires the arms and legs to work separately and together. In ballet, the same challenge is found with the tendus, stretching and pointing the feet while executing complementary arm movements Lowering and lifting the heels on the Reformer with the legs straight is identical to a relevé in ballet, except that you are standing instead of lying down.

Extension of the spine on the Ladder Barrel, bending backwards, stretching out, bending back, stretching out, and then rounding over to start again is almost exactly what a dancer does standing at the barre. In both cases the spine is completely lengthened and supported fully by the abdominal wall before extension back ever takes place. The abdominals, gluteals, hips, lower back, and inner thighs contribute to all movement, whether it is ballet or Pilates. But Pilates teaches you how much each of these muscles must be activated to get the smoothest, most complete movement possible.

The Leg Springs in Pilates are comparable to a dancer's executing difficult steps in the air. When he jumps, a dancer has virtually nothing to help him except his body posture and core strength. Nothing. Not only that, he has gravity and inertia going against him, as well.

The Leg Springs can help. They allow a person who is supported by a mat to execute very precise movement of the lower body, lifted by and resisted by these large springs. The springs want you to go one way, yet the exercise asks you to work against them. You have no choice but to employ your powerhouse or be pulled off track by the springs. It is a perfect and safe way for a dancer to understand exactly what must be engaged in order to perform in the air. I have seen and felt this so many times in Pilates work that I have actually wanted to put it into practice. This would be foolish at 53, since my body is well past its ability to sustain a good landing anymore, but is it something I teach? You bet. Any dancer who does not realize that Pilates is the answer to unlocking the vault that holds him back in his dancing is mistaken. As I have said before, "Ballet needs Pilates. Pilates does not need ballet."

Similarly, the Jump Board improves a dancer's ability to leap in the air. Unfortunately, it is not used nearly as much as it could be used. How brilliant to be able to jump without actually jumping, your body weight going horizontally rather than vertically. Especially in ballet, you can regain the feeling of what it's like to push through your legs and feet to spring in the air, without actually leaving the ground or absorbing the impact of your full body weight as you land. The springs bring you back in, and, of course, that's all adjustable. You're lying on your back, level with the floor and you have a certain amount of spring tension. At whatever speed you want, you're able to push through your legs and feet and extend your body at its full length, replicating exactly the same thing you would do if you were standing.

Many other exercises in the Pilates repertoire can prepare a dancer for movements in the ballet repertoire. The Push Through Bar is wonderful for young, male dancers who are learning to lift their partners. With one spring and later two springs on the bottom, they push the bar up a few times at first, just pressing the back into the mat. Then they lift the body without the legs, eventually lifting the entire body into Teaser position. Later, they can work different mechanics with the legs, while sustaining the bar, then working the roll down, which is so important. This sequence is strikingly similar to lifting or lowering a partner from overhead to the stage floor in a controlled manner.

It is important, however, to note one critical difference in all of these comparisons: ballet requires complete turn out from the hips, causing the toes to go in completely opposite directions. Pilates uses only the natural amount of turn out from the hips (sometimes not at all). I think the key word here is natural. Pilates is absolutely natural for the body to acquire. Ballet is completely unnatural for the body and requires years of attention and physical prying open of the joints to obtain the beautiful lines in the body associated with classical work.

I believe anyone can do Pilates. Not everyone can become a ballet dancer of note.

The Pilates method of body conditioning is a very natural way of getting the body to understand how it was meant to function, how it can function in its most natural state. And the truth is, for a person to do anything extremely athletic, it is much more helpful for them to understand how their bodies work in the more natural sense that Pilates teaches, without all the extreme turn out of ballet, or the intense rotation of throwing a baseball, or the incredibly complex athletic movements in mixed martial arts. Training in the Pilates method gives a person the kind of awareness that is critical for the type of extreme athleticism that can injure the body. Although athletic pursuits are great to watch and great to participate in, they really can be physically very damaging at professional levels.

Other than Pilates, there are no training methods available that are precise and connected enough to combat this wear and tear on the body. I know, because I have tried most of them in an effort to be fit outside of dance. Nothing ever felt as complete as Pilates. At one point, I trained on Cybex machines, which at the time were state-of-the-art. This type of machine builds muscle in such a way that the stronger you get, the more pressure you exert on the Cybex and the more resistance it provides. So if you start out very weak, it isn't very hard to improve your strength by increasing intensity. The problem is that it is only effective in strengthening isolated muscle groups. What is really important is to work the entire body. In fact, the entire body is what is used for any athletic endeavor or modality.

Some of the more recent fads in fitness are downright crazy. The PX90 or P90X workout boasts that a person can go from fat to ripped in 90 days. This is completely unhealthy. But even in 2012, people are still looking for the magic pill. Joe knew there wasn't one. What he did was devise something which is great for you individually, physically and athletically, but it's really bad for business. It takes time. It simply takes time. And the more time it takes for you to get through various levels of his method of body conditioning, the better athletically you become.

Instinctively, Joe must have known that to achieve true fitness you had to go from A to B, and B to C, and C to D, not A to Z. And you can see the progression in complexity from the more basic workouts to the intermediate workouts, eventually leading to the advanced system, which is very athletic. Even then there are modifications to those exercises that are still more demanding.

The demands in the professional world of athleticism and dance are high, as well; you're expected to be able to do things supernaturally in many ways. But it takes a toll. A dancer has a very narrow window of opportunity to wrap his arms around as many different ways of moving as possible, to master the different aspects of dance in a young, short lifetime. That's not the way a person who's studying Pilates or working in Pilates has to go about it, and I think that's the beauty of it for the individual. If they're willing to take the time, they can get just as strong as possible in both body and mind.

As a dancer, I was drawn to the athleticism in Pilates. I believe we are all drawn to certain things as we're growing up, adapting to the world. If you relate to the world in an athletic way, this natural physical energy is always present. You try to find that thing that gives you the most satisfaction for that release of energy. By all accounts, Joseph Pilates had an extremely intense energy level, relating to the world in a physical way. Perhaps this is why he gravitated toward boxers, dancers, and other athletes, who then inspired him to find more and more ways to refine his method. Every day, I am grateful for the brilliant body of work he produced, which enables me to function with grace, strength and balance. Thank you, Joe.

About Carl

Co-founder of the Pilates Fitness Studio in Montgomery, Illinois, Carl studied The Method with renowned teacher trainer Juanita Lopez, receiving his Pilates certification in 1999 from The Pilates Studio in New York City. After a 20-year performing career with the Joffrey Ballet, where he rose to the position of assistant Ballet Master, Carl became Ballet Master and resident choreographer for the St. Louis Ballet. He continues to be a guest artist, teacher, and choreographer to ballet companies and universities across the United States; and he is currently a year round faculty member for State Street Dance in Geneva, Illinois.

The Dancer's Edge

By Davorka Kulenovic
Translated by Virginia Schildhauer

> *...Pilates helps dancers get to know*
> *their own bodies even better;*
> *it improves their balance, stability,*
> *and ease of movement...*

"Physical fitness is the first requisite of happiness. Our interpretation of physical fitness is the attainment and maintenance of a uniformly developed body with a sound mind fully capable of naturally, easily, and satisfactorily performing our many and varied daily tasks with spontaneous zest and pleasure." -Joseph Pilates, *Return to Life Through Contrology.*, *p.6.*

I have been fortunate that both of my professions, ballet and Pilates, have also been my passions. More than anything else, I have been blessed to learn the Pilates method of body conditioning from Romana Kryzanowska. The time I spent with her was an enlightening experience, and she taught me so much during my course of independent study in New York. Years of ballet dancing left me with two herniated discs and arthrosis in my hips. I had been looking for an exercise system that would help me. My employer at the time, Ursula Bischoff-Musshake, told me about Pilates, which was just gaining popularity in Europe. Ursula, in cooperation with the city of Stuttgart, organized a seminar and invited Romana Kryzanowska to Germany to conduct a three-day workshop. I was able to take a private lesson with Romana, after which she proposed that I come to New York to train as a Pilates instructor. I took her advice and haven't looked back since.

Now I have been teaching Pilates for 14 years. Personally, I am a devoted practitioner, and my enthusiasm prompts me to impart the beauty of Pilates to others. Thanks to The Method, I live without pain, and I enjoy being able to move my body easily and freely. I'm absolutely convinced this would not be possible without Pilates.

Everyone has his own personal and professional history, and it goes without saying that this is also true for Pilates instructors. This history surely affects our style of teaching. I most certainly have been influenced by my career as a solo ballet dancer; and I am sure that my way of looking at clients is different from that of, let's say, a physical therapist. I know that Pilates is a method of body conditioning and not an art form. Nonetheless, aesthetics or elegance is a significant part of Pilates, which follows its own specific principles, one of which is flow of movement; and, for me, this is the aesthetic element of Pilates. Naturally, technique takes first place and needs to be perfected, but I am never fully satisfied until the exercises are beautiful to watch, until they are performed gracefully and elegantly. It is difficult to achieve this with all clients, but with my students I strongly emphasize this aspect and strive towards elegance. When dancers begin Pilates training, they already move gracefully. Students who do not have a background in dance have to learn this at the same time that they are mastering the technique of Pilates. It is a long process, but I am generally quite proud of them.

I teach all my students through independent study, which means that I work very closely with each of them, observing them keenly. Based on this intensive instruction and close personal contact, I can tell when a student is ready to move on, not only in terms of execution of the exercises, but also regarding personal and emotional development as a student of Pilates. I am careful not to overwhelm students by conveying too much information at the beginning. The path to success needs to be taken step by step, and an individual approach is needed for every student. In general, I try to limit the training period to two years (70 private lessons and 600 observation hours) because I believe that continuity and regular training are important. This time frame seems to work very well, since many of my students train part time, have jobs, families, and/or other responsibilities. Thus, I cannot stipulate that they have to spend 20-30 hours a week at the studio. I am quite tolerant in this respect; however, since quality is the most important aspect of all, I have to see that a student is training and learning continuously as well as making progress steadily.

The atmosphere in the studio is very important to me, as well, since it contributes significantly to the success of our work. My teaching style is collaborative, minimizing competition between my students;

I encourage them to help one another and to accept each other's limitations and skills. A good Pilates trainer should not be defined by remarkable physical abilities, such as how high one can lift one's leg or whether one can do a full split. Although it is very nice to watch someone perform the exercises in a beautiful manner, we should not forget that the most important point is how an instructor works with clients. Moreover, Pilates should not be characterized by competition because it is a form of body conditioning for everybody; and since we all have our own individual anatomy and different prerequisites, it does not make sense to compare people.

Good instruction in the authentic Pilates tradition enables a trainer to use Pilates meaningfully for many purposes and many different bodies because it provides a remarkable range of exercises. This means that anyone—dancers, children, seniors—can do Pilates and stay physically fit. A body conditioning program can be individualized according to the needs of a client and still remain true to the exercises and principles developed by Pilates, adhering to the tempo, transitions and order. Even when teaching a group of older people or a client with an injury, trainers can still work with the classical Pilates method because it offers so many exercises, variations, and modifications.

The foundation of classical Pilates is the flat back. Of course, normal lordosis is the natural form of our spine, and we need to maintain it in our everyday life. While sitting upright in an office chair or car seat, the spine should have a slight curvature. However, it should not be lordotic while performing Pilates exercises, as this causes the muscles in the lumbar region to contract, stretching the stomach muscles slightly and making it impossible to stabilize the pelvis without placing strain on the spine. By maintaining a flat back, pelvic stabilization can be achieved. This is extremely important, because the pelvis is our center, holding all torso and leg muscle attachments. Thus, we can only safely execute an exercise such as Double Straight Leg Stretch in an advanced form if we work with a flat back. The sacrum and lumbar region should press into the mat, allowing the lower back to open and broaden. Otherwise, considerable pressure is imposed on the lumbar region, leading to back injuries.

The pelvis is in a neutral position when we stand upright casually, and this position of the pelvis affects the form of our spine and its anatomical lordosis. These various incorrect postures can often be corrected with Pilates. By using a flat back for Pilates exercises, the spine elongates and straightens. In response, the pelvis will shift somewhat, too. That is the ideal position for learning the Pilates technique. It is the same body posture through which dancers achieve the stability needed to maintain body balance in any position. The upright position and stability of the pelvis significantly affect the quality of movement. This means that the pelvis is always stabilized in one direction, enabling free movement in another direction. For torso movement, part of the abdominal muscle attachments in the pelvis have to be stabilized, but the attachments of the torso muscles have to allow freedom of movement. Torso movement is also ensured by stabilizing the attachments of the leg musculature in the pelvis. Hence, the placement and stabilization of the pelvis are central elements of ballet training. Even very young ballet students have to learn this position from the very beginning, since the entire technique of classical ballet is based on an upright pelvic position. If the pelvis is not in an upright position, it is not possible to turn the legs outward (en dehors); this is absolutely necessary in classical ballet.

This pelvic placement taught in Pilates sessions helps dancers to achieve proper placement in their balletic movements. Twice a week, I give a 45-minute Pilates exercise class to members of the ballet company at the State Theater of Stuttgart. The dancers have to master an extensive repertoire, as well as daily training and rehearsals. Their working day usually lasts at least 6-8 hours and involves strenuous physical work. For these dancers, Pilates is a kind of warm-up and preparation for the subsequent training; it prepares them for the rehearsal and, accordingly, the rehearsal is preparation for the performance in front of an audience. Pilates helps these dancers improve their technique, which, in turn, is the instrument through which they can express the art of dance. Hence, the focus of the training is on precision of movement. Dancers need Pilates to balance their muscles, since muscular effort frequently is biased toward one side of the body, depending on the parts being danced at the time. Contrary to many types of sports, as well as ballet, Pilates always works the whole body symmetrically: both sides of the body, as well as the entire body.

Classical Pilates helps dancers get to know their own bodies even better; it improves their balance, stability, and ease of movement and teaches them to use their strength effectively to avoid overexerting their bodies. My own experience as a student of Pilates is proof of The Method's effectiveness. Although I discovered The Method at 38, quite close to the end of my career, Pilates enabled me to dance with considerably less exertion despite my age.

Dancers have a considerable range of spine mobility when bending backward, but not necessarily forward; they sometimes find it hard to round their backs. Thus, it is important to focus on opening the lower back in Pilates sessions. Otherwise, this lumbar hypermobility results in a loosening of the ligaments; the nucleus pulposus and verte-bral joints become deformed, resulting in a very short career. Instead, dancers should initiate the backbend (cambré) from the thoracic spine, lifting the chest and creating a long line starting in the lumbar region. This then is the flat back that we use in Pilates exercises. The fixation of the spine in an upright position through the deep back and abdomi-nal muscles allows dancers to move the hip joints freely. Simultane-ously, the abdominal muscles are pulled to the spine and upwards, creating a kind of muscular corset. This type of training helps protect the lumbar region and prevent injuries.

Dancers can gain forward spine mobility and stretch their spines; by performing exercises such as the Roll Up, Spine Stretch Forward and rolling exercises, they gain space between the individual verte-brae. Since they have very flexible backward spine mobility, Swan Dive should be executed in a less exaggerated form so that the lumbar region is not subjected to strain. It is much more important that the body stays compact.

Commonly, the back problems affecting many dancers can be traced back to the extreme movements to which a dancer's spine is exposed: strong movements alternate with very slack posture. While dancing, the spinal joints are moved quickly in different directions over an extended period of time; and then, in stark contrast to this, the body is relaxed all of a sudden. As a result, the soft tissue surround-ing the joints is stretched excessively in all directions. When a joint subjected to this kind of strain alternates between extreme positions, deformities or shifts of the disc or nucleus pulposus may arise and this, in turn, is frequently the cause of back problems. When exercis-ing regularly with the Pilates method, body awareness is increased. Moreover, the small, deep stabilizing muscles are strengthened, which helps prevent overly slack posture after physical effort.

A Pilates exercise routine involves stretching and contracting muscles, which adapt more effectively to physical strain through systematic training. Pilates prevents injuries and warms up the muscles for their ballet training. When muscles are not warmed up sufficiently, there is always a risk of pulling a muscle. Primarily, this affects the adductors, the muscles that come to the front when the legs are turned out, the inner side of the thighs. However, these muscles are worked very hard in Pilates exercises. Preparing mentally for rehearsals and performances is also important, and it is precisely this intertwining of body and mind in Pilates that appeals to athletes and dancers, in particular.

Pilates is also an effective modality for injured dancers. In the past, an afflicted limb was placed in a cast for several weeks, during which time the mobility decreased significantly. Today, we know that joints must retain their mobility and strength; consequently, care is taken to keep the injured limbs in motion. This is where Pilates comes in: following medical treatment and physical therapy, Pilates exercises can help dancers regain strength and physical fitness within a short period of time without putting undue strain on the affected limb. Unlike physical therapy, which focuses on and treats a specific physical problem or part of the body, Pilates works the entire body. Jay Grimes alluded to the restorative aspect of Pilates; when asked what to do with an injured client whose physician recommended Pilates training, Jay replied, "Just do the basic Pilates program."

There are so many options in the repertoire. For example, when a dancer with a foot or knee injury resumes training, he can practice jumps on the Reformer with one spring, and eventually, two springs before executing jumps in the ballet studio again. For a client with unstable ankle joints, exercises like Pumping or Pumping with One Leg, Achilles Stretch and Pumping Standing on the High Chair help achieve stability. Exercises on the Foot Corrector and Footwork on the Reformer improve foot alignment.

When training dancers, attention to foot placement is essential. The feet are our connection to the earth. Since they anchor us, the shape and movement pattern of the feet reveal any instability. Ballet dancers often place too much weight on the outer edge of the foot (you can see this by the wear on the soles of their shoes). Consequently, the adductors do not work hard enough. To balance the foot musculature, pressure is applied equally to the ball of the big toe, small toe and heel. It is not uncommon for dancers to be plagued by knee injuries, often caused by hyper-extended knees. Since much of the ballet repertoire requires balancing on one leg, the standing leg must bear the weight. Overextending that supporting leg, however, does not work the leg muscles. Instead, it strains the knee joint. If, however, the leg muscles do the work, then the knee is relaxed. The leg being lifted can be straightened completely since the knee joint does not have to bear the body weight. Pilates can reduce knee strain, teaching the dancer to work from the powerhouse, using the muscles and not the joints.

In addition to its rehabilitative function, Pilates is an ideal form of body training for developing long, lean musculature: when executed correctly, it will never exhaust muscles or increase muscle mass. This is important for dancers, as over-developed muscles are not considered aesthetically appealing. Male dancers who turn to resistance equipment in gyms to strengthen their upper bodies learn this all too quickly. Although they see results in a short period of time, unless they work out at only 60-70% capacity, they experience a substantial increase in muscle mass. In dance training, as well, the teacher must reduce repetitions and follow an exercise routine that alternates between muscle groups in order to increase muscular strength without developing muscle mass.

Dancers benefit, as well, from the connection between breath and movement taught in Pilates. Many dancers breathe shallowly. Pilates teaches them diaphragmatic breathing, expanding the ribcage laterally and keeping the stomach flat as they breathe. It is a far more effective way of gaining stability when dancing than breathing into their stomachs. Stomach breathing prevents the muscles from receiving sufficient oxygen and, consequently, dancers will tire very quickly.

Clearly, the benefits of Pilates are recognized in the dance world. Numerous ballet schools and academies have incorporated it in their curriculum. It should be offered, as well, to young ballet students, who begin with modified exercises. Children younger than 13 years of age should only do Mat work. From 13-14 years on, they can train on the Reformer with two springs. Teaching Pilates to children makes the dance teacher's task easier. It is very difficult to teach young children how to execute ballet exercises precisely. Pilates enables them to increase their strength and stability, allowing their bodies to progress more quickly in the program. Just imagine how difficult it is to teach a young child an arabesque, standing on one leg and extending the other leg behind the body. Because the spine is so pliant, it bends directly in the lower back without the child being able to support this movement with the abdominal muscles. This may injure the spine. The original Pilates method helps children become aware of and strengthen their abdominal muscles. Then they can support the backward flexion of the spine more effectively.

Before and after adolescence, the growth zones of a young person's body have limited resistance; and, consequently, excessive strain should be avoided during a young dancer's ballet studies. Stretching exercises can help prevent injuries during this time, but physical strain and muscular elongation need to be achieved carefully. For this reason, doing Pilates together with ballet training helps children gain stabilization without putting undue strain on their joints.

Classical ballet movements in their perfected form are intended for adult bodies. Ballet training, however, starts when the dancers are young and still growing. Teachers need to be familiar with the growth phases of children and take into consideration the individual state of development of each child, even though this may prove difficult in a class of 6-10 children. Again, here is where Pilates is helpful. It is a suitable tool for strengthening the muscles of children as they experience spurts of growth. During this time, their arms and legs grow quicker than the spine, and children find it hard to hold themselves upright: the muscles become weaker and cannot keep up with the bone growth. In their ballet classes, they have to learn to turn their legs outward; and frequently they exaggerate the movement, even though the hip joint cannot execute the rotation yet. Consequently, their feet sink onto the large toes or inner sides of the feet. The knees necessarily follow this movement and turn inwards. This incorrect position of the knee joint may cause pain.

Ballet teachers have a great responsibility when teaching the extensive spectrum of ballet exercises and technique to children, and they must ensure that the movements are executed with precision in order to prevent injuries. The ideal solution would be Pilates classes three times a week for 45 minutes each. When the children have absorbed the Pilates exercises, every ballet class could be started with a 20-minute Pilates routine to warm up and gain stability.

From the very beginning children love to move. Pilates helps to keep this joy alive. Based on my observation and 14 years of experience as a Pilates instructor, I know that people who regularly exercise with Pilates become friendlier, enjoy their lives more, find pleasure in movement, and gain substantial motivation because they feel good and can tell that their bodies are undergoing a change for the better—a more defined and erect figure—through Pilates. This is the essence and brilliance of the classical Pilates method.

About Davorka

Davorka began her ballet training at the National Theater in Sarajevo, continuing her studies at the Vaganova Academy of Ballet in St. Petersburg. She danced as a soloist at the National Theater of Sarajevo in Spilt and Zagreb and gave solo performances in Yugoslavia and Europe. Emigrating to Germany, she taught ballet and worked as a soloist at Telos-Tanztheater in Stuttgart. In 1997, Davorka began studying Pilates with Romana Kryzanowska. Eight years later, she opened her own Pilates studio and certification institute in Stuttgart, where she works with members of the Stuttgart Ballet. She is an avid tango and salsa dancer.

Classical Pilates and the Golf Connection

By Natasha Madel

> *...Pilates exercises reflect grace and balance in the golfer.*

In my early years as a Pilates teacher, Basil Blecher, a South African expat who was working for Gratz Pilates Equipment, tracked me down in Johannesburg and told me that if I wanted to be a really good Pilates teacher, I should go to New York and train with Romana Kryzanowska. So I did. It was during my apprenticeship with Romana that I met Peter Fiasca at a dinner. Peter was also busy with his apprenticeship, and our dinner conversation soon turned to Pilates and Romana and her strict insistence that each of us develops devotion, humility, passion, individuality and artfulness. We discovered we were like-minded souls, sharing a true passion for the original Pilates method, reveling in the grace and skill required to execute a perfect Pilates workout. Before the evening was over, we had arranged to train together, having a duet in the re:AB studio in New York in the following months. I became hooked on the energy of those sessions, and my passion and devotion for Pilates grew stronger. I knew I had to take that passion to South Africa, a country full of its own passions—one of which is golf.

Home to nearly 500,000 golfers, South Africa is fast becoming a mecca for the sport. While there is a new and exciting generation of professionals emerging from these numbers, the vast majority are weekend warriors. It's the sport of gentlemen (and women), a place for business deals and networking, governed by rules and etiquette. More and more frequently, couples are opting to play as an enjoyable leisure activity. But, according to recent sports medicine reports, 40% of average golfers suffer from at least one injury during the golf season.[1]

Golf is a sport, a serious sport, no matter what the player's level. It requires a certain degree of physical fitness not only to play better, but also to prevent injury. Sadly most golfers are unfit and lack the understanding of the impact their physical condition has on their game, or how improved physical conditioning can vastly improve their performance.

But they are passionate about their game! Early on in my Pilates career, I found myself training a number of golfers. They spoke constantly about wanting the ever-elusive hole-in-one, wanting to hit the ball further and with more precision and generally aiming to be better golfers. I began using classical Pilates as a technique to improve their functional fitness, and eventually their golf game. The feedback was encouraging, and over the years I have fine-tuned this knowledge into a Pilates for Golfers course.

The game of golf is technically challenging, requiring strong mental skills and specific physical mechanics to prevent injury, while constantly improving technique. This provides a host of challenges to fitness professionals who train golfers. Pilates is the perfect tool for this type of training. The Method teaches physical and practical skills, addresses the mind-body connection, and positively influences the quality of a golfer's game, as well as the longevity of his playing life. It is an exercise program that coordinates the mental and the physical realms, enabling one to support the other on the path to overall fitness—developing "a sound mind housed in a sound body."[2]

The nature of the golf swing is inherently unhealthy for the spine, as the forward motion, combined with the rotation and twisting, creates significant stress on the spine and surrounding muscles. This includes the discs and ligaments, as well. Add to this the four to five hours in a bent-over stance, repeating the same-sided twisting motion over and over, and it's no wonder golfers end up with sore backs!

Core strength and flexibility training are the two best things a golfer can do to prevent or minimize back pain. Having strong muscles in the stomach, lower back, inner thighs, and gluteals not only develops a more powerful, controlled swing but protects the spine from injury.

Each of us has the ability to take control of our own well-being. It begins by becoming aware of our bodies as an integrated part of our creative minds. We are all born with that power. Sometimes we only need reminding, and The Method is just such a reminder to all Pilates teachers of their own power. And what could be more powerful than showing a client how to creatively blend the power of the mind with the movement of the body in a way that is both efficient and extremely enjoyable?

Correctly executed and mastered to the point of subconscious reaction, these Pilates exercises reflect grace and balance in the golfer. Indeed, "Contrology exercises will build a sturdy body and a sound mind, capable of performing everyday tasks with ease and perfection. They also provide tremendous reserve energy for sports, recreation and emergencies."[3]

Injury: any sport participant's worst nightmare. But why do injuries occur? Common causes are overtraining or undertraining, thus keeping the whole body from actively participating in a chosen sport. All too often we ignore the cost of getting ourselves ready and plunge in all set to go: new this, new that, reading specialty magazines, watching DVDs, talking, fantasizing. This is only the start.

However, in order to succeed at golf, Gary Player and other golfing greats all acknowledge that they follow an overall fitness regime that includes both mind power and body strength. Player says, "We create success or failure on the course primarily by our thoughts."[4] The sheer magic of the body and mind working in unison is what we observe on our TV screens when we watch the professionals play. It looks so easy, and we delude ourselves into believing there are short-cuts to a great golf game.

Golf Fantasies vs. Reality

Fantasy #1: Golf is a game of technical skill rather than an athletic sport.

Reality: An understanding of the biomechanics needed for a good golf swing might cause us to throw our hands up in despair, as we recognize moving from a sedentary lifestyle to active participation requires a total commitment from both the mind and body.

The muscular activity required for a good golf swing depends on nearly every joint between the tips of our toes and the ends of the fingers. All the joints together create the unbroken chain of movement required for the perfect golf swing.

Why Pilates? Pilates is the art of Contrology. The focus is on mind and body working in unison. The apparatus helps to realign the body, evenly distributing and developing muscular strength. The personal instructor is the conduit to assess the client's specific requirements, ensuring both strength and cardiovascular development.

Fantasy #2: Pain and injury related to golfing are due solely to a poor swing.

Reality: The body has two sides, but if one side works more than the other, the muscles tire and compensate with unnatural moves, and the cellular memory of the body kicks in to remind us of past injuries. New injuries and poor performance on the golf course are the result. Adjusting the golf swing each time is like applying a Band-Aid and does not address the underlying cause of poor performance.

Why Pilates? Pilates participants should not experience any pain during their sessions; if it hurts, don't do it. We need to listen to our bodies. The proper physical condition for peak performance, no matter what your age, will enhance not only a golf game, but overall mobility. This is a lifestyle choice.

Fantasy #3: A conditioning regime that focuses on strength will improve driving distance.

Reality: Weight training, cardiovascular exercise, and other fitness modalities are all valuable training tools. The requirements for a great golf game also include overall stamina, flexibility and range of motion. The art of a perfect swing is flowing motion with no hesitation.

Why Pilates? Pilates is a discipline that allows our bodies to go beyond what we believe we are capable of. The development of the core or "powerhouse," cardiovascular training, and controlled stretching with strength balance the body and facilitate freedom of movement.

What Is Required for the Perfect Swing?

Mind and body must be in total synergy. Golf coaches stress that a good golf swing requires concentration, centering, control, precision, flowing movement and breathing. Sound familiar? These are the six basic principles of Pilates. All movement in Pilates requires focus on these core fundamentals, which can benefit golfers in everyday life:

Concentration: In Pilates, body movement originates from the mind. Focus and concentration are required to use the apparatus and the muscles. The mind is the coach, and the muscles of the body, the team. The mind wills the body to action, giving golfers the requisite mind-body connection.

Centering: The center is the physical point between the sternum and the pubic bone. Pilates improves strength and endurance in this area. The various apparatus and exercises will reveal a dominant side of the body or a weak "powerhouse," the large group of muscles in our center. Physical energy is exerted from the center to coordinate movements. This builds a strong foundation for all movement and is highly beneficial to golfers, even assisting them to sit upright at their desks or in front of their computers for longer periods of time. In turn, this encourages correct breathing.

Control: All movements are performed with control while maintaining a strong, firm center. Learning correct postural control ensures correct execution of the exercises, thereby avoiding injury during other activities. No sloppy or haphazard movements are allowed, since that can lead to injury. Each movement serves a function, and control is at the core.

Precision: Work smarter, not harder. This is the integration of centering, control and coordination. The ultimate reward is to do the exercises precisely and to achieve visible results. Muscles have a memory, so it is important to always be precise; otherwise, the same errors will be repeated, and there will be no improvement.

Flowing Movement: Work smoothly and efficiently. During exercise, only the muscles needed for the activity should be recruited. The movement must flow so that there is no strain that might cause injury. Intuition is essential; listen to your body and use any modifications that will develop your body optimally.

Breathing: Specific breathing is needed to maximize abdominal control and strength. Breathing correctly and using the breath to connect to your core will assist in relaxing you. It enhances the ability to do the exercise correctly, enabling you to connect with the powerhouse of energy. Breathing assists golfers, as oxygen is needed for muscles to work efficiently. All exercises require breathing to be a focal point, expanding the lungs and increasing the golfer's breathing capacity.

Pilates is not just about attaining body shape; it is a tool for everyday living—a lifestyle choice. What is learned in the exercise sessions has impact outside the studio, enabling the golfer to achieve grace, balance and ease, thus reducing stress levels. Pilates should be practiced in conjunction with other sports for a healthy, all-round approach to physical well-being. Incorporating the principles of Pilates into daily existence can lead to a lifetime of good health and fitness, as well as improved athletic performance.

But what turns an athlete into a super athlete? Different factors influence this transition: super athletes have an understanding of the essentials and a solid foundation; they never stop learning and never stop believing that there is room for improvement; dedication is key. Tiger Woods is an excellent example of this kind of dedication. Approximately two years into his professional career, he left the game to go back to basics to revamp his approach to his swing. What did he use to achieve this? Pilates!

At this point you may be asking: How will Pilates improve my clients' golf game? Pilates will teach them to engage properly and to use the powerhouse. It will unleash energy and strength they never knew they possessed, and it will lead to improved concentration, thus enabling them to achieve maximum control and precision.

Our goal as Pilates instructors is to help golfers reach their full potential. Few golfers ever achieve a level of success equivalent to the amount of hard work they put into their game. More often than not, their lack of success is the result of physical limitations which prevent them from performing at a level required to excel. Conventional strength training, core conditioning, and other fitness disciplines have not resulted in golfers achieving their perfect swing. Conventional strength training has limitations because flexibility is not stressed. Flexibility training on its own is not enough either, because strength is also needed to swing a golf club well. By sensibly combining various movements from Pilates, we can give golfers the optimum combination of strength, flexibility, and speed—all essential to developing the golf swing fully. Pilates provides the best combination possible for both strength and flexibility training and is beneficial to golfers of all handicap levels: professional, low or high handicap, or even beginner level. It is the perfect complement to golf.

Multiple Pilates exercises address every part of the golf swing to help increase and strengthen the hip and shoulder turn, improve rotation in the arms, strengthen wrists and forearms, and improve cardiovascular fitness. This approach results in more consistent play, a faster swing, improved ball striking ability and trajectory, increased driving distance, and better contact and directional control of the ball. Most importantly, Pilates helps limit potential injury.

The main aim of the exercises is to create balance in the body. It is a low-stress method of physical and mental conditioning designed to cater to the needs of each individual. The specific combination of these exercises works to correct any muscle imbalances through the use of Contrology. This involves both mental and physical control to attain maximum conditioning. Each exercise is synchronized with a corresponding breathing pattern and is performed with either a rhythm or melodic rhythmical expression, creating gentle or vigorous cardiovascular-aerobic stimulation, depending on the intensity and speed of the execution.

Special attention is paid to increasing the functional capacity of the spine, resulting in a superior and well-proportioned body that is significantly less prone to injuries. It also reduces long-term accumulation of micro-trauma and assists in neuromuscular rejuvenation. Joseph Pilates wrote: "The slouch position upsets the equilibrium of the body resulting in disarrangement of various organs, including the bones and muscles as well as the nerves, blood vessels and glands...Proper carriage of the spine is the only natural way to prevent against abdominal obesity, shortness of breath, asthma, high and low blood pressure and various forms of heart disease."[5]

Following, I endeavor to provide the transfer of skills and the physical requirements of the golfer. Then exercises are suggested to address particular issues: muscle balance, flexibility, coordination, strength, endurance, and range of motion. The benefits to the golfer are many: muscle tone is enhanced; concentration is optimized; coordination, posture, balance and alignment are improved; the vestibular system is strengthened; injury is prevented through core strengthening; muscle flexibility and joint mobility are increased; sleep is improved due to enhanced proprioception.

The first level of learning is to understand the three ways in which the body moves: locomotor, nonlocomotor, and manipulative. Loco-motor movement allows for moving around an area and includes eight basic movements: walk, run, gallop, slide, jump, hop, leap and skip. Locomotor skills are influenced by the golfer's age, lower-body strength, balance, and neurological development from childhood. Nonlocomotor or axial movement includes 13 stationary movements: bending, stretching, twisting, turning, pushing, pulling, rising, callus-ing, swinging, swaying, dodging, spinning, and balancing. Manipu-lation is movement in which the hands or the feet use equipment to perform fine motor and gross skills. Fine motor skills use the hands and fingers and include tying shoe laces, using scissors or writing. Gross motor skills use the large muscles of the legs and arms and are skills used primarily in games and sports such as rolling, kicking or dribbling a soccer ball.

Pilates emphasizes the importance of correct posture in order to maintain a strong spine and ease of spinal movement. Joseph Pilates is known for saying, "If your spine is inflexibly stiff at 30, you are old; if it is completely flexible at 60, you are young."[6] Proper posture also affects the breath, movement efficiency, and energy. In golf, posture influences body concept, energy and emotional state. When the body starts to slump, and the shoulders round forward in a slouch, the chest and heart space cave in, stressing the cervical vertebrae as the head droops forward. The body becomes fatigued as its ability to receive oxygen is diminished in this closed-off, rounded posture. Starting with younger golfers, it is important to understand good posture mechanics. This can be emphasized while sitting at a computer or at a desk doing work. Students should be aware of how they walk and carry books or backpacks that are extremely heavy and cause injury. Teaching correct lifting mechanics is also important. Developing proper posture, espe-cially at a young age, is essential for life-long health.

Address the golf stance with proper posture. Bend from the hips, chest arched, neutral pelvis, and head on top of spine. Employ the correct stance for the chosen golf club, stance square, suction feet with arms hanging, reaching through the club line. Balance is important. Maintain the correct distance from the ball, shoulders down, neutral grip. Make sure the ball is in the correct position for woods and irons, and the feet are placed properly. Feel grounded by slightly pulling up the toes.

Opposition in the legs supports the rotation/coil: primary left leg in the back swing and right leg during the down swing. Narrowing the pelvis creates stability and balance. Movement starts in the hips for both back swing and down swing. Focus on weight shift, scissoring of the legs, and correct hip and knee motion. The legs help balance centrifugal force, and correct foot action supports balance. The legs must completely support the rotation of the spine, and the feet support the movement of the hips and knees.

Maintain the arch and width of the chest during the rotation or cross of the chest. Movement starts in the hips for both back swing and down swing, and the pelvis remains narrowed and neutral. Focus on closing the rib cage, connecting the upper body to the lower body. The center of gravity stays in one place throughout the swing, head and tail stacked on top of each other. To maintain posture, avoid any up, down, forward, or backward movement. There should be contrast between head and tail during the swing, and the rotation is the main power source.

Common mistakes made during the rotation include losing the correct curvature of the spine, losing the width and length of the spine, tilting of the spine and losing the correct angle of the spine. The benefits of twisting include physiological benefits to the circulatory system and internal organs, structural benefits to the musculoskeletal system and benefits to consciousness. The organs are compressed during a twist, pushing blood filled with metabolic by-products and toxins. On releasing the twist, fresh blood flows in, carrying oxygen and the building blocks for tissue healing. The twist involves the spine, hips and shoulders. This is affected by a sedentary lifestyle, which causes shortening of soft tissue. Muscles, tendons, ligaments, and fascia or connective tissue need to be stretched a few times a week to prevent shortening and to improve joint mobility. Twisting also helps to maintain the health of the discs and facet joints.

Focus on the scooping of the humerus or upper arm bone, reaching through the club, allowing rotation of the arms. The shoulders stay down and the arms always remain in front of the body through the completed swing, wrist cocked instead of hinging. The right arm bends during the back swing, while the left arm bends during the down swing. The arms stay connected to the torso throughout the entire movement.[7]

Breathing revitalizes the body, steadies the emotions, and creates clarity of the mind. Since your state of mind is reflected in the way you breathe, it follows that by controlling the breath, you can learn to control your state of mind. This is important to golfers. Joseph Pilates suffered with asthma as a child and believed full, deep breathing was essential for energy and vitality. He developed a system of full lung breathing with activation of the deep abdominals during deep exhalation. In Pilates, diaphragmatic breathing is encouraged by cueing deep inhalation, expansion of the rib cage, and navel-to-spine emphasis on the exhalation. This engages the tranversus abdominus to assist with full and complete exhalation.

Breathe in, breathe out. How simple it sounds! We think we are breathing efficiently until we are in a situation that requires concentration. Then what do we do? We forget to breathe...sound familiar? Stress is part of life; the breath is the primary stress modulator and stabilizer, and, within limits, can be controlled both consciously and unconsciously. It is the lead horse in the team of horses called the autonomic nervous system. Deep breathing, in through the nose and out through the mouth, connects you with your core. This has a profound effect on every aspect of overall health and well-being. Physically, breathing sustains the natural metabolic process of the body. Psychologically, breathing keeps the mind calm and focused.

In corporate or business environments, when we are stressed, our breathing varies considerably, depending on the situation facing us and external influences like air-conditioning. So how do we regulate or control stress? Perhaps with a round of golf! Imagine a sunrise filled with color: bold reds, yellows and oranges, excitement and adventure, the call of the fish eagle, the sounds of wide open spaces, steaming cups of coffee washed down with ginger nuts. It's amazing how breathing changes with one's thoughts.

Golf courses are designed with precision and forethought. They are havens of tranquility with trees boldly lining fairways of adventure and discovery, with bunkers, ponds, beckoning greens, and breathtaking views. The physical environment fosters excitement about the day, the game, life, those sneaky bunkers and ponds that are not going to interfere with the perfect swing straight down the fairway onto the green. Approaching the first tee, however, the vision fades; breathing becomes erratic. The concern now is the ball, the address position, the swing, and one's body. Cellular memory conjures up images of past mishaps.

Stop. Breathe in with a deep breath through the nose—all the way, fully expanding the lungs. Pause. Breathe out gently and slowly through the mouth. Connect with the core, just as in Pilates sessions. The upper body will expand and relax, arms will relax, and the muscles all the way down the back will relax. The arms should feel more comfortable and move more freely than before.

Then remember to focus on the following before every golf swing: stand a comfortable distance behind the ball; see where your target is, and, in your mind, visualize your perfect shot; while doing this, slowly and deeply inhale through the nose, and gently exhale through your mouth to relax your body; now assume your address position; look down at your ball; slowly and deeply inhale and exhale; relax your arms, and soften the muscles in your upper body; slowly inhale as you go into your backswing; slowly exhale at the top of the back swing, rotating further, and continue exhaling as you move through your downswing and follow-through.[8] Just as breath coordinates with movement in Pilates sessions, so, too, breathing patterns coordinate with the golf swing.

It goes without saying that working the golfer through a Reformer or Mat routine will improve overall strength, flexibility, balance and control. Imbalances and weaknesses will be ironed out using specific exercises on the apparatus. Keep progressing the golfer client, and include a variety of stable and unstable surfaces. Conventional training generally looks at stable surfaces, whereas our training includes unstable surfaces for golfers so the body can work harder, improving balance, control and stability. The functional training program I pre-scribe for golfers includes closed kinetic chain exercises; this means that one limb is in a fixed position and in contact with a surface. These closed kinetic chain exercises ensure faster results, with more power, strength, balance, and stability compared to open kinetic chain exercises.

Playing golf may look like a relatively slow-moving activity, but it actually places a lot of strain on the body. Picking up the golf bags, swinging a golf club, constantly twisting the upper torso and bending to place and pick up golf balls are all responsible for causing pain in the golfer's back, shoulders and wrists. The holy grail of all golfers is to correct the golf swing. Following are some exercises that can be given for each aspect of the swing.

Problems associated with the back swing include limitation in shoulder and neck rotation, tightness in the hamstrings, and limited side flexion. Several Pilates exercises address these problems. Pelvic Lift improves segmental control in the lumbar spine by lengthen-ing the latissimus dorsi, tibialis anterior, rectus abdominus, quadri-ceps, psoas, and erector spinae, as well as strengthening the gluteals, deep abdominals, quadratus lumborum, latissimus dorsi, hamstrings, adductors, and soleus. It is good for lower back pain, ankle inversion injury, stress fracture, hamstring strain, trochantic hip pain and shin splints. To perform the movement, lie on your back with your knees bent and feet flat on the floor, hip-width apart. Arms are lengthened at your sides, shoulders wide, and shoulder blades elongated down your back. Engage your lower abdominals and slowly curl from the base of your spine. Allow each vertebra of the spine to curl up, one by one, under and away from you until you reach the tips of your shoulder blades. Hold and slowly reverse the movement to return to the start-ing position. Repeat and aim higher through the lumbar spine. When you reach your optimum movement, hold and allow your shoulder blades to drift down your back. Raise your arms up and back, keeping the arms close to the sides of your head. Stop when your chest and ribs start to rise. Leave your arms behind as you as you roll the spine back down. Then float the arms back to the sides. Avoid curling too high. Keep your tailbone curled under. Don't rest your weight on your shoulders or raise your arms too high. Your chest and ribs should stay on the floor.

Also great for the back swing, Standing Mermaid elongates the sides of the body, lengthening latissimus dorsi, obliques, and side flexors in the neck and strengthening obliques and quadratus lumborum. This exercise is good for lower back strain, rotator cuff pain, biceps tendonitis, patellar-femoral pain and hamstring strain. Stand with your feet hip-width apart, hands loosely at your sides. Slowly raise one arm above your head while allowing the opposite arm to slide down your leg. Keep your raised arm in line with your body and avoid twisting your trunk. Stretch your arm as far as you can to open your side. Don't twist your body when reaching. Ensure that your arm is over your head and not across the front of your body.

Problems associated with the down swing include limitation in thoracic spinal rotation and tightness in the hamstrings. Short Box, Side to Side strengthens the powerhouse, legs and buttocks, and lengthens the sides, legs and spine. After Short Box, Flat Back, remain in the same starting position and lean slightly forward until your shoulders are just in front of the area where your thighs meet with your hips. Pull your powerhouse in and squeeze your buttocks. Inhale and reach over to your right as far as you can while keeping the opposite hip down. Squeeze your buttocks again and return to the starting position as you exhale. Repeat to the other side. Most importantly, reach tall from the base of the spine up through the crown of your head. It is important to sit up tall and keep your spine long throughout the movement. Keep your arms equidistant from your head. Don't let your shoulders hike up or your arms move towards your ears. Lock your elbows and knees or bend your knees if it helps you sit up taller. Keep the shoulders down.

Short Box, Twist and Reach strengthens the waist and powerhouse, and lengthens the spine and legs. Omit this exercise if there are any neck, shoulder, hip or back problems. After Short Box, Side to Side, sit up tall, reaching your arms straight towards the ceiling. Squeeze your buttocks and pull your powerhouse in and up. Exhale and twist your torso at the waist to rotate to the left. Inhale and reach back, keeping your buttocks squeezed, and stretch out long. Exhale and return to an upright position. Then inhale to rotate back to the start position. Repeat three times on each side. Keep your spine tall without arching. Don't let the arm lift change the shape of your spine. When you twist your torso, keep your stomach in and let nothing below your waist move. The spine rotates, but the hips must stay anchored and not shift.

Difficulty with acceleration ball strike is frequently associated with tightness in the shoulder rotators, particularly externally. Two exercises in the system reduce this tightness, improving acceleration ball strike. Pulling Straps on the Long Box strengthens the arms, legs, back, buttocks, and powerhouse and develops flexibility of the spine. Lie on the box holding the straps and reach out in front of you with loosely clenched fists facing each other. Look at the floor, pull your powerhouse in and engage your buttocks without lifting your feet. Inhale and pull your fists alongside your body until they are behind you, simultaneously lifting your chest up off the box. Hold your breath in this position for a second or two. Contract your fists, arms, back, buttocks and powerhouse, squeezing your legs together. Exhale to return to the starting position.

Pulling T Straps on the Long Box strengthens the legs, buttocks, back, arms, and powerhouse; and it opens the chest and stretches the shoulders. After Pulling Straps, remain on the box in the same face-down position. Bring your arms out to the sides, keeping your neck long. Your body should resemble the letter T. Inhale, pull your powerhouse in, and squeeze your buttocks. Pull your arms back and together, keeping them parallel to the floor as you lift your chest into the air. Hold this position for a second or two. Exhale and return to the starting position.

Problems with follow-through are associated with tight external shoulder rotation. There are several Pilates exercises that correct this problem. Swakate on the Mat strengthens the arms, shoulders, back, buttocks and powerhouse. Kneel on the Mat, knees slightly apart, and hold your body upright in one straight line from your head. Keep your left arm down at your side and lift your right arm to chest height, lightly touching the chest with a loose fist. Keep your shoulders down. Inhale and straighten your right arm out to the side, tightening your right fist, arm, powerhouse, back and buttocks. Exhale and return to the starting position. Repeat three times on the right side and then the left.

Criss-cross strengthens the obliques and quadratus lumborum. Lie on the Mat with your knees up, feet hip-width apart, hands clasped behind your head, and elbows open. Engage your powerhouse and draw your right shoulder towards the opposite knee. Your chest, not your elbow, should be aimed toward your knee. Keep your elbow open. Continue to curl up until both your shoulder blades are off the floor. Hold this position. Then lower your upper body slowly to the Mat. Repeat on the other side.

What is Balance? Newton's Third Law of Motion states, "For every action there is an equal and opposite reaction." Balance unites opposing forces. Balance is the tension between standing up and falling down. Balance is an invisible center between the left foot and the right foot. If we don't breathe in, we can't breathe out; this, too, is balance. The more fully we move, the more fully we relax—also balance. Holding on and letting go, thinking and doing, laughing and crying—opposing actions are tempered by balance.

To develop strength and balance, teach the Standing Arm Series while standing on small balls. This provides an effective strength and balance workout that exercises both the upper and lower body, at the same time improving the golfer's sense of balance.

The simple classical exercise Rolling the Beanbag can be taken a step further by adding the unstable surface of a foam roller. This exercise will develop better body awareness and improve postural security, ocular control and visual discrimination. Begin standing with good Pilates posture behind the foam roller. Then step on top of it. With control, slowly unwind the cord, lowering the Beanbag towards the floor by simultaneously releasing your right hand and bending the wrist backwards as you curl your left hand forward and away from you. When the Beanbag reaches the bottom, reverse the action. To get the most from this exercise, really work the forearms, wrists and hands, and articulate all the joints as you unwind the weighted bag. Breathe in and out with a natural rhythm, maintaining your scoop. Don't allow the shoulders to help the action. Be aware of your posture at all times during the Beanbag exercise, standing with your feet rooted firmly on the foam roller. Keep your stomach scooped in and your hips over your feet. Just balancing on the foam roller will provide a challenge! If the exercise is too difficult for you initially, you have several options for modifying it. You can reduce the weight of the bag, or eliminate the bag altogether in order to concentrate on winding and unwinding the dowel with powerful, effective movements. Over time you can slowly increase the weight of the bag.

The brain and the endocrine, nervous, and immune systems all play a part in our emotional well-being. When we have a thought or feel an emotion, the brain releases neuropeptides that translate that emotion into a physical state. Teach adult golfers that Pilates really can make a difference when it comes to controlling mood swings, as well as help with learning how to ground and center oneself on the green. Pilates can help to balance hormones, elevate the spine, and move oxygen through the body. Energy always follows thought, and in so doing, increases functional strength, flexibility, hormonal balance, focus, and a much stronger mental game.

I use the pre-class exercise Connecting the Circle. Seated in a circle, golfers are asked to rate their emotional electricity on a scale of 1-10. They determine whether they are wired, calm, or somewhere in-between and what emotions control them on and off the green. Once they have established what the emotions are that keep them from achieving their personal best in tournaments, they can move on to the next step, connecting and balancing out the left and right hemispheres of the brain and drawing the connection between the mind and body both on and off the green. This can all be achieved with the following Pilates workout.

The Hundred: breathing techniques increase blood flow to the brain. Arm Circles: adding a greater range of motion to the shoulder joint is key to a more powerful swing. Reach on the Short Box: reach for your dreams. Connect with your vision and long-term golf goals. Push Through: release stress. Let go of frustrations, making space for new avenues of improvement in your game. Pilates Stance: focus, concentration, and determination help to ground oneself through the feet and legs, connecting solidly with the green. This serves one well when teeing off and even more so afterwards. The use of silent affirmations improves the overall mind-set, resulting in a new and improved golfer and game. Backward Arms: create greater flexibility in the joints, resulting in a deeper rotation enabling the golfer to strike through a swing with greater power. Twist: in the follow-through, torso rotation increases the range of motion in the hips and lower back. These movements energize the spine, sending increased blood flow to the brain, stimulating and balancing hormones. Mermaid: asymmetry in golf, as in all one-sided games, develops more muscles on the dominant side. This exercise helps stretch out the back, hips, and shoulders, thereby balancing the body. Side Bend: if held longer on the weaker side, this exercise helps to compensate for any imbalance. Rolling Like a Ball: this incorporates aspects of the five abdominal series and rejuvenates the whole body.

Use visualization and imagery to do what I call "Golfing through the Pilates Body." As you conduct a full advanced Reformer workout, lead your client through a guided visualization that scans the body from head to toe. Imagine playing a round of golf on your favorite golf course. Take note of the sensations and feelings that wash over you as you perform each exercise with a minimum of motion, just as you "play" that golf ball. You will feel completely different—more invigorated, energized and alive. Use your Reformer workout to work through all those negative thoughts and feelings, like frustration, fatigue and anxiety, which do not benefit you as a golfer or as a person. As you do a final think-through, reconnect with your power swing as you sink that last ball in the 18th hole. You have what it takes, so use the original Pilates workout to be the best at your game!

Annika Sörenstam, the world's greatest woman golfer, extols the virtues of exercise in her new book, *Golf Annika's Way*:

> I have worked hard to craft a swing that's simple and re-peatable, but my workouts have also contributed to my success. My newfound strength gave me endurance to win eight LPGA titles in 2001, eleven in 2002 and six more in 2003. My strength gave me the power to drive the ball more than 270 yards and the confidence to compete against the world's best male players at the 2003 Colonial. The results have been amazing. I now hit three of every four par-5's in two; 10 years ago I hit one of four. I ranked in the LPGA's top five in driving distances for the first time in 2002, and then led the category in 2003. And I got longer without losing my trademark ac-curacy because my training program not only made my golf muscles stronger, but also improved my balance, flexibility, and rotational power.[9]

To many, golf appears to be a relaxing sport, played at a leisurely pace with little or no physical exertion. But in reality, golf can be rough on the body, especially the back, says golfing legend Gary Player. He has won 163 tournaments around the world, traveled more than 14 million air miles, and is one of only 5 golfers to have won the Grand Slam. Gary knows all too well that a golfer swings in one direction all his life and never balances the opposite muscles, putting tremendous pressure on the lower back. Swinging a weighted club with both the left and right hands is recommended to improve flexibility and balance to both sides of the body. Player believes it is the strengthening of the core muscles that makes it easier to generate club head speed and maintain ability through the golf swing.[10] One of the best core strengtheners is the front plank or Pilates Balance Control Front.

In addition to a strong torso, Player believes powerful legs are critical to success on the course and help develop a swing that will take a lesser toll on the body. A strong lower body gets you through the ball well and creates leverage so you gain distance. Squats against the wall using a big ball are recommended. Shoulder muscles are also often neglected—rotator cuff muscles are a common injury for golfers. To build stability and strength to protect the rotator cuff muscles, shoulder stabilizing exercises should be done. Pulling Straps and T-position on the Reformer address this issue.

Ernie Els, South Africa's favorite golfing son, is only the third South African after Bobby Locke and Gary Player to be honored by the World Golf Hall of Fame in May 2011. In 1994, at the age of 24, he won the biggest tournament in the world, the US Open. The highlights of his career include being ranked No. 1 in the world, winning two U.S. Opens, a British Open, a record seven World Match Plays and the World Cup in 2001 with fellow South African Retief Goosen as his partner. For two straight years, 2003 and 2004, he topped the European Tour Order of Merit. In 2010, he became Europe's all-time leading money earner, even though he plays most of his golf on the US PGA Tour and won twice last year, along with the Grand Slam of Golf and the SA Open. In 2007, he celebrated 700 weeks in the top 10 in the rankings, and in 2009 he set up the Els for Autism Foundation, as his nine year-old son Ben is autistic. His history as a golfer goes back to South Africa in the early 1980s when Gary Player was an inspiration for him on the pro tour and he won the World Juniors at 14. Although The Big Easy has a swing that seems effortless, he knows first-hand the importance of exercise: "Preparing my body and mind helps me deal with the pressure of competition. As a result of my increased stamina, strength and flexibility, and the confidence that comes with them, I perform better on the course."[11]

Younger golfers on the circuit seem to have learned this lesson at an early age. South Africans across the country cheered as they watched a new golfing hero pull on the sought-after green blazer from the Masters and pocket $1.44 million in prize money. This dramatic victory ensured Charl Schwartzel 11th position on the world rankings, three positions above his mentor, Ernie Els. Now his name is the latest buzz word in golfing circles in South Africa and further afield. He is the third African to win the Masters, after Gary Player in 1961, 1974 and 1978 and Trevor Immelman in 2008. In an interview with Martin Park, Schwartzel reflected on the new generation of golfers: "I think the lifespan [of a professional golfer] will be a bit longer now because I think the guys, the youngsters, are exercising more than the previous generation used to do."[12]

Most golfers believe that it is the set of golf clubs that plays the golf and not their bodies! Golf-teaching professionals can try all they want to adapt the swing to the golfer's lack of body biomechanics, but the golfer will continue to compensate and this will eventually lead to injury. Golf is an athletic sport that requires a conditioned body. A trained Pilates instructor specializing in Pilates for Golfers can assess firstly what the golfer's ineffective movement patterns are and then address them with appropriate corrective exercises and movements. The outcome is a ball that travels farther (every golfer wants this) and straighter, while ensuring that the golfer stays pain and injury-free. It's the safer and more effective way of lowering your handicap!

Although golf is growing at a fast pace among women, the majority of golfers in South Africa are still males over the age of 40. They tend to have more body strength, but it is not integrated into their bodies. Their legs, hips, backs, and shoulders are tighter than females, placing more stress on joints, ligaments, tendons and muscles. Pilates works for these men, regardless of age—whether they are senior golfers, active golfers, or golfers recovering from injury.

I am fortunate to have had the top amateur golfer in South Africa train with me at my studio since 2005. Daniel Hammond is a 19-year old Springbok player, who aims to turn professional at the end of 2011. Daniel can't say enough about how Pilates has improved his game:

I have been doing Pilates with Sandra for the last six years, and it has helped me in the following ways: core stability, which is essential for a good golf swing; flexibility, which creates a bigger arc and X factor (coil); fitness, strength and most importantly concentration. Since I have been doing Pilates, my golf game has improved to the point where I frequently finish in the top ten or win tournaments.[13]

Summary

There are many Pilates exercises that enhance lower limb strength superimposed on a stable core; this could help to prevent the upper limb overuse injuries. Injuries are not uncommon among the world's best golfers, and many are plagued by chronic injuries, particularly in the latter years of their careers. Greg Norman and Jack Nicklaus have chronic hip injuries. Back injuries to players such as Fred Couples and Davis Love III have been well documented. Younger players such as Tiger Woods have had devastating knee injuries.

The more mature golfing population is particularly susceptible to neck, back, hip, and shoulder injuries. Golfers often tell me that they know exactly what the golf pro wants them to do as far as the golf mechanics are concerned, but either they lack the range of motion (poor trunk or neck rotation) or they feel pain when they attempt to correct their swing, and this ultimately results in playing badly. On assessing these players, they often have one of the following: limitation of joint range of motion, either due to stiffness or pain; muscle imbalances which also cause limitation of movement and pain; lack of stability, which causes either overuse or substitution movements to compensate for this lack of control issue.

The golfer has to be thoroughly assessed and all the underlying limitations need to be addressed. This is the easy part. The difficult part is to be able to prevent reinjury and to get the player back on the course playing regularly. Pilates enables golfers to maintain their flexibility, balance, and strength as a means to prevent injuries, as well as to improve the quality of their game. A. A. Milne writes, "Golf is so popular simply because it is the best game in the world at which to be bad."[14] But it's so much better if you are pain-free, so stay fit using Pilates principles. And watch your golf game improve!

About Natasha

On completing her schooling as an all-rounder and head prefect achieving honours with distinctions in her finals, Natasha was presented with a world of opportunity. Her innate physical intelligence, however, housed her true passion; and naturally she continued her life of dance, acquiring many a noteworthy accolade. Through her travels internationally as a ballet dancer, she was exposed to the Pilates method, training with Romana Kryzanowska. Today, a pioneer of both Pilates and Gyrotonic® in South Africa, Natasha still values a simple approach to the pleasures of health and physical well-being. In her leisure time, she enjoys running.

REFERENCES

[1] B. Brandon and PZ Pearce, "Training to Prevent Golf Injury,"
Current Sports Medicine Reports (May-June 2009); 8(3): 142.

[2] Joseph Pilates, *Your Health.* (Incline Village, NV: Presentation Dynamics, Inc., 1998), 135.

[3] Joseph Pilates, *Return to Life Through Contrology.* (Incline Village: Presentation Dynamics, Inc., 1998), 14.

[4] Gary Player, http://www.1-famous-quotes.com/quote/1300471.

[5] Joseph Pilates & William John Miller, *Your Health: A Corrective System of Exercising that Revolutionizes the Entire Field of Physical Education.* Originally published in 1934. Current edition, Philadelphia, PA: Bainbridge Books, 2000, p. 44, in *The Complete Writings of Joseph H. Pilates*, editors Sean Gallagher and Romana Kryzanowska.

[6] Joseph Pilates & William John Miller, *Return to Life Through Contrology.* Originally published in 1945. Current edition, Philadelphia, PA: Bainbridge Books, 2000, p. 58, in *The Complete Writings of Joseph H. Pilates*, editors Sean Gallagher and Romana Kryzanowska.

[7] David Rassmusen, Gyrotonic® Application for Golf manual, September 2005, 11-12.

[8] Deanna E. Zenger, "Pilates,"*Golf Fitness Magazine*, September/October 2008, 28.

[9] Annika Sörenstam, *Golf Annika's Way.* (Penguin Group, 2004), 247.

[10] Lorie Parch, "Fit for Golf,"*Resort Living*, 33-34.

[11] Ernie Els and David Herman. *Guide to Golf Fitness.* (Random House, Inc., 2000), 8.

[12] Martin Park, interview with Martin Park, 13 July 2011.
http://www.pgatour.com/2011/r/07/13/schwartzel-transcript/index.html

[13] Sandra von den Berg, personal interview, 18 April 2011.

[14] A.A. Milne, "The Charm of Golf," 1920. *Quotidiana*, Ed. Patrick Madden. (19 Jan 2007), http://essays.quotidiana.org/milne/charm_of_golf/.

Pilates Technique and Body Awareness

By Junghee Won

Pilates reformed the quality of life through balance of mental and physical exercise...

There are many ways to understand the Pilates technique. We can learn it through practicing, watching, teaching, and taking lessons and workshops just like other movement techniques. We can add more knowledge from body function in anatomy and kinesiology, as well. How about emotion and imagination? I think these elements can be very useful in diving deeper into the work and further exploring the Pilates technique. When I visited Kathy Grant, a student of Joseph Pilates, in her studio at New York University, a picture of a cat in a stretching pose was on the wall. I understand that she often used this image to deepen the understanding of movement. It is more than just a change in place or position. Think about movement with timing, effort, and direction. For example, there are many ways to lift arms. Are you going to lift arms firmly with muscular action or with less effort? Are you lifting your arms slowly or quickly? Are you lifting your arms to the side or forward? Do you like to lift your arms with an arc line or directly up? Do you use imagination and emotion as well for the action?

My approach will focus more on Pilates as movement, as a system larger than the sum of its technical aspects, muscle action, and prescribed technique. Pilates technique requires quality of movement. Pilates is an exercise, and it is joyful movement. Why do we love Pilates? Because it is a unique, fun method that gives us a strong, healthy, beautiful body. Pilates is more than just simple exercise.

Experiencing body awareness helps us to understand the technique and absorb work into our bodies. For example, dancers train and develop their bodies for many years resulting in heightened body awareness. Conversely, a body without years of movement study may have a disconnect between body and mind. For these people, can awareness be developed and well-integrated into their lives? Absolutely. Through time and diligent practice of Pilates, anyone can improve body awareness. Even though I was a trained dancer, Pilates enhanced my body awareness. Without the connection of body and mind, understanding movement is difficult, and you cannot reap the full benefits of the Pilates technique.

Laban Movement Analysis (LMA) is a wonderful tool to better understand movement, and it will also help to improve Pilates technique. The scope of this essay cannot focus on the study of Laban in its entirety, but there are elements that can enhance the way you explain and observe movement as an instructor, as well as enable you to become a more skilled practitioner.

My early formal training includes Ballet, Modern, and Korean traditional dance. I came to the United States from Seoul, Korea, in 1992 to further my education and major in Dance and Dance Education at New York University. I chose this program because I wasn't sure if I wanted to be a dancer/choreographer or if I wanted to do something else related to dance. During my first semester, I enrolled in a "Dance Alignment" course, which was Pilates. This was followed by an "Effort Shape" course in LMA. During this course, I learned how to pay attention to every aspect of a movement. This class helped me develop an eye for examining movement with regard to direction, timing (quick and slow), quality, and effort: all the components of a movement. I even learned to read and sense the movements inherent within still photographs from magazines and museum drawings. I did not need to rely solely on watching people's movement in the park or seeing a dance concert in the theater. At the time, this was a fun new discovery and exciting for me, as it deepened my understanding of Pilates' work.

I fell in love with Pilates when I first saw the Cadillac, one of the many pieces of wonderful Pilates apparatus. Everyone has a different story about how they first encountered the Pilates method. My first experience with that love was just about the Cadillac. I think I liked the cube shape, which is essentially an open space. I could imagine so many movements within the frame of the Cadillac. I wanted to move in that cube. I was also inspired by watching older people with gray hair at True Pilates studio in New York (formerly Drago's Gymnasium), where Romana Kryzanowska, who was also one of Joseph

Pilates' students, was working. I was very surprised to see the older people move so well. I was determined to learn this technique.

Over the 10 years I have been a certified Pilates teacher, practicing my own workouts, I have regularly taken lessons every week and workshops with many wonderful teachers. Fortunately, I lived in Manhattan when Romana was in the studio every day. That was a huge influence on my practice as well as my teaching skills. She often spoke about timing, quality of movement, and bringing expression into the movement to perform better. I always thought about what I learned from my "Effort Shape" class at N.Y.U. It really is the same, just without the terms of LMA. I discovered later that Joseph Pilates and Laban worked together when they returned to Germany at some point after World War I.

Rodolf Laban was born in 1879 in Bratislava when it was part of the Austro-Hungarian Empire. His father worked as a field-marshal and military governor of Bosnia and Herzegovina. As a young boy, Laban travelled abroad with his father where he witnessed first-hand the folk dances of Yugoslavia, Turkey, and Germany, and the ballroom dances of Vienna.

Laban, a philosopher, scientist, mathematician, and theoretician, was also a celebrated artist, architect, dancer, choreographer, and dance designer of colossal vision. Like all good teachers, he never stopped learning. Among his already numerous skills, he was also a crystallographer, topologist, pianist and composer.

Joseph Pilates and Rudolf Laban both had an unwavering passion for the work they did. Laban believed that everyone should dance. His energy and magnetism were boundless, although he often struggled financially. As a result of the family's suffering, his wife left. These hard times eventually left him in poor health.

Laban very much enjoyed working with amateur or "ordinary" people. There were a lot of choir performances in Germany and other countries at that time. Laban organized performances of amateur dancers and movers using professionals to lead them. He continually sought ways to free dance from the restrictions of music, believing that the natural rhythms of the body were more inherent than metric rhythms. Laban wrote books and published many articles. And he also worked tirelessly on his great project, dance notation.

Laban was very good at creating grand effects with large numbers of people. One of his major achievements was a vast procession in Vienna, involving 20,000 participants. Like many others, Laban was not happy about having his work controlled by the Nazi regime.

Laban later had to flee the country and eventually arrived in Paris. He was then brought to England by Kurt Jooss and Lisa Ullmann. With the help of the Joose Ballet company owners, Leonard and Dorothy Elmhirst, Laban was finally free to do his work. Lisa Ullmann was a student of Laban and was able to smuggle some of Laban's papers out of Germany. Together they worked teaching physical educationalists and dance teachers. Little by little his work was beginning to be accepted. Soon Laban's views on movement analysis (and the fact that he could notate any movement of the human body) would prove invaluable and help revolutionize future work in the fields of industry and agriculture.

Laban died in 1958. Many people are influenced by his work without even realizing it. His philosophy was based on the belief that the human body and mind are one.[1]

There are four efforts in Laban Movement Analysis: flow, weight, time, and space. Flow describes movement which is unimpeded and continuous. Emotion plays an important part in all movement expression, and through its inward and outward streaming; it establishes relationships and communication.

In Pilates each exercise has its own flow. The repeating arm movement up and down in the Hundred is flow motion with a metric rhythm. Roll Up on the Mat is also flow motion through the articulation of the spine. All Pilates exercises have flow. Breathing in a particular exercise has flow, too, as in the Saw.

Flow also serves as one of the Pilates principles. Pilates is technique in motion, movement with placement; it should not focus upon overanalyzing or overindulging body position. Motion with flow involves using your mind with control; Romana Kryzanowska says, "You can say what Pilates is in three words: stretch with strength and control, and the control part is the most important because it makes you use your mind."

Weight by definition is "the force of gravity acting on a body."[2] Laban observed that some people indulge in gravity and others tend to resist it. Where do you put most of your weight in Hands Back in Stomach Massage Series on the Reformer? Your hips are fighting gravity to sit up tall, and your hands on the shoulder blocks add support to enable you to sit up even taller. Your main weight is on the hips, and the secondary weight is on the arms. I mention this because you often see people putting weight more on the arms than the hips.

The Reformer's springs are also a gravitational force. In Footwork, Toes, the force of the springs is on the toes. But the force of gravity is actually on the back. So you have to think about two forces on the Reformer. In each exercise you need to think about what the main force of gravity is. For example, in Front Split on the Reformer, part III (kneeling), the front toes are working against the forces of real gravity as well as the force of the spring tension. The back knee, therefore, does not have too much pressure on it from either force, actual gravity or spring tension.

Think about our body kinesphere. We can stretch our arms, legs, and even fingers all the way out, reaching as far as we can, moving with a big, spread-out motion. We can use all our joints to curl up into a small ball, too. We can stand up straight and move, or we can kneel down and move. We can walk forward and backward. We can move side to side. Think about where you want to move. Reach up diagonally, or reach down diagonally. You can section the space into a high level, a middle level, and a low level. Use space clearly when you work out. Be aware of which direction you move in space. Where is the starting point of the movement? Be clear. On the Reformer, the carriage is always moving; therefore, your kinesphere is also moving, resulting in better balance.

Laban tells us that rhythm is the lawless law which governs us all without exception. It is always around us and within us and reveals itself everywhere, but only a few are familiar with it.[3]

Time can be simply divided into quick and slow (Laban uses the term sustain). When we practice Running on the Reformer, is it quick or slow? Think about following your heartbeat. It makes sense to do the exercise Running in time with Laban's idea. Knees Off in the Knee Series has a very intense up-tempo, which makes your heartbeat increase. The next exercise, Running, should still be up-tempo until your heartbeat slows down. Remember one of the purposes of Running is to cool down. Like a runner crossing the finish line, you slow down gradually.

Think about Down Stretch in the Long Stretch Series. The breath is a crucial aspect of this exercise. Romana says, "Empty the lungs." The action of emptying the lungs takes extra effort to do completely. It has to be slow and sustained. This is also true in the Saw on the Mat, when you are wringing out the lungs.

There are another two components in time, regular (metric) and irregular (free) rhythm. More expressive or dynamic interpretation makes free rhythm. Think about the intention of each Pilates exercise and how you can apply the appropriate rhythm. Rolling down and articulating through the spine must take time, which is free rhythm as in Short Spine Massage on the Reformer. However, Footwork on the Reformer must be with regular rhythm. Breathing and stretching-related exercises need more time, like yawning.

Even with the right technique, if you do not have body awareness, you cannot apply these elements. That's why learning technique requires repeated practice. Repeatedly studying brings about gradual awareness and can even create subconscious muscle memories. When a pianist gets a new music score, he has to practice for the concert by reading, and the fingers memorize the score. The pianist doesn't need the music score for the concert.

I have been teaching Pilates for over ten years and have had clients of many different body types. Some are very easy to teach, and some are very hard to teach. As a former dancer and dance teacher, I was familiar with dancers but found it challenging to teach non-dancers, or the average person. Some people are coordinated with movement while others do not understand how to curl the tail bone under, or are unable to stretch the arms up without lifting the shoulders. I came to realize that it is not only a limitation of the body, but also a lack of body awareness. I was surprised that one could have such limited body awareness. I don't mean to sound insensitive, but at the time this was very foreign to me, yet interesting that these individuals still enjoyed doing Pilates. Somehow Pilates really worked for them, they liked it, they felt good after the sessions, and it helped them with the issues they have in their bodies. I felt good about their appreciation of Pilates despite my struggles to teach them. I started to pay more attention to how to teach these people and learned effective methods and better explanations to guide them to move better and make them understand technique with their bodies and minds.

After a few years teaching and practicing Pilates in New York City, I went back to Seoul, Korea, in 2002 to attend Kyunghee University's Ph.D. program. I opened the very first Pilates studio in Seoul, Korea, and also founded their first Pilates Teacher Training Program. Being surrounded by members of the dance community gave me an idea for my research. Dancers have amazing body awareness. They use their bodies more than anyone else in a variety of ways: jumping, balancing, turning, lifting, and holding a still position. Integrated into this strength and flexibility is the emotion required for performance. Can these wonderful dancers acquire even greater body awareness by doing Pilates? The answer is a resounding yes, they can. Moreover, I wanted to quantifiably prove that Pilates can foster body awareness, can strengthen the connection between mind and body, and can facilitate coordination of movement. I wanted to prove this through scientific research.

My Ph.D. dissertation provided research that became a precedent for studies in Pilates. It was published in 2005, when much of what was available was redundant and/or specific to functional physiology. This dearth of research gave me a chance to embark on an original study for my dissertation, which contains not only the experimental stage and results, but also Joseph Pilates' history and principles, Pilates apparatus history, genealogy, Pilates trademark history and techniques.

My research study is titled, "The Effect of Pilates Method on Dancers' Cognitive Style and Body Awareness." The main purpose of my study was not only to examine the effects of the Pilates method on dancers' cognitive style and body awareness when the Pilates exercise program is applied to them, but also to describe the relationship between cognitive style and body awareness. This research was conducted through ideal case selection, using eight selected dancers (two male and six female dancers), and conformed to the selection of qualitative research. The Pilates exercise program was structured into twelve sessions (two times per week and 55 minutes per session) with beginner and intermediate level systems of Power Pilates. All data was collected through three in-depth oral interviews, twelve sessions of participant observation, and twelve instances of self-journaling. The collective material employed domain analysis and taxonomical analysis. Because qualitative research is based on researcher's subjectivity and prejudiced opinion, the reliability and validity of the research results were confirmed with triangular inspection and the investigation of community and specialist meetings.

In accordance with the results of this qualitative research on the collected materials and the effects of participating in the study, Pilates exercise offers the experience of cognition, the transformation of cognitive problems, and developing an understanding of the stages of the body, such as, cognition of muscle function, correction of posture, weight loss, improved concentration, confidence, flexibility, relief of lower back pain, stress relief, and improved health of the inner body which cannot be realized easily in normal life. These experiences have a variety of effects in normal life, such as at school and at work.

The essential content resulting from this research included (1) dancers' cognitive style; (2) transformation of action through body awareness; (3) the relationship between Pilates exercise and cognitive style and body awareness. Three types of results yielded through this research suggest that:

Pilates exercise produces a response that changes the participant's perception of his inner body and field-independent cognitive styles, as well as perception through self-experience rather than field-dependent cognitive style concerning the problem of movement action.

Pilates exercises improve body awareness through an inner coordinative perception style about the body and the process of change within the inner body. The improvement of body awareness contributes to understanding the body in areas such as muscle function cognition, corrected posture, weight loss, improved confidence, flexibility, relief of lower back pain, stress relief and health improvement.

Pilates exercise has an advantage over cognitive style which makes analytical and objective decisions on the inner body. These cognitive styles may promote a closed relationship to inner body awareness, whereas Pilates requires a psychophysiological process integration and facilitates the process of inner body awareness.

The result of this research supports the philosophical beliefs of Joseph Pilates on health. Pilates reformed the quality of life through balance of mental and physical exercise, and his method has been established for over 100 years. Considering the deficiency of prior research on the Pilates exercises, practical research activity, and quantitative research and the development of training methods, it is then necessary to establish a theoretical system that offers proof of the relationship between Pilates exercises and mental health.

About Junghee

In 1999, Junghee received her certification from Pilates, Inc., under the tutelage of Romana Kryzanowska. She has also studied with Sari Mejia-Santo, Bob Liekens, Ton Voogt and Stephanie Beatty. Junghee is also certified by the Pilates Method Alliance and Power Pilates, for whom she is a teacher trainer. She holds a M.A. in Dance and Dance Education from N.Y.U. and Kyunghee University, where she received her Ph.D. in 2005. Her dissertation explores "The Effect of The Pilates Method on Dancers' Cognitive Style and Body Awareness." Currently, she is a teacher trainer for the United States Pilates Association and she teaches Pilates at CAN DO Fitness/Edgewater.

REFERENCES

[1]Hearn Newlove and John Dalby, *Laban for All* (London, England: Nick Hern Books, 2004), 11-16.
[2]*Webster's New World Dictionary* (Riverside, NJ: Simon & Schuster, 2003), 671.
[3]Hearn Newlove and John Dalby, 127.

Chapter V

Pilates and Academia

Preserving Classical Pilates

By Marianne Adams and Rebecca Quin

*...five principles that we believe to be
common and imperative...*

Since the loss of the trademark almost a decade ago, it seems time
to call for a unified organization in the field for the continuing body
of practitioners who have stayed with the lineage that came to them
from Joseph and Clara Pilates through Romana Kryzanowska. We
have faced many challenges since the disbandment of the guild; the
splintering of philosophies and practices has led the way for the development of a variety of commercial teacher training programs. In addition, public misconceptions over the trademark battle and misuse of
the terms "Classical, Authentic, or Traditional Pilates" have muddied
the field. We hope that the commonalities that we share with lineage
through Romana are greater than our differences.

Could we, the classical, traditional, and authentic Pilates teachers
start a Guild again? A strong alliance organization, with skilled and
experienced teachers, to meet and share regularly for continuing education, develop applicable standards for the field, including the final
training of apprentices? Of course, we realize this may be an idealized
dream, as Romana Kryzanowska's teaching was the heartbeat of the
Guild for most of us, and that font of passion, knowledge of tradition
and exuberance does not exist as it did in the past.

Now, there are slight differences in the exercise system that was
created over 80 years ago, and there are a wide variety of programs
claiming to be classical. However, the legacy is strong and as evidenced, the passion and interest in The Method continues to flourish
25 years after Joseph Pilates' death. We would like to propose a possible philosophical framework that could begin to deepen the dialogue
and strengthen the alliance and an adherence to a classical, traditional,
and authentic lineage.

Of course, those of us who had lengthy study with Romana saw many variations and perhaps even witnessed some Romana-isms. And so, we must ask ourselves the difficult question: when and where should the line be drawn to say The Method itself has been corrupted? And who is to be the rightful judge? Can there be a rightful judge years after Joseph Pilates' death? More importantly, what are the philosophical principles that we can still agree on and adhere to? What is really central to our core practices and theories?

Here are five principles that we believe to be common and imperative to an authentic, classical, and traditional approach to Pilates:

- The Pilates system is whole, indivisible, and unblended.
- The Pilates method works with the whole person.
- The oral tradition of teaching Pilates is imperative.
- In Pilates, the client must be kept moving.
- Pilates teachers must always see the person before them.

I. The Pilates system is whole, indivisible and unblended

Of course this assertion is sticky as many training programs today currently offer piecemeal approaches. However, there are fundamental losses to those who study The Method in this way; the divided parts rarely add up to the rich, interconnected whole. There are too many teachers from piecemeal programs who never invest the time or money that it takes to be a comprehensively trained and certified teacher. So they advertise as a "classically" trained Pilates teacher, and know only the Mat I, or the Reformer I or II. However, anyone who does not know and work on all the apparatus really cannot have an overall concept of the interwoven nature of the entire Method. And most likely, a divided approach will entirely miss smaller components such as the Foot Corrector, the abdominal series on the Wunda chair, the Beanbags, and the Magic Square.

As an example of the important principle of interconnectedness, let's look at the Teaser. It is one of the most recognizable exercises in The Method, and it is often quoted as a nemesis for those struggling to master it. Most all varieties of Pilates classes or lessons have a version of the Teaser. But to understand why the Teaser is such a hallmark of The Method, let's look at a partial list of how the Teaser is woven within four apparatuses and the Mat, from basic to super advanced. This example is given to illustrate a perspective that would be difficult to really understand from a piecemeal program.

Here is a possible sequential order in which the Teaser exercises could be woven into lessons ranging from basic to super advanced:

- Wunda Chair: Press Down Teaser and Teaser Stretch
- Cadillac: Teaser (preparation, shoulder stretch and upper body rollup)
- Spine Corrector: Teaser I, on the step, facing the Barrel
- Mat: Teaser I, with instructor assistance, (Romana would also have us work with the Swedish Bars)
- Reformer: Teaser on the Long Box, seated, without straps, adding legs straightening and straps
- Spine Corrector: Teaser II & III on the step, torso facing away from the Barrel
- Wunda Chair: Reverse Swan/Teaser I & II
- Mat: Teaser I, adding II & IIII
- Reformer: Teaser from layout position, add arm circles, forward and back
- Spine Corrector: (Instructor Assisted) Teaser Stretch
- Cadillac: Teaser, adding Teaser II & III
- Reformer: Teaser, from layout position, arm circles forward and back, add Shaving
- Guillotine: Teaser I-III
- Mat: Teaser into rocking Swan, repeatedly, then reverse directions

Within the classical Method, this exercise is introduced and worked on in many, many levels and on a wide variety of apparatus. Although one would vary the sequence of this list for a particular individual, this is a general interrelated list that would be studied and its logical development understood. Within the general progression of the exercises, there exists a basic framework or map guiding how to work on, and truly benefit from the Teaser exercises.

While the Teaser works on building strength in core flexion and homologous coordination, the Swan is another exercise that recurs frequently throughout the system, building on the core strength, increasing back extension and adding spinal flexibility in a similarly methodical way, as evidenced by this progressive list using five different apparatuses and the Mat:

- Mat: Neck Roll for Swan Preparation
- Ladder Barrel: Modified Swan/Swan
- Wunda Chair: Flying Eagle
- Cadillac: Half Swan
- Ladder Barrel: Backward Hang, since this exercise simply changes the plane of the backward extension and uses the pull of gravity for increased stretch of the back, the case could be made for including it in this list as well
- Mat: Rocking Swan
- Cadillac: Full Swan
- Wunda Chair: Swan/Swan Dive
- Cadillac: Flying Eagle could be included, which adds the challenge of three dimensional arm circles and rotator cuff ROM or shoulder rotation, to add more strength and stretch to the upper body and arms
- Spine Corrector: Swan, which adds more precise balance challenges
- Reformer: Swan on the Long Box
- Mat: Rocking Swan into Teaser
- Reformer: Breaststroke could be included as well, based on a similar rationale as used for the Cadillac Flying Eagle

Of course, similar progressions could be studied and explored to develop and understand lateral flexion, side bends, spinal rotations, twists, or to focus on the development of the upper body, lower body or contralateral strength, flexibility and awareness. A comprehensive training approach offers the apprentice the possibility of understanding the interrelatedness of The Method on this level, effectively demonstrating that changing the apparatus can add challenge or offer help. Other concepts that are explored in depth are the benefits of working in a variety of planes—sitting, lying, or standing. Several other conceptual advantages arise from changing conditions such as adding straps/springs, working on a spatially restricted surface, or the introduction of working on a moving apparatus. Revisiting related but different exercises all test and deepen the overall understanding of The Method and the purpose behind each exercise.

The cross-pollination between levels that happens when a person studies the whole system comprehensively is never accessible if someone only studies the Reformer, or the Mat, or if the person has had exposure only to the basic or intermediate material. Not to understand the Pilates method as a deeply related and indivisible whole is to miss much of what the trademark wars were fought over.

It is part of the genius of Joseph Pilates that there are many such exercises that are cousins. In the hands of a skillful teacher, these related exercises have great capacity to offer endlessly diverse, sequentially challenging lessons to help clients truly progress. For this reason, the exercises that are taught are not "Pilates-based"; they are simply chosen from the vast array of Pilates exercises that Joseph Pilates developed and taught on apparatus made in the tradition of Joseph Pilates.

Most practitioners who try to combine Pilates with other methods, like Yoga, Alexander Technique, swimming, don't do the Pilates method justice; we don't know of a classical teacher who teaches the Pilates method from a blended approach. We know many teachers (including ourselves), who cross-train and teach in different body ways since many body practices are complementary to one another; however, true depth of understanding and mastery is needed in each, and most who blend within lessons, don't have enough depth to draw on.

II. The Pilates method works with the whole person

How do you work the whole person? Romana Kryzanowska said over and over, "Start with the core and work outward to the limbs," not bogging down in anatomical language or lengthy focus on a particular area of injury or weakness. This is not to suggest that traditional teachers do not take a careful history and assess thoroughly which exercises are to be given and which might be initially omitted until further observation and strength are built. It does imply that practitioners can find ways of working thoroughly, systematically, and methodically with the whole body since they have a full array of exercises in which they are completely versed.

The language used is simple, directive, and brief. Over time, anatomical knowledge is imparted and feedback is given in increasing levels of sophistication. However, at the onset it is important to spend time making a relationship in an active way—moving.

A repeated criticism that we have heard of the "classical" method is that it is too strict and rigid, without leeway to modify when needed for injury or rehabilitation. This statement signifies a lack of understanding of the whole interwoven system of the Pilates method. Most of the modifications needed are in the range of apparatus that Pilates so brilliantly devised. While one apparatus adds challenge, another apparatus or variation gives a beginner or rehab client a needed simplification.

It is inherent in the classical method to start with the whole body/ whole person, and not fixate on the broken parts. If we start with strengthening the core, and then systematically move outward to the limbs of the body, many of the presenting problems, such as "bad back, bum knee, bad shoulder, and sciatica," often begin to disappear. New skills, thinking patterns, and physical behaviors arise to replace the limited self-image of the client, instead of merely being a person who is "injured."

It is in this aspect that the classical approach is strength-based, both physically and mentally. The client is taught as a whole person, building on strengths, and gradually rebuilding more effective patterns of movement.

This is not unrelated to new paradigms of thinking in the fields of Positive Psychology and Expressive Arts, both of which recognize the idea of "life coaching." As Pilates instructors, we have used the term "PMA" or positive mental attitude thousands of times to encourage clients to develop a positive mental attitude to recognize small steps toward fitness or their progress in healing. When the whole person is encouraged toward health, injuries and/or limitations are pieces of the whole, but they are not the whole focus.

Central to this principle is that even a beginner, or a client with limited mobility, works through a whole body progression. Whatever the level or focus of the day's lesson may be, it is important to complete a sequential progression on an apparatus in order to ensure that the whole body is addressed. Thus the client learns that he can move beyond his limitations, via a guided comprehensive progression, safely and with limited repetitions.

This way the complete body is engaged and the mind stimulated, not getting bogged down on one specific area or limitation.

III. The oral tradition of teaching Pilates is imperative

Our teacher's voices, both good and bad, ring in our ears. We call on them when we are tired, unimaginative, or uninspired. We also call on them when we are feeling energetic, imaginative or inspired. The passion of our teachers lives within our hearts, our brains, and resonates within our bodies. When we hear our teachers say, "I don't know, but I can find out," we know that we can be life-long learners. Often, when we first witness our teachers make a mistake, we wish we hadn't recognized it; we want to keep them on a pedestal. Later, we realize that they are human, and we begin to know that all teachers make mistakes and they can still be good teachers. The oral tradition is shortened in many programs, as it is labor intensive and, therefore, not cost-effective in the short term. Of course, the long-term benefits of the oral tradition are enormous—the wisdom from master teachers, the studio lessons, the time observing, the Q&A times, the workouts, and the endless hours teaching; those memories remain etched and embodied within us, while book study fades.

Part of the oral tradition is getting to know someone as a mentor or as a student for an extended period of study. Quality programs offer both close supervision for rapid apprentice progress and extended experiences for apprentices to gain perspective on both their teaching and learning skills relative to others. If apprentices have been given carefully crafted lessons constructed for systematic progress, most apprentices begin to intuitively know how to start a client through a progression that makes sense; however, verbalizing what they know, and taking authority as a teacher for the first few times can be daunting.

When young teachers first begin giving verbal cues and feedback to their clients, they are most likely parroting what they have heard, over and over. Although a student might start by mimicking their teachers' familiar phrases, within the first 10 lessons that the apprentice teaches, a client will say in response to the phrase that has made sense, or worked for the apprentice, "What do you mean?" or "That doesn't make sense to me. I thought you were referring to xyz." In this way, each client teaches us how to attend, fine-tune, cue, or give feedback a little differently. Each client helps us to find a new image, explore another layer of explanation, or find a new dimension to the exercise. Teaching and learning are a powerful and interconnected loop of feedback, not unlike a Möbius strip.

Very quickly, the apprentice learns the need for judicious and sincere praise. Our clients need to be able to trust the timing, timbre, and focus of our praise. Without an extended teacher training which provides a mindful and consistent eye toward the details of what could be improved, the young teacher might tend toward inauthentic praise. Finding the courage and willingness to correct for deeper understanding of the exercises helps the client to listen to their own internal cues, and to trust the accuracy of the teacher's observations.

In any teaching situation, but particularly in the 1:1 setting, we are making a relationship. And it is imperative that our instructions are professional, to the point, knowledgeable, positive and honest. And that comes from an oral tradition of teachers teaching teachers, passing down knowledge both physically and verbally, not via YouTube, the Internet, or by correspondence courses.

IV. In Pilates, the client must keep moving

Romana often said, "Don't stand there and talk about it, get the client moving. Explain as you go." The real work of teaching is not giving out exercises, but in seeing how quickly you can aid your clients in becoming more efficient, balanced, and at ease in their daily movements. If after teaching the nuts and bolts of a particular exercise to beginners, it feels like you are in a rut, then you probably are. If you find you are giving the same cues over and over without seeing progress, you are most likely bored with your own teaching, and the client most certainly is. If what you are saying becomes scripted, the client will sense that you are not fully present or working with their unique physique and psyche. How do you begin to help each client to glimpse his or her own movement potential? And how do you assist each client in becoming a more confident mover?

We all respond well to undivided attention. And focused attention is really a rare treat in today's multitasking world. A good teacher is always striving to multitask on teaching. For example, a teacher's eyes must not just see flaws but also see how to keep the client moving while asking if they can focus on "xyz." At times, a teacher may need to redirect a client's expressed insecurities or doubts into positive actions toward fitness. Other times, a teacher may need to coach or direct the client: for example, "Can you twist while finding space in the waist, finding length between your pelvis and the ribs?" At other times, a teacher may need to find an internal focus or intention (for themselves) when they are feeling fatigued or distracted by problems outside the studio. In these times, we find it most helpful to embody the actions that we are asking of a client, at least partially indicating in our bodies how to pull up, reach, twist, bend sideways, etc. A teacher's full presence can greatly affect the client's willingness to give 110%.

As we practice the teacher-client relationship, the client begins to recognize the positive benefits of regular lessons. Feeling the aeration of the lungs, the pliability that gradually returns in our muscles and our spines, the endorphin high that comes from exercise, and the relaxation that comes from gentle fatigue, are all ways that we return to our senses. Naturally, we remember our human urge to move and our wish to move with agility and with full range of motion.

And so, as teachers and as models for our clients, we must remember to move daily. It is our committed daily practice that keeps our teaching fresh and refuels our passion for The Method. Daily practice is important to stress early on with clients by giving the Mat work and assigning it as homework in between lessons. It will also serve to reinforce for the client the principles that underpin the Pilates method and help them to be assimilated into their other daily life practices.

Also, no matter how jam-packed our days become, as teachers, it is imperative that we continue our own daily practice of Pilates. This is a discovery time, a time to understand ever more deeply, a time to be in our senses, a time to feel ourselves alive with the joy of movement! The Method requires trust, the tortoise mentality (faith in the long haul), patience and perseverance. And those reasons are precisely why so many individuals enjoy Pilates as a life-long fitness practice; it is both mentally exciting and physically adaptable.

V. Pilates teachers must always see the person before them

A prerequisite to seeing the person before you is to know the content material so deeply that there is no anxiety about "what to teach." What to teach is right there before you—it presents clearly within the client's body. A good teacher always sees the individual who is before them and is constantly probing for ways to better benefit their learning: what step can the client take next? What information can the client grasp at this moment?

What pattern, habit, or sensation can the client realize that would facilitate his progress at this point? What is the next step towards efficiency? Could the client benefit from more mindfulness, PMA, or a clearer sense of habitual patterns? What is their next step in terms of physical mastery? As a teacher, paying close attention is what encourages the client to pay attention to the information that his or her own body is presenting. Concentrating on the client's particular needs also helps to teach the client to concentrate.

This is a skill that comes with practice, and some teachers are better at it than others. As a teacher's confidence grows from practice, young teachers can really start to trust their own intuition. What sequential pattern would the client benefit from, which new exercises could be introduced? Or, perhaps the question becomes how to clean up and deepen the exercises that the client already knows. Or how to positively and sincerely reinforce progress; there are infinite directions that could be explored. Many classically trained teachers will use their intuition and imagination within the development of the lesson, however they do not need to be creative in making up new exercises if they have studied the classical repertory thoroughly; the roadmap for variations and modifications already exists. Part of seeing the person before you is meeting the human nature that is before you.

When a new teacher repeatedly gets stuck at the same point with clients, saying, "They aren't listening to me," or "I don't know how many more ways to say use your deep abdominals," they are missing many ways of truly seeing the individual before them. When the teacher can begin to read the smaller cues, such as paying attention to eye contact, breath inconsistencies, patterns of holding tension, and relate their observations, a dialogue of engagement is invited. Although the content of the lesson is physical, sometimes there is an emotional limitation that is holding someone back; sometimes a client simply needs recognition and acknowledgement of their efforts. At other times, the client may need encouragement to accept the fact that there are natural plateaus in any fitness regime.

Sometimes what the teacher is ready for the client to do and what the client is ready or willing to do are two different things. What worked beautifully for the last five clients may not be the path for this client. And that is where the relationship that you establish with your clients is of primary importance. Sometimes the biggest learning in the lesson is about give and take, how to "dance" with this partner, or about how to listen more deeply to your client's needs. The most successful teacher-client relationships are built on listening carefully to one another and trusting that there is not just one path for unique, individual progress.

VI. Developing a new training model

When the Pilates Guild disbanded in 2001, we faced many questions from our students interested in further training and comprehensive certification programs. In turn, we realized we had many questions about the direction of the field. The umbrella organizations that have arisen, such as the Pilates Method Alliance, have not seemed equally representative of "East Coast" models or unbiased in their theoretical viewpoints. Other large training programs have begun offering piecemeal certifications or buy-ins to previously certified classical instructors. These types of approaches led us to shy away from alliances and the politics of the field and to dream of starting a new teacher-training model based in academia. In light of the values stated above, we developed our program with the support of the university in 2005. Appalachian is a mid-sized, state university in the rural, Blue Ridge Mountains of North Carolina. When the Pilates trademark was lost, there was a vacuum of training opportunities for those seeking classical, comprehensive teacher training programs in a remote area.

We have structured our program requirements to ensure at least a year of study in the Pilates method before apprentices are able to apply to the spring/summer intensive training. We have found that this approach allows time for the apprentices to begin to integrate the immense amount of physical and mental material before they make the transition to working with clients. Our goal is to offer a thorough grounding in the principles that have historically guided The Method. The University underwrites the 675-hour program by providing the facility and the fully-equipped Pilates studio. For more information about our program: www.dance.appstate.edu/pilates

Summary

In conclusion, we are interested in the alliances that could be made as we look to the future of Pilates, Pilates education and teacher training programs. We are curious and open to other's ideas about educational models, in both commercial and academic settings. We are interested in the common values that are needed to begin an alliance or guild. How can we find ways to support and trust our colleagues, network with other like-minded professionals, and preserve the grand tradition of Joseph Pilates' Method? We look forward to being in the dialogue.

Excerpts of this chapter were previously published in an earlier format and are used by the author's Permission. Adams, Marianne, and Quin, Rebecca. *The Pilates Teacher Training Manual.* (2007). The Hubbard Center, Appalachian State University, Boone, NC.

About Marianne

Romana Kryzanowska certified Marianne Adams after intensive Pilates study that began with Alycea Ungaro in 1996. Marianne co-founded The Appalachian Pilates Teacher Training Program, a comprehensive, yearlong training program in 2005. She holds an M.F.A. in Choreography and Performance from the University of North Carolina and an M.A. in Clinical Psychology from Appalachian State University. As a professor and Chairperson of the Theatre & Dance department at A.S.U., she teaches dance, bodywork and expressive arts.

She is also certified in Gyrokinesis® and Gyrotonic®. Her recent publications have been in the areas of Somatics, mindfulness, and dance education.

About Rebecca

Rebecca Quin has an extensive background in Pilates, dance, and Expressive Arts therapy. She holds a M.A. and N.C.C. in Community Counseling with an emphasis in Expressive Arts. She completed a 700-hour apprenticeship to receive certification in the Authentic Pilates Method through the Pilates Studio in N.Y.C. Quin has taught classes for the cast of *42nd Street* in New York City, Platinum Pilates, Batchelor Chiropractic, Wellspring Chiropractic, Rippling Waters Yoga Studio, Neighborhood Yoga, and Linville Ridge Country Club. She is also certified in the Gyrokinesis® method of bodywork and is an adjunct faculty at Appalachian State University.

Pilates: Its Place in Education

By Elizabeth Lowe Ahearn

...students need fitness that is fun,
effective and appropriate.

Educating Our Youth the Pilates Way

As traditional instructors of the Pilates method of body conditioning, we are dedicated to keeping The Method alive. Historically, Pilates has been passed down from teacher to pupil in Pilates studios or in gyms "grounded in a tradition of instructors communicating Joseph Pilates' values, movement qualities, technique and history to one another, and to their students."[1] These students are generally adults, rather than secondary or postsecondary pupils. However, Pilates himself wrote about the need to educate the child first and actually dedicated and titled a chapter of his book, *Your Health*, "First Educate the Child!" That section of his book discusses the benefits of learning Pilates at a young age and the importance of forming good habits.

Joseph Pilates believed that the "proper development of body and mind, through the new science of 'Contrology,' is what must be taught the child."[2] As instructors and stewards of The Method, I believe, like Joseph Pilates, we should deliver the values and principles of Pilates to our youth and educate them about the unique system of exercise that we have had the honor and privilege to learn and study. As a professor at Goucher College and an instructor of dance at Carver Center for Arts and Technology, it was only natural for me to address the needs of our dancers, as well as the needs of all of the students at each institution of learning. In 1995, when I received my Pilates teaching certification, Joseph Pilates' vision of educating youth had not come to fruition. This was partly because certified teachers had no connections to the county school systems, colleges, or universities. Yet, I was in a unique and ideal position. Already employed by two highly respected and pioneering schools, I knew first-hand the benefits of Pilates. It was my dream to share Pilates with my students, as my mentors had shared it with me, and as I knew Joseph Pilates would have wanted.

I wished for my pupils to physically and intellectually gain the benefits of the Pilates method. I also felt strongly that the study of Pilates should be included in academia. Is it not a science, based on anatomy and kinesiology, and an art that is orderly and systematic? Is it not a clearly defined and functional body of knowledge that embraces curiosity, discipline, creativity, and productivity? Is it not cross-disciplinary in nature? I needed only to convince the administration at Goucher College and the principal at Carver Center for Arts and Technology of the validity of Joseph Pilates' work and the overall benefits of a system that had yet to be introduced to the populations of either institution. The adventure I embarked upon was exciting, educational, and often wearisome, but it resulted in additions to the curriculum of each institution that left a positive and indelible mark on the students and advanced Joseph Pilates' mission and goals without disrupting or altering the traditions of his work.

The Pilates Method – The Benefits

There are countless articles and books which address the benefits of the Pilates method. According to Peter Fiasca, "Pilates addresses the wellness of the individual as a whole."[3] The ordered sequence of exercises may be modified to address a variety of physical limitations, weaknesses, imbalances, and symptoms and is, therefore, accessible to a broad range of participants—from the young to the elderly and from the agile to the impaired. Results from research by Michelle Olsen and Carrie Myers Smith in 2005 indicated "that Pilates workouts at the intermediate and advanced levels meet the requirements for promoting general fitness when performed with high enough frequency and duration."[4] Their research also concluded that Pilates Mat exercises, "if done at an intermediate to an advanced level, can provide a moderate cardio stimulus similar to that provided by some lower-impact activities like walking, but in a more interval-like way."[5] According to a study funded by the American Council on Exercise and conducted by Stefanie Spilde and John P. Porcari, Ph.D., the average caloric expenditure of two 50-minute Pilates workouts at an intermediate level is 75 calories and the average caloric expenditure for an advanced routine is 254 calories.[6] Their research confirmed the effectiveness of much of the Pilates Mat exercises on the abdominal muscles, noting that Pilates remains one of the most "challenging and effective means of building core strength and stability."[7] A study by Neil Segal, M.D., Jane

Hein, P.T., and Jeffery R. Basford, M.D., Ph.D., concluded that Pilates training resulted in improved flexibility. "Flexibility may contribute to improved physical performance, reduced energy requirements for movement of joints (because of reduced tissue tension), and reduced likelihood of soreness or injury with physical exercise,"[8] determining that the improved flexibility from Pilates is an important health benefit that deserves further study. In summary, professionals have found that the mental engagement and concentration innate to the work provide a full body workout unlike many other systems of exercise, including but not limited to increased flexibility, improved posture, prevention of injuries, improved cardiovascular conditioning and coordination, mind-body awareness, and improved strength and endurance.

Pilates and Dance – A Perfect Partnership

The combination of exercising the mind and the body while developing and improving strength, muscle and joint range of motion, posture, and coordination initially attracted a number of talented dancers to Joseph Pilates' original studio at 939 Eighth Avenue. These dancers included such "well known figures as Hanya Holm, Ted Shawn, Jerome Robbins, Rudolf von Laban, George Balanchine, Pearl Primus, Suzanne Farrell, and Martha Graham."[9] My own personal experience and subsequent analysis for my article published in *The Journal of Dance Education* had revealed that "Emphasizing correct breathing, body alignment, and pelvic stability, Pilates uses the abdominals, lower back, and gluteals as a power center, enabling the rest of the body to move freely, creating a healthy, rigorous, and symmetrical workout for all muscle groups. The result is a leaner, stronger body and a valuable core or center."[10] The outcome for dancers is improved alignment, increased muscle flexibility and strength, and more balanced development of the musculature.[11] Research by Robin L. Kish supports these outcomes, concluding, "the Pilates method improves the alignment of dancers and increases the functional flexibility of the adductors and hip flexors."[12] It should be noted that Pilates is not dance, although certainly those with a background in dance have the physical skills and "knowledge of coordination, balance, precision, stamina, and the ability to translate a teacher's verbal instructions into specific movement."[13]

Clearly, a dancer's background supports the principles of Pilates and facilitates advancement in The Method, but dancers also need Pilates to counteract the injurious effects of their performance art and to prevent injury. Lisa Marie Bernardo and Elizabeth Nagle find, "Published anecdotal evidence supports the use of Pilates in dancers sustaining injuries and requiring rehabilitation or physical therapy."[14] Recent research by Tânia Amorim, Filipa Sousa, Leandro Machado, and José Augusto Santos also suggests that Pilates training has "a positive effect on muscular strength."[15] Their 11-week study produced specific changes in "the technical skills penché and développé back,"[16] clearly illustrating the positive influence of the Pilates method on their experimental group's performance. Moreover, the dance profession's long history with Pilates has allowed it to experience and understand first-hand the benefits of Pilates. Consequently, dancers have been in the forefront of The Method's growth and popularity from its beginning. As dance transitioned to college as a major in 1926, dance faculty introduced a variety of courses into their curriculum that were considered cutting edge and innovative, educating their dancers and eventually spreading the news of The Method to the general exercise population. Teachers connected to academia had greater access to the resources and staffing needed to introduce and implement Pilates into their programs than did traditional dance studios. But how does Pilates benefit the wider population, and why should it be included in the curriculum of secondary and postsecondary schools?

Pilates in Secondary and Postsecondary Schools — Passageways for Our Youth

Secondary and postsecondary schools are considered passageways to adulthood, prime paths and time frames to develop good habits. Nationally, colleges and universities are devoted to the physical, mental, and emotional well-being of their students and student athletes. It is commonly known that exercise reduces stress, depression and anxiety, and improves self-esteem and sleep patterns. According to Kelly Slavko, Fitness and Wellness Director for T.C.U. Campus Recreation, "participating in a regular exercise program has been shown to reduce risk for cardiovascular disease and certain cancers, decrease blood pressure and resting heart rate, help a person lose weight, improve functioning of the immune system, reduce risk of having a stroke, and improve the body's ability to uptake oxygen and deliver oxygen to the working muscle."[17] For secondary and postsecondary students, these benefits are sought-after assets. Therefore, recreation and sports centers in many secondary and most postsecondary schools are now equipped with state-of-the-art equipment and trainers. They are now interested in offering a variety of classes from which students may choose, including aquatics, fitness (strength training, yoga, tai chi, Pilates), martial arts (Judo), outdoor recreation (hiking, cycling), and more. Significant financial investments have been made in facilities that provide increased opportunities to stay physically active with choices far beyond traditional team sports.

Educational institutions realize that their students need fitness that is fun, effective, and appropriate. A pilot study published in *Preventative Medicine* in 2006 followed thirty 11-year-old girls who took Pilates Mat classes 5 days a week for 1 hour per day over a 4-week period. After four weeks of participation, researchers found marked improvement in body mass index percentile and found Pilates a promising method of reducing obesity.[18] Furthermore, participants noted their personal enjoyment with the activity, which is crucial for longevity of interest. The investigators also concluded that "Pilates Mat classes can play a valuable role in improving the health and fitness of young girls."[19] Since mats were the only equipment used in the study, the introduction of Mat work was cost effective as well, which is an important factor when requesting funding and support for the introduction of Pilates into a program's curriculum.

Due to demand, and supported by research, Pilates is now being included in the course offerings of both dance departments and physical education programs of secondary and postsecondary schools. Secondary schools like McLean High School in Virginia, Trinity High School in Illinois, and Falmouth High School in Maine have jumped on board. Additionally, many dance companies and dance schools, such as Ballet British Columbia and The National Ballet School, have introduced their dancers to the Pilates method.[20] Danielle Bullen notes, "In a survey of 1,477 American College of Sports Medicine members, Pilates was ranked ninth on the list of the top twenty fitness trends for 2010."[21] Research, although slim, confirms what many Pilates practitioners have known for some time—Pilates is good for you.

Improving the Health of Our Youth—Contrology at Work

Joseph Pilates would be distressed to learn that "during the past 20 years there has been a dramatic increase in obesity in the United States."[22] Data confirms that "one in three American adults, aged 20-74, is overweight and one in every five children, aged 6-17, is overweight"[23] and that an "estimated 16.9% of children and adolescents, aged 2-19, years are obese."[24] The health of the current youth population clearly reflects the health of our nation, and the implications for the future of our country are profound. In response to the current trends, the U.S. Surgeon General issued a call to action in 2001. As a result, "Healthy People 2010 identified overweight and obesity as 1 of 10 leading health indicators and called for a reduction in the proportion of children and adolescents who are overweight or obese."[25] Yet, sadly, the United States has made little advancement toward the target goal to reduce obesity. It is common knowledge that physical activity is a protective factor in long-term health, and habits developed in childhood can improve future health.

Regular exercise, such as Pilates, can help adolescents build and keep healthy bones, muscles, and joints, improve sleep patterns, reduce stress, control weight, reduce blood pressure, raise HDL cholesterol, reduce the risk of diabetes and some cancers, and improve psychological well-being. Secondary and postsecondary schools and their faculty have the knowledge, skills, tools, services, and support to promote physical activities that improve the health and general well-being of adolescent Americans. They can play a key role in addressing our nation's public health challenge. I am certain Joseph Pilates would stand by his dream to help our youth attain physical fitness and maintain their health in their formative years. He would want them to achieve and enjoy "health and happiness."[26] An examination of one secondary and one postsecondary school that embraced Pilates illustrates how incorporating The Method into the curricula can make this dream a reality.

Pilates in Postsecondary Education—
The Goucher College Model

Upon completion of the Pilates Teacher Certification with Romana Kryzanowska in 1995, I taught Pilates from my home. The response and demand for instruction was overwhelming. At the time, no one else was teaching Pilates in Maryland. When I began the certification process, I was teaching dance at Goucher College. It was my hope, upon completion of my teacher certification, to be able to teach people from the Baltimore community, as well as dancers at the college. I knew first-hand the benefits of The Method for dancers—increased strength, flexibility, core strength, and improved posture and alignment. It was also a useful tool for stress relief, prevention of injury, and rehabilitation.

Regretfully, students were unable to get transportation to my home studio to work with me. Their schedules were complicated, and I had a wait-list of non-student clients that was growing rapidly. So I spoke to Romana Kryzanowska, protégé of Joseph Pilates and my beloved teacher and mentor, and Sean Gallagher, founder and director of Performing Arts Physical Therapy and at that time owner of the trademark to Pilates, about developing a direct relationship between the Pilates® Studio in New York and Goucher College. I proposed offering classes in Pilates to the Goucher community and opening a training center at Goucher College. The chair of the dance department and the academic dean of Goucher were supportive of my efforts, but much had yet to be accomplished to make the center a reality.

These first steps unleashed a flurry of steps that followed. I decided first to pursue opening what would become the Pilates Center at Goucher College. After submitting a business plan and a budget to the college, Goucher offered me a stipend to serve as director of the center and provided me with space and equipment. After agreeing to reimburse the college with income earned by the program, I was able to purchase at least one of every major Pilates apparatus. I designed a brochure and worked with the college's communications office on an advertising campaign.

The studio opened in the summer of 1997, and for the first several years, I personally taught all of the Mat and private classes. Since the college was providing the space, my expenses were small. They included a yearly licensing fee to Sean Gallagher, so that we would be allowed to use the trademark that was required at the time. Classes were open to the Baltimore community and to Goucher students and faculty (at a reduced charge), but regrettably at that time, our students were not receiving academic credit for their endeavors. In my opinion,

Pilates is a discipline worthy of academic study that fits perfectly into the curricular offerings of a dance department and a college. It was time to draft requests to the college's Curriculum Committee.

My initial request was for two courses to be incorporated into the curriculum—an apparatus class that would register a maximum of six students and a Mat course that would accommodate a larger number of students. It was proposed that these classes would serve as a complement to the dancers' conditioning program, separate from and augmenting their daily technique classes. The classes would be open to the entire student body. As part of my request, I was required to describe the contribution of the courses to the dance department and to the college. It was important that my proposal support the dance department's curriculum and philosophy, but I also wanted the potential courses to appeal to the entire student body.

The format—comprised of lectures, discussion, required readings, observation, and applied instruction—was designed to pose questions encouraging anatomical self-evaluation. The first course, "The Pilates Method of Body Conditioning I," was an elective 1.5 credit course in which students studied and applied the Pilates method of body conditioning. The maximum cap of six students allowed special attention to be given to exercises performed on the five major pieces of apparatus, guaranteeing safety and precision. My proposal discussed the capacity of the course to address dancer and athlete injuries and its application in rehabilitation. It also addressed how majors with a Dance Therapy concentration could apply the knowledge gained to their various patient populations and how our students with a Dance Science concentration would have the opportunity to study a body therapy that would aid them in their future endeavors in Dance Science, Physical Therapy, and Sports Medicine. The Pilates method was a natural supplement to the intensive dance training offered at Goucher and preparation for the multi-faceted world of dance. Additionally, the course was an ideal venue for scholarly research that could provide Goucher students with an opportunity to pursue teacher certification through the Pilates® Studio in New York. The contribution of the course to the college curriculum addressed Goucher's philosophy and commitment to the education of the entire student—body and mind. It was clear that "The Pilates Method of Body Conditioning I" fit Goucher's concept of wellness by encouraging students to develop attitudes, skills, and resources for life issues that augment and enhance each student's academic experience. It is important to note that at the time of the request, there was only one other institution of higher education in the U.S. that offered students the ability to pursue teacher certification and to participate in Pilates classes. It was my hope that this fact would intrigue the Curriculum Committee.

The second course proposed was titled, "The Pilates Method of Body Conditioning Mat." This non-credit course was devoted to the study and application of the exercises that were developed by Joseph Pilates at the turn of the century, with special attention to the Mat exercises, Magic Circle series, and Arm Weight series. Unlike the apparatus course, this course was designed to fulfill a physical education (PE) requirement. The proposal focused on the uniqueness of the course. First, Goucher would be the only college in Maryland offering such a course in the curriculum. Second, there were no physical requirements in the current Goucher curriculum at the time that were similar to the proposed Pilates Mat class. Third, the course complemented and enhanced classes in the dance department (technique, anatomy, and kinesiology), in the physical education department (strength training, principles of training, care and prevention of athletic injuries), and in the chemistry department (nutrition). Fourth, the Pilates Mat class was an ideal introduction for those students interested in pursuing the Pilates apparatus course for which I was also requesting approval. Last, the Pilates Mat course fit perfectly into Goucher's vision of wellness. Students would be able to link their minds and their bodies and, in turn, gain greater self-understanding as they pursued the Mat workout.

Both courses were approved for the spring semester of 1997, and were quickly filled during registration. As I look back on the 1997 and 1998 rosters, it is interesting to note that two students later continued their studies with Romana Kryzanowska and became certified instructors. One pursued a post-graduate degree, focusing on dance science, and three became dance teachers who regularly reference and utilize Pilates in their personal training of dancers. The courses, once exclusively dominated by Goucher dancers, are now populated by a large number of non-dancers who are not only reaping the physical benefits of The Method, but also engaging in the culture of the dance department in a way that is positive, supportive, and meaningful. It is also important to note that student interest in advancement prompted the implementation of a second, more advanced apparatus class titled, "The Pilates Method of Body Conditioning II." This course allows students to progress to the intermediate level and requires a prerequisite of the level I course.

Eventually, the Pilates Center at Goucher College became large enough, and the demand for academic courses great enough, that the college agreed to hire a second certified instructor to assist me in the teaching of classes and the day-to-day running of the studio. At this writing, The Pilates Center at Goucher College employs four full-time instructors and three part-time instructors and offers approximately 26 Mat classes per week, ranging from introductory to advanced levels. The center serves approximately 190 Mat clients and 104 private clients per week from Baltimore County and the surrounding communities, as well as a large population of college students. It connects the campus community with a greater population outside of Goucher, mutually benefitting students, faculty, staff, and the Baltimore community at large. The center also hosts continuing professional education workshops (CPEs) and other guest teacher events that bring instructors from the surrounding areas to the campus for educational endeavors. I had no idea what the results of my efforts would be or how much the program would grow. Reality far exceeded my dreams.

Carrying on the Torch—Recruitment of Qualified Instructors

As the need for more instructors increased, and the program became financially self-sufficient, I inquired about the possibility of offering a scholarship for a Goucher student to participate in the certification program. At the time, certification course fees were rather costly and the closest certification program was in New York City, an expensive city in which to reside for any period of time. The costs were prohibitive for most interested and talented undergraduate students to pursue certification. Again, I approached the dean with the possibility of offering tuition scholarships to eligible students in order to supplement their education and to nurture and groom qualified teachers for the Center. The dean approved the expenditure, and I developed a process for students to apply for funding. In order to address our need for qualified and devoted teachers, the recipient of the funding was required to teach at Goucher for a period of time after his or her training was complete. This guaranteed a qualified teacher for the college, helped Goucher graduates with their post-graduation job placements, and insured Goucher's place in continuing the tradition of The Method for the next generation.

Since the inception of the scholarship program, and at this writing, we have provided scholarships to approximately 10 Goucher students and have employed 16 instructors. All full-time instructors receive an annualized salary, plus benefits, in accordance with the policy of the college. Salaries are eligible for an increase, subject to satisfactory performance, and benefits include a retirement annuity, Social Security, health insurance, life insurance, and long-term disability insurance. Full-time instructors are required to work 33 hours per week, which includes office work assigned by the director. This balance of work load allows staff to teach both private and group classes, assuring income for the college, and reducing the need for additional administrative assistance. Staff also feel a significant connection to all aspects of the center and, as a result, are sincerely committed not only to their teaching, but to the design and structure of the Pilates Center.

Upon finishing their scholarship commitments to the college, Pilates instructors have the option of either continuing full-time or part-time or leaving the college. Those who continue full-time may do so indefinitely. Those who have chosen to leave have done so in order to pursue graduate school, to teach Pilates closer to their families in another state, to pursue performing careers outside of Baltimore in Pennsylvania, New York, and California, or to open their own facilities. On the other hand, those who have chosen to continue or remain part-time have done so to pursue other interests, including motherhood, creative endeavors such as choreography, or dance instruction. Part-timers are hired as independent contractors and are compensated on an hourly basis for a stipulated number of hours per week (usually between 19-21) or as part-time employees teaching no more than 990 hours per year. The work schedule of a Pilates teacher is ideal, allowing instructors the time to devote to other endeavors while also earning a solid income teaching something in which they deeply believe. One of our part-time instructors, a graduate of Goucher, teaches two academic Pilates courses and an academic ballet course, as well as a reasonable load of private and group Mat classes. At Goucher, she has been able to successfully balance her mutual love of dance and Pilates

The scholarship program has served the Pilates Center at Goucher College well, providing us with teachers who already are devoted to Goucher as alumni, who have the appropriate coursework to pursue successful teaching, and who have completed one of the most rigorous Pilates teacher training programs in existence. We plan to continue administering the scholarship program with the goal of averaging approximately one scholarship per year to students who illustrate the devotion, skill and commitment to Pilates that Romana desires in all of her apprentices.

Several students have also taken advantage of internship opportunities connected to Pilates as part of their teaching certification. For example, I served as an Internship Advisor to several students at Drago's Gym. The three-credit internships allowed the students to develop their personal skills in Pilates with the expert guidance of the staff at The Pilates Studio in New York, now known as True Pilates. The intense study of The Method through an internship model enhances their technical work in ballet and modern dance by providing a better working knowledge of the body as an instrument. Additionally, they develop an eye for creating individualized workouts for clients, learn to maintain Pilates equipment, and increase their knowledge of the history and theories behind Pilates. As part of their apprenticeship, they receive daily feedback on their performance and are assessed through written and practical exams administered as part of the certification process. Written work may include a journal and a practical exam administered by the Internship Advisor. In addition, on-site supervisors complete performance evaluations of the intern that address performance, attitude, and human relations. Internships allow students to obtain academic credit for their Pilates studies while also pursuing teaching certification.

Secondary Education—The Addition of Pilates at George Washington Carver Center for Arts and Technology

After the program at Goucher was sufficiently established, I felt it was time to provide the opportunity for Pilates to become an integral part of the curriculum at Carver Center for Arts and Technology, a Baltimore County public magnet school, offering college preparatory academic curricula for students in grades 9-12. I was already incorporating the work in my intermediate and advanced ballet classes, but I wanted the Pilates units to become a significant and permanent part of the curriculum for the dancers during their four years in the magnet program. Integrating Pilates required creative and detailed planning.

The gifted and talented dance curriculum at Carver Center offered the resources and schedule parameters for Pilates Mat to be added to the existing ballet technique classes. I decided to gradually incorporate Pilates exercises prior to ballet barre over the course of four quarters and then evaluate its success based on assessments made throughout the year. Beginning my classes with Pilates Mat work allowed "students to bring their minds to class, to find their centers, and to increase circulation, all of which aid in the warm-up of their bodies prior to standing work."[27] In this way, objectives could be pursued and cross-referenced as each unit was introduced and transfer of learning across disciplines could be facilitated. Practical objectives included:

- Increased awareness of the body's capacities and limitations
- Maximized muscle efficiency (strength, flexibility, control, and stamina)
- Pronounced prevention of injury
- Improved technical ability
- Enhanced dynamic posture and alignment
- Accelerated rehabilitation when applicable
- Prolonged longevity of career

Prior to introducing students to the Pilates method kinesthetically, students completed units on "Anatomy" and an "Introduction to Pilates." Basic anatomy and terminology were introduced, structural differences and limitations were discussed, and the history and six principles of Pilates were examined. Upon completion of the units, students were ready to kinesthetically experience the Pilates Mat work. Exercises were modified, as needed, and they were dissected with special attention to the benefits and goals of each exercise. Upon completion of Mat work, the transition from supine and prone exercises on the Mat to standing barre work was particularly crucial. Therefore, barre began with a plié combination that had already been mastered by the students: "This allowed the new sensations and knowledge gained from the Pilates exercises to be assimilated into preliminary barre work with as few distractions as possible."[28] The process allowed dancers to find their center (powerhouse), address personal imbalances, and enhance their performance. As dancers mastered beginner work, new Mat exercises were added to their repertory, and previous and new exercises were detailed.

With time, dancers were able to "self-correct errors in placement and performance and, most importantly, to avert them."[29] By the time students progressed to the last quarter of their studies, they understood the Pilates method's ability to improve muscular strength, balance, mental and physical control, and muscular flexibility, prerequisites for classical dancers. They even began to find relationships and correlations between the Pilates Mat exercises, proper placement, and the classical vocabulary performed in class. Ideally, such a course should be taught by a certified instructor, but instructors without extensive knowledge of Pilates can apply the six principles to Mat exercises, as well as to barre and center work. Introducing Pilates at Carver addressed many postural and alignment problems, muscular imbalances, lack of strength, and insufficient muscular flexibility that our students had acquired prior to enrollment.

The movements performed in a Pilates class support the movement objectives of a dance technique class, facilitating determination of alignment inconsistencies in both the lower and upper extremities. Ann McMillan, Luc Proteau, and Rose-Marie Lèbe find, "The weekly regimen creates references (recall and recognition schemata) of correct alignment that can be used during execution of movement in ballet class."[30] Also, "Technical faults, areas of weakness, and anatomical discrepancies can be easier to recognize in students lying supine than in students standing in first position at the barre."[31] I found that Pilates, partnered with significant and informed knowledge of ballet technique, can be used to detect inefficient movement patterns and to increase the awareness of the body, allowing me to develop dancers who are less prone to injury and are better able to engage in dance activities for years to come. Because of the success of Pilates in my courses, Carver Center included Pilates as a unit of study required by the students in Ballet III courses, making it a permanent feature of the curriculum. The Department of Health, Recreation and Dance also provided its teachers with workshops and trainings in the Pilates method and now has a Pilates Training program on Safari Montage, a classroom lesson presentation tool, which is designed for the use of teachers in their classrooms. This unique video program, scripted and narrated by myself, was created for Baltimore County Public Schools with my assistance. The video is successfully bringing Pilates to a more general student population, just as Joseph Pilates wanted.

A Distinctive Home—Pilates in Education

Now there are many colleges and universities besides Goucher College that offer Pilates classes to their students, including La Roche College, Shenandoah University, the University of Oklahoma, Muhlenberg College, Southern Methodist University, and University of Florida. Fullerton College offers a two-year certificate program in Pilates, and S.U.N.Y. Purchase offers a certificate program in Pilates Mat Instruction. DePauw University, Boston University, and Ithaca College offer Pilates classes to their student body through their recreational sports programs. Specifically, at Appalachian State University, a Pilates teacher-training program, sponsored by the Department of Theatre and Dance, has been added to the curriculum. The 675+ hour training program "begins with 6 credit hours of academic work in Pilates and culminates with a summer intensive, exams, and a full-time apprenticeship leading to certification."[32] Academic courses provide students with a solid foundation in The Method, as well as their initial observation and teaching experiences.

Other dance programs, such as the one at Indiana University, are preparing their students for careers outside of dance by providing them with marketable Pilates skills that go beyond performance. These dance programs understand that their graduates need alternative and marketable skills in order to support and sustain their careers as dance artists, since performance careers are relatively short. Results of recent research on the work patterns of dance artists found that "two-thirds of a range of performing and visual artists were found to include work outside of their art form or outside of the cultural sector altogether."[33] For example, at California State University Long Beach, many dance majors are seeking careers in dance or dance fitness, pursuing a B.A. degree in Dance with a Dance Science emphasis. According to Karen Clippinger at C.S.U.L.B., many students decide the dance world is too competitive and therefore "opt for another direction, such as being a personal trainer or Pilates instructor."[34] Therefore, the Dance Science curriculum at C.S.U.L.B. prepares dance majors for the competitive job market and also provides students, through applied and practical experiences, with the "background information to make them better teachers - to understand how to prevent injuries, and how to design a better class."[35]

Classes in Pilates are an integral part of the program. Additionally, Shenandoah University's Kim Gibilisco began a Pilates Mat certification at the school. The curriculum is "designed for a student population (ages 19-25) who may not have had experience with The Method."[36] Until 2007, the program enrolled mostly dance majors, but in 2009, registrants included majors from other programs, Shenandoah University alumni, and members of the community. Shenandoah's unique Teacher Training Program is an elective course of study that can fulfill a dance elective requirement, therefore serving a large population of the student body.

Colleges and universities, often spearheaded by dance departments, are beginning to incorporate courses in Pilates into their curriculum. Needless to say, upon obtaining Pilates teacher certification, there are a variety of career paths one may choose. Teachers may work in a health or wellness center, resort, Pilates studio, university or college, or in rehabilitation. Earning potential ranges from an hourly wage of $15-$100 per hour or more. Dance programs understand the demand to provide their students with a multitude of possibilities that will maximize their strengths as non-performers, and provide them with the opportunities for careers that are both rewarding and exciting.

The Future with Pilates – A Balanced Body, Mind, and Spirit

Pilates is definitely here to stay. In 2010, "CNBC reported that Pilates is the nation's fastest growing activity, with 8.6 million participants."[37] According to Nora St. John, education program director of Balanced Body® University, this is due to "its long-term appeal."[38] I have certainly seen evidence of this personally and also with clients who have been with me since I began teaching in 1995. As Pilates merges with educational programs, it is important that the instructors employed are qualified, equipped with a strong foundation in anatomy, an understanding of the biomechanics of movement in general, and in Pilates specifically. The education programs that exist must require a sufficient number of hours to prepare competent teachers and to educate consumers, so they can tell the difference between qualified and unqualified instructors. Quality must take precedence over quantity. Perhaps one day schools in the United States will not only offer credit-bearing courses in Pilates, but degreed programs, as well.

While I believe the future of Pilates has yet to be fully realized, I am confident that Joseph and Clara Pilates would be happy with the expansion of the Pilates method into academic programs across the country. Surely they would be pleased with the positive impact it has made on so many students in our schools nationwide. In *Your Health*, Pilates states that his "work will be established and when it is, I will be the happiest man in God's Universe. My goal will have been reached."[39] Joseph Pilates' work is clearly established, thriving in a way that he likely never imagined. We who follow have only to continue to implement our knowledge and our imaginations. Joseph Pilates must surely be looking down upon us, smiling as his work is disseminated to the youth of our country by instructors and educators who have embraced his teachings and his work and by those of us who are dedicated to "retaining its purity and integrity for generations to come."[40] I challenge the reader to seek the trinity of a balanced body, mind and spirit that Joseph Pilates so eloquently describes in *Return to Life through Contrology*, and I encourage teachers of the Pilates method to continue their efforts in feeding the Pilates flame so that our youth of today may reap the benefits of The Method tomorrow.

About Elizabeth

Elizabeth is Chair of the Dance Department at Goucher College and faculty member at Carver Center for Arts and Technology. She earned her B.F.A. and M.F.A. from New York University's Tisch School of the Arts and, in 1995, she completed her Pilates teacher certification under the tutelage of Romana Kryzanowska and Sari Mejia-Santo. Her most recent article "The Pilates Method and Ballet Technique- Applications in the Dance Studio," published in the *The Journal of Dance Education*, is an extension of her work as Founding Director of the Pilates Center at Goucher. Ahearn serves on the Executive Committee of ACDFA as the Vice-President for Regional Planning.

REFERENCES

[1]Peter Fiasca, *Discovering Pure Classical Pilates*, 2nd ed. (n.p.: Classical Pilates, 2009), 30.
[2]Joseph Pilates, *Your Health*. (Incline Village, NV: Presentation Dynamics, Inc., 1998), 42. Originally Published by J.J. Augustine, 1945.
[3]Fiasca, 10.
[4]Michelle Olson and Carrie Smith, "Pilates Exercise: Lessons from the Lab," IDEA, (2005): 4.
[5]Olson and Smith, 4.
[6]John Porcari and Stefanie Spilde, "Can Pilates Do It All?" *Ace Fitness Matters*, (November/December 2005): 10.
[7]Porcari and Spilde, 11.
[8]Neal A. Segal; Jane Hein; Jeffrey R. Basford. "The Effects of Pilates Training on Flexibility and Body Composition: An Observational Study." *Archives of Physical Medicine and Rehabilitation* vol. 85 (December 2004).
[9]"The Great Balancing Act." *Elle*, (October 1991): 110, 116, and 120.
[10]Elizabeth Ahearn, "The Pilates Method and Ballet Technique: Applications in the Dance Studio." *The Journal of Dance Education*, vol. 6, no.3 (2006): 92.
[11]Amanda Anne Parrott, "The effects of Pilates technique and aerobic conditioning on dancers' technique and aesthetic." *Kinesiology and Medicine for Dance* vol.15 no.2 (1993): 49.
[12]Robin Kish and Janice Gudde Plastino, "The functional effect of Pilates training on college dancers." (Thesis-M.S., California State University, Fullerton, 1998). Retrieved from www.nureyev-medicine.org/articles/the-functional-effects-of-pilates-training-on-college-dancers.
[13]Fiasca, 19.
[14]Lisa Marie Bernardo and Elizabeth Nagle, "Does Pilates training benefit dancers? An appraisal of Pilates research literature." *Journal of Dance Medicine and Science*, vol. 10, no. 1-2 (June 2006): 46-50.
[15]Tânia Amorim, Filipa Sousa, Leandro Machado, and José Augusto Santos, "Effects of Pilates Training on Muscular Strength and Balance in Ballet Dancers." *Portuguese Journal of Sport Sciences* 11 supl. 2, (2011): 147.
[16]Tânia Amorim, Filipa Sousa, Leandro Machado, and José Augusto Santos, 148.
[17]Andy Halerin, "Exercise helps college students maintain health." *TCU Daily Skiff*, November 12, 2003.

[18]Russell Jagol, Marielle L. Jonker, Mariam Missaghian, and Tom Baranowski. "Effects of 4 weeks of Pilates on the body composition of young girls." *Preventative Medicine*, vol. 42, no. 3 (March 2006): 177-180.

[19]Shirley Archer, "Pilates Improves Youth Fitness." *IDEA Fitness Journal*, vol. 3, no 9 (October 2006).

[20]T. Crowell, "No Pain, No Pain." *Dance Connection*, (Summer 1993): 26.

[21]Danielle Bullen, "Proper Form: Using Pilates effectively as a rehab treatment option for college athletes." *Advance for Physical Therapy and Rehab Medicine*, vol. 21, issue 25 (2010).

[22]Centers for Disease Control and Prevention, "U.S Obesity Trends."(September 2010). www.cdc.gov/obesity/data/trends.html.

[23]Christine Romani-Ruby, "Why Pilates?" *ClubSolutions*, (2007) :19.

[24]Cynthia Ogden and Margaret Carroll, "Prevalence of Obesity Among Children and Adolescents: United States, Trends 1963-1965 Through 2007-2008." Centers for Disease Control and Prevention (June 2010). www.cdc.gov/nchs/data/hestat/obesity_child_07_08/obesity_child_07_08_.htm.

[25]Ogden and Carroll.

[26]Pilates, 64.

[27]Ahearn, 94.

[28]Ahearn, 94.

[29]Ahearn, 94-95.

[30]Ann McMillan, Luc Proteau, and Rose-Marie Lèbe. "The effect of Pilates-based training on dancers' dynamic posture." *Journal of Dance Medicine and Science* vol. 2, no. 3 (September 1998): 107.

[31]Ahearn, 98.

[32]"Pilates Teacher Training." http://www.conferences-camps.appstate.edu/adult/pilates.php.

[33]Dawn Bennett, "Careers in Dance: Beyond Performance to the Real World of Work." *The Journal of Dance Education* vol. 9, No. 1 (2009): 29.

[34]Victoria Looseleaf, "Dance with a practical edge: some college dance programs train students for a second career." *Dance Magazine* (September 2010): 51

[35]Looseleaf, 50.

[36]Jessica Cassity, "Pilates Goes to College." www.articlesbase.com/yoga-articles/pilates-goes-to-college-717209.html.

[37]Mary Monroe, "The Pilates Phenomenon: Where Do We Go From Here?" *IDEA Fitness Journal* vol 7, no. 7 (2010), http://www.ideafit.com/fitness-library/the-pilates-phenomenon-where-do-we-go-from-here.

[38]Monroe.

[39]Pilates, 55.

[40]Fiasca, 2.

WORKS CONSULTED

Berardi, Gigi. *Finding Balance: Fitness and Training for a Lifetime in Dance.* Princeton: Dance Horizons/Princeton Book Company, 1991.

Fitt, Sally Sivey. *Dance Kinesiology.* New York: Schirmer Books, 1988.

Gallagher, Sean and Romana Kryzanowska. *The Joseph H. Pilates Archive Collection: The Photographs, Writings and Designs.* Philadelphia: Bainbridge Books, 2000.

Pilates, Joseph H., and William John Miller. Pilates' *Return to Life Through Contrology.* Incline Village: Presentation Dynamics Inc., 1998.

Authentic Pilates & Psychoneuroimmunology

By Peter Fiasca

Joseph Pilates' exploratory research served him well, allowing all of us to benefit from the fruits of his studies...

This chapter explores psychoneuroimmunology and Authentic Pilates, while providing empirical evidence for understanding the interconnections between the two disciplines. Psychoneuroimmunology is an area of study that emphasizes unity and integration of body-brain systems—that is, mind-body interaction—in contrast to neurology and neuropsychology, which focus upon the study and treatment of pathologies. More specifically, neuropsychology is often associated with the study of brain dysfunction, behavioral dysfunction, and perceptual dysfunction.

Neuropsychological symptoms and their determinants have been observed, interpreted, and studied for centuries.[1] Psychoneuroimmunology is a more recent discipline, emerging over the past five decades from the results of new empirical research methods and scientific discoveries. This field of scholarship has been developed by many thinkers, most notably Solomon & Moos (1964) as well as Ader & Cohen (1975).[2]

Psychoneuroimmunology is clearly associated with physical health and well-being. In a broad sense, psychoneuroimmunology involves complex interactions among several medical areas such as neuroscience, psychology, immunology, medicine, sociology, genetics, and endocrinology, all in the service of understanding and maintaining health.[3] Specifically, psychoneuroimmunology examines "...how mental events and processes modulate the function of the immune system and how, in turn, immunological activity is capable of altering the function of the mind."[4] In a more direct way, psychoneuroimmunology comprises "...the interactions amongst the mind, nervous system, and immune system."[5] Psychoneuroimmunology offers significant evidence that our immune system and nervous system are inextricably connected, and shows how their interactions affect overall behavioral health.

Through the lens of psychoneuroimmunology, it is possible to scientifically substantiate one of Joseph Pilates' central claims: Contrology—defined as the complete coordination of body, mind, and spirit—improves the performance of our central nervous system, our immune system, and their relation to brain function. Illustrating this point, Pilates writes, "By reawakening thousands upon thousands of otherwise ordinarily dormant muscle cells, Contrology correspondingly reawakens thousands upon thousands of dormant brain cells, thus activating new areas and stimulating further the functioning of the mind."[6] Pressing his point further, Joseph Pilates indicates the reciprocal connection between mind and body that, in our modern era, we take for granted. As he states, "One of the major results of Contrology is gaining the mastery of your mind over the complete control of your body...the brain itself is actually a sort of natural telephone switchboard exchange incorporated in our bodies as a means of communication through the sympathetic nervous system to all our muscles."[7]

It is striking that Joseph Pilates would allude to the interconnectedness between the central nervous system (CNS) and the immune system approximately 20 years before Solomon & Moos (1964) first began describing the emerging discipline of psychoneuroimmunology. Pilates presumed the importance of CNS and immune system interactions, even though he did not have access to psychoneuroimmunological research on the subject. Suffice it to say that he was at least aware that our CNS and immune system are both functionally and anatomically integrated. It is not a coincidence that Joseph Pilates names the sympathetic nervous system, for its functioning is integral to maintaining homeostasis of the body, mobilizing the body's stress response, and regulating the body's internal organs.[8] His well-known statement, "If your spine is inflexibly stiff at 30, you are old; if it is completely flexible at 60, you are young,"[9] confirms his awareness of the interaction between the sympathetic nervous system and psychoneuroimmunological function, as do various passages in his two books, *Your Health* (1934) and *Return to Life Through Contrology* (1945).

Joseph Pilates' awareness of the interaction between the sympathetic nervous system and psychoneuroimmunological function was crucial in helping him develop Contrology. Yet there has been an extraordinary amount of new research completed since his death in 1967, as well as a major scientific paradigm shift that includes experimental studies demonstrating the interconnectedness of CNS and immune system functioning. According to University of Hawaii professor of neurobiology, Adrian J. Dunn, there are four points of experimental evidence that substantiate CNS and immune system interactions:

1. Alterations in immune responses can be conditioned;
2. Electrical stimulation or lesions of specific brain sites can alter immune function;
3. Stress alters immune responses and the growth of tumors and infections in experimental animals; and
4. Activation of the immune system correlates to altered neurophysiological, neurochemical, and neuroendocrine activities of brain cells.[10]

Joseph Pilates' exploratory research served him well, allowing all of us to benefit from the fruits of his studies and his creation of an integrated system of mental and physical conditioning called Contrology. In a major research study by Elenkov, Ilia J., et al., interactions between the brain and immune system were analyzed to understand how the two systems "talk to each other."[11] The study produced many significant findings. For example, it found that the brain and the immune system are the two major adaptive systems of the body; and during an immune response, they communicate with each other in a process that is essential for maintaining homeostasis. Two major pathway systems are involved in this cross talk: the hypothalamic-pituitary-adrenal (HPA) axis and the sympathetic nervous system (SNS). It is noteworthy that the study focuses on the role of SNS in neuroimmune interactions, an area that has received much less attention over time. Elenkov, et al., point out that evidence accumulated over the last 20 years suggests that norepinephrine is a primary neurotransmitter active in lymphoid organs. Thus, primary and secondary lymphoid organs receive extensive sympathetic innervations. The study observed that norepinephrine is discharged from sympathetic nerves in lymphoid organs, and that target immune cells convey adrenoreceptors. Furthermore, through receptor stimulation, norepinephrine affects lymphocyte transmission and propagation, in addition to adjusting cytokine production and lymphoid cell activity. The Elenkov study shows that although there is sympathetic nerve activity in bone marrow, especially in thymus and mucosal tissues, knowledge about the effect of the sympathetic nerve activity on development of blood cells, generation of T lymphocyte cells, and mucosal immunity is restricted. This research study concluded that subluxation reduces signal transduction between neurons, which can result in loss of inhibition of the sympathetic nervous system. The consequence is overactivity and the release of more hormones produced by the adrenal glands. This increase in hormones reduces systemic type 1 (Th1) immune system response. Since the Th1 immune system response essentially fights infections, there is a greater probability of illness or death from infection. It has been found that adjustments using chiropractic or osteopathic techniques may increase systemic Type 1 (Th1) immune system response.

Comparisons with Chiropractic Medicine

The previous paragraph provides scientific evidence of CNS and immune system interaction, which encompasses chiropractic intervention. Briefly recall Joseph Pilates' claim that his system of Contrology improves performance of CNS and immune system function as well as brain function. To achieve a more complete picture of this assertion, it will be useful to explore research from chiropractic medicine.

There are significant commonalities between the two disciplines. For example, both chiropractic medicine and Authentic Pilates address the fundamental relationships between musculoskeletal structure and functioning as related to the CNS. Similarly, both chiropractic medicine and Authentic Pilates consider CNS activity and immune system activity in relation to overall body functioning. The two disciplines involve systematic spinal variation based upon an integrated set of principles and techniques that preserve and enhance health, emphasizing spinal alignment, spinal conditioning, and optimum spinal range of motion. Finally, chiropractic medicine and Authentic Pilates have a beneficial impact on the functioning of our CNS, immune system, and brain. All CNS fibers convey electrochemical impulses of sensation and movement between larger systems such as respiratory, circulatory, renal, gastrointestinal as well as the brain, spinal cord, organs, muscles, and skin tissue. Therefore, it's illustrative to conceive of proper spinal alignment, spinal conditioning, and optimum spinal range of motion as collectively being a necessary, but not sufficient, condition to enhance connections between CNS, immune system, and brain functioning.

There is growing evidence suggesting that spinal manipulation through chiropractic medicine—and by implication the Authentic Pilates movement—can reduce inflammatory processes as a reaction to tissue damage and pain in some subjects.[12] Other research suggests that spinal manipulation through chiropractic medicine—and by implication the Authentic Pilates movement—can improve proliferation of immunoglobulins (antibodies) and production of cytokine IL-2, which is an immunoregulatory protein that attracts white blood cells.[13] These research studies conclude that spinal manipulation can improve immunoregulatory processes as well as contribute to decreased inflammation and pain. In a recent study by Teodorczyk-Injeyan, et al.,[14] the authors explore interactions between CNS and immune system as related to immunoregulation. Their conclusions indicate that immune system internal stability and coordinated responsiveness pivots upon communication with the CNS system through the specific activity of cytokines (a protein secreted by lymph cells that affects cellular activity and inflammation) and neurotransmitters. Furthermore, there is electrochemical communication between autonomic nerve terminals and macrophages (cells that remove waste products, harmful microorganisms, and foreign substances from the bloodstream) as well as lymphocytes (cells that produce antibodies that attack infected cells, including cancerous cells). The authors conclude that CNS and immune system interaction between nerves and immune cells helps sustain metabolic homeostasis.

From the research cited above, we might infer that spinal manipulation based upon chiropractic medicine has the potential to promote psychoneuroimmunological health. On a parallel track we might ask: Can the practice of Authentic Pilates movement occasion similar psychoneuroimmuniological health benefits as chiropractic medicine? If we were to temporarily entertain this question, Authentic Pilates technique might be construed as a movement system of "manipulations" and "adjustments," however, without the high velocity movement of actual chiropractic medicine technique.

There are obvious and striking differences and similarities between Authentic Pilates and chiropractic medicine.

DIFFERENCES show the greater range of possibilities with Authentic Pilates:

- In Authentic Pilates, movement depends upon self-initiated energy, intention, and action to achieve a complete body workout, unlike chiropractic medicine, in which the practitioner conducts the manipulations;
- Authentic Pilates has varying rhythms and dynamics, and is rarely abrupt like chiropractic manipulations or adjustments;
- The spinal range of motion in Authentic Pilates can achieve a far greater degree of rotation, extension, flexion, and side bending than does chiropractic manipulation;
- The 500+ exercises in Authentic Pilates far exceed the number and variety of chiropractic medicine manipulations or adjustments; and,
- Authentic Pilates trains individuals to improve overall stability, strength, stretch, control, precision, breathing, balance, coordination, and flowing movement, whereas chiropractic medicine is primarily focused upon subluxation.

SIMILARITIES lie in the fact that both disciplines accomplish the following:

- Have the ability to correct structural distortions;
- Enhance proper alignment of the body's musculoskeletal structure;
- Assist the body's natural healing capabilities without medication or surgery;
- Help prevent and reduce pain;
- Restore, sustain, and increase joint mobility;
- Offer non-surgical approaches to help individuals develop health and well-being; and
- Contribute to increasing the body's nerve supply, which is a critical factor in overall health.

Developing the idea further that benefits of chiropractic medicine might be gained through consistent practice of Authentic Pilates, let's turn to a list developed by Dr. Steven G. Yeomans:[15] The sensory and motor effects of a chiropractic manipulation include:

- Increased joint range of motion (ROM) in all three planes, along with reduction of pain;[16,17]
- An increased skin pain tolerance level;[18]
- Increased paraspinal muscle pressure pain tolerance;[19] and
- Reduced muscle electrical activity and tension.[20]

Sympathetic nervous system effects of a chiropractic manipulation include:

- Increased blood flow and distal skin temperature (fingertips);[21]
- Blood pressure reduction; [22,23]
- Differences in distal skin temperature in the fingertips. Dr. Yeomans explains that blood flow in the fingertips may rise or fall with specific chiropractic adjustments to the spine. For example, the distal skin temperature has been shown to rise (signifying increased blood flow) following a chiropractic adjustment to C1-C7 and/or L4-L5. The temperature fell (less blood flow) when the chiropractic adjustment was made to the area between T1-L3.[24]

Blood chemistry changes after a chiropractic manipulation include:

- Increased secretion of melatonin. Secreted by the pineal gland in the brain, melatonin helps regulate other hormones and maintain circadian rhythm (the 24-hour cycle that determines when people fall asleep and wake up).[25]
- Increased plasma beta endorphin levels. Endorphins are the body's natural pain killers; when increased, they help humans manage pain.[26]
- Elevation of Substance P and enhanced neutrophil respiratory burst. Referring to the rapid release of oxygen species, respiratory burst is an important reaction in the degradation of internalized cells and bacteria.[27]
- Pupillary diameter changes. Changes in diameter of the

pupil (which range from 2-8mm) are often associated with different levels of fatigue and mental workload.[28]

In light of previous paragraphs describing health benefits of chiropractic medicine, it seems reasonable to suggest that Authentic Pilates technique—the integrated whole body system of neuromusculoskeletal movement developed by Joseph Pilates—may indeed provide similar health benefits to those of chiropractic medicine. Since there is an increasing amount of fascinating research in the categories of chiropractic medicine and psychoneuroimmunology, it will be useful to review aspects of immune system fortification.

Immune System Fortification

One obstacle in researching health is that empirical analyses most frequently define health as a reduction in or absence of symptoms, rather than defining the positive conditions of health. Although research focusing upon the indicators of dysfunction has clearly led to beneficial applications in various disciplines, disease-model experiments tend to yield few conclusions that can be applied to health, vitality, and well-being. Therefore, let us focus our attention on research associated with psychoneuroimmunology and immune system fortification.

Jorge H. Daruna, professor of psychiatry and neurology at Tulane University School of Medicine, claims "…that a variety of personal beliefs and practices, including social activity, expression of emotion, relaxation habits, physical exercise, and nutritional choices, have beneficial effects on immune function."[29] Beliefs, suggestions, and expectations contribute to the effects of preventative medicine practices, as well as response to intervention, which can contribute to either immune enhancement or stress. In addition, psychoneuroimmunological function can be found in the placebo effect and nocebo effect. The former is defined by ways in which beliefs or expectations influence symptom reduction; the latter is defined by ways that beliefs or expectations influence symptom increase.

Expectation plays a pivotal role in the placebo effect. For example, in a research study titled, "Placebo effects and the common cold: a randomized controlled trial,[30] the authors studied participants in four groups: "(1) those receiving no pills, (2) those blinded to placebo, (3) those blinded to Echinacea, and (4) those given open-label Echinacea...Participants randomized to the no-pill group tended to have longer and more severe illnesses than those who received pills. For the subgroup who believed in Echinacea and received pills, illnesses were substantively shorter and less severe, regardless of whether the pills contained Echinacea."[31]

In a well-known study, "Psychological variables in human cancer,"[32] a patient named Mr. Wright had severe lymphosarcoma, which is cancer of lymph nodes. His condition included tumors larger than grapefruits, the necessity of regular fluid removal from his lungs, and administration of oxygen so that he could breathe normally. After learning that his physician, Dr. Klopfer, was researching a substance called Krebiozen—which is composed of creatine and mineral oil—Mr. Wright requested this potential cancer treatment. The patient's condition exhibited a dramatic reduction in lymphosarcoma, and he was able to return to adequate functioning in daily life. However, the American Medical Association (AMA) and U.S. Food & Drug Administration (FDA) later began publicizing reports about Krebiozen being a useless and ineffective drug. After hearing these news reports, the patient's lymphosarcoma returned. Dr. Klopfer decided to tell Mr. Wright that he would be given a newly enhanced and stronger dose of Krebiozen. Instead, Dr. Klopfer actually gave his patient injections of sterile water. Strikingly, Mr. Wright's lymphosarcoma remission was even more complete than before: his cancer tumors dissolved, and he returned to managing daily responsibilities and avocations. Therefore it was solely the placebo effect, caused by Mr. Wright's belief that his supposed "medication" was successful in producing recovery from illness, that restored him to health. Unfortunately, after approximately two months Mr. Wright became aware of subsequent AMA and FDA reports citing the fact that he was injected with sterile water, not Krebiozen. Soon his lymphocarcoma returned, and he died.

Beliefs, suggestions, and psychological expectations are also related to personality traits. In *Personality and Human Immunity,* by Cohen, Janicki-Deverts, Crittenden, and Sneed, the authors review research investigating connections between personality traits and immune function.[33] They focus on the "Big Five" aspects of personality: "...extraversion, agreeableness, neuroticism, conscientiousness, and openness to experience."[34] As they note, personality and immune strengths are complex subjects to define and measure. Personality is often measured by categorizing a group of behaviors into one or more of the above categories, then researching various dimensions, such as recreational activities, vocational interests, social behavior, dating behavior, motor skills, impulsivity, and satisfaction.

The immune strengths that are most often related to personality studies include "...leukocytes, antibody response to immunization, natural killer (NK) cell cytotoxicity, mitogen-stimulated lymphocyte proliferation, delayed-type hypersensitivity (DTH), antibody level to herpes viruses, stimulated production of pro-inflammatory cytokines, and circulating markers of inflammation."[35] Selected research studies of extraversion indicate that this personality trait is associated with less susceptibility to developing flu virus and greater lymphocyte production and NK cell cytotoxicity.[36] With regard to neuroticism, several studies show a decrease in antibody responses as well as poor lymphocyte propagation, "...NK cell cytotoxicity, phagocytosis, chemotaxis, and stimulated IL-2 production."[37]

Turning to immunology research and its relation to conscientiousness as personality trait, results are scant. As it turns out, though, lower amounts of conscientiousness are linked with higher amounts of inflammation. For example, "Amongst HIV patients, conscientiousness has been associated with slower increase in viral load and, inconsistently, with slower decline in CD4+ cells."[38] Similar to the construct of conscientiousness—as a personality trait—the concept of agreeableness was associated with some research results indicating greater resistance to cold susceptibility. However, other research studies did not show any connection between agreeableness and immune function. In the three research studies that have investigated openness to experience as a personality trait, none have indicated association with immune function.[39]

Another area of supporting evidence for psychoneuroimmunological function can be found in research studies that explore social engagement and stress reduction.[40] Although some research results are mixed, constructs associated with social engagement and social support indicate increased lymphocyte production of white blood cells known as "natural killer cells" (NK cells), which supply quick immune system response to cells that are infected by a virus and have begun tumor formation. In addition, social engagement and social support improve "...cell-mediated immunity, as indexed by diminished herpes simplex virus (HSV) antibody titers."[41] It is useful to note that professional massage practice has been shown to increase the proliferation of NK cells.[42]

Stress leads to many physical manifestations such as migraine headaches, tension headaches, sexual dysfunction, hypertension, asthma, various physical pains, and gastrointestinal problems. Stress can also worsen existing diseases such as HIV/AIDS, cardiovascular disease, breast cancer, and chronic fatigue syndrome. Cognitive-behavioral stress management (CBSM) techniques have been used successfully to improve psychoneuroimmunological function in relation to these diseases.[43] Since the 1990s CBSM has proven effective "because stressors, cognitive appraisals, coping strategies, and interpersonal processes (e.g., social support) may influence psychological adjustment, biobehavioral process, and physical health status..." in individuals with the diseases listed above.[44] CBSM techniques are based on the premise that certain types of unclear or inaccurate thought patterns occasion hurtful and distorted emotional-behavioral and psychoneuroimmunological patterns. If we learn how to think more clearly and accurately, then we can improve emotional-behavioral and psychoneuroimmunological response patterns. Some research has shown that through cognitive restructuring and the use of exercises such as deep breathing, meditation, and relaxation, "...there is a strong trend for these psychological changes to parallel neuroendocrine changes that relate to improvement in immunological and viral biomarkers of disease progression."[45] Although research results vary, the preponderance of data supports the use of CBSM in improving mental and physical outcomes.

There is another area of supporting evidence for psychoneuroimmunological function: expression of emotion. A majority of relevant research studies indicate that verbal disclosure of traumatic events and negative emotions is associated with improved health as a result of immune system activity.[46] Parallel to the positive effects of social engagement and stress reduction, verbal description of negative emotions also contributes to higher levels of NK activity, as well as to lymphocyte production. While social engagement can overlap with verbal description of negative emotions, the two functions can certainly remain independent of, and diverge from, one another.

In his chapter titled, "Emotional Expression and Disclosure," Roger J. Booth begins to describe the importance of expressing emotion by citing several fundamental aspects of our human experience. Starting with the fact that we are social animals who express ourselves in meaningful linguistic ways, he notes that communication always implies the presence of another human being. Mr. Booth further explains that our bodies respond and adjust in psychoneuroimmunologically important ways to help sustain valuable relationships, that our structures of psychoneuroimmunology naturally adapt to events in our lives, that our reflections and narratives constitute cognitive representations connecting events and emotions, and that recalling events occasions an emotional context wherein we may prefer to remember or not remember.[47] Booth writes, "Following any sort of emotional experience, people generally talk about the experience, and the rate of sharing is often very high and remarkably similar across different cultures."[48]

Since the early 1980s, research has confirmed the positive benefits of verbally conveying or writing about negative experiences. For example, in a research study by Zech (1981) that asked over 1,000 college students whether talking about an experience was a source of relief, 89% answered affirmatively.[49] In 1986, Pennebaker and Beall completed a research study in which subjects were asked to identify, explore, and write about very stressful events in their lives, setting the stage for a wave of continued international interest in the subject of expressing emotions.[50] Because of the success in helping individuals achieve relief from "writing therapy," various research studies began to assess more than mood changes as they entered the realm of psychoneuroimmunology to include cardiovascular, autonomic nervous system, cortisol, immune system, and endocrine changes. Many research studies measured salivary (sIgA) concentration, T lymphocyte production, proliferation of NKs, and CD8 T levels.[51] The results indicated a positive relationship between writing therapy and improved psychoneuroimmunology.

In their chapter titled, "Positive Emotions and Immunity," Sarah Pressman and Lora Black examine in detail research paradigms and specific studies related to immune function and experimentally induced emotions.[52] Pressman and Black conclude that there is a relationship between positive affect and higher immune function. They write, "Overall, studies show that both high and midarousal PA [positive affect] induction is associated with higher immune function (as measured by sIgA, NKCA, NKCC, and pro- and anti-inflammatory cytokine levels)."[53]

Let's take a quick look at their terminology. SIgA is the short form of secretory immunoglobulin A in saliva, which is an essential antibody that protects against infections. NKCA refers to Natural Killer Cell Activity, which is a rapid immune system response against abnormally stressed, microbe-infected or malignant cells; and NKCC is Natural Killer Cell Cytotoxicity, which is how natural killer cells target and kill abnormal, infected, or malignant cells.

With regard to results from naturalistic studies, Pressman and Black cite additional conclusions suggesting positive affect (PA) is connected with immune functions such as "...higher NK cell number and activity, better control of latent EBV [Epstein-Barr Virus], faster wound healing, and increased cytokine responses to live influenza virus and cancer treatment."[54] Some studies are showing PA as a factor in decreased allergic responses and improved skin healing. PA is also linked to proliferation of cytotoxic T cells and NK cells in people who have herpes.[55] Even though these associations are certainly worthwhile, Pressman and Black acknowledge research limitations between naturally occurring PA and induced PA, which could constitute two different conceptual classes and could produce two different kinds of arousal. Much of the existing research was based on small sample sizes or control groups that were less than ideal; many studies neglected to assess negative affect (NA) for comparison to PA; and some studies did not include "manipulation measurement" to assess for gradation, amounts, or levels.

Psychoneuroimmunological function also relates to sleep and relaxation.[56] One example of proper immune system activity is inducing sleep to mobilize antibodies that counter infection. When infections persist, sleep often becomes interrupted. As a result, inflammatory disorders such as fibromyalgia, chronic fatigue syndrome, and rheumatoid arthritis can worsen, though not consistently. For example, there are some mixed research conclusions in the area of relaxation and immune system support, showing that relaxation generally helps to reduce stress as well as reduce cortisol levels in the body. So, too, relaxation tends to increase sIgA, an antibody crucial for mucosal immune function.[57]

In *Psychoneuroimmunology of Fatigue and Sleep Disturbance: The Role of Pro-Inflammatory Cytokines*, by Shamini Jain, Julienne Bower, and Michael R. Irwin, the authors specifically focus on research that analyzes cytokines, which are immunomodulating proteins and glycoproteins secreted by white blood cells.[58] After citing research acknowledging the prevalence and cost of fatigue and sleep disturbance in the United States—approximately 30-40% of the general population, $136.4 billion dollars in lost productivity, and $92.5-107.5 billion in direct health costs—the authors describe cytokines as responding to local immune responses as well as having an active role in the CNS. They state, "…it is now known that cytokines are secreted by certain classes of brain cells, including microglial cells and astrocytes,"[59] adding that cytokines "…have been found in hypothalamus, basal, ganglia, cerebellum, circumventricular sites, and brainstem nuclei."[60] Although cytokines are too large to cross the blood-brain barrier, there are secondary paths involving secondary messengers, as well as cytokines having the ability to affect peripheral afferent nerve terminals, indicating that cytokines can actually affect the CNS.[61] There is significant research that suggests cognitive-behavioral and mind-body treatment approaches are effective in reducing proliferation of pro-inflammatory cytokines that may contribute to fatigue and loss of sleep. It is useful to consider, however, that pro-inflammatory and anti-inflammatory cytokines can mutually inhibit each other. We should also acknowledge that proinflammatory cytokines contribute to inflammation that aims to destroy or restrict the damaging cause, to begin repairs, and to restore body tissue to its original function levels.

Another area of research that illumines psychoneuroimmunology function is physical exercise and body conditioning.[62] It was well-established decades ago that physical exercise and body conditioning increase leukocyte proliferation, including NK cells, while also improving levels of "…epinephrine, norepinephrine, gonadal steroids, corticosteroids, ß-endorphin, and growth hormone."[63] In contrast, however, physiological responses to exercise or body conditioning appear to exhibit some effects similar to psychosocial stress, trauma, and infection. In this way, physical exercise and body conditioning seem to have a paradoxical result with regard to certain acute-phase proteins, antibodies, and cytokines, in that there are simultaneous pro-inflammatory and anti-inflammatory physiological increases in cyto-kines, Interleukin-1, as well as mutually neutralizing effects of higher cortisol and catecholamine levels. The crucial difference between physical exercise or body conditioning on the one hand and psycho-social stress, trauma, and infection on the other is that the former are positively correlated with improved energy and longevity.[64] Of course, physical exercise and body conditioning are associated with benefits such as controlling weight, improving sleep, enhancing sexual arousal and pleasure, reducing risk of stroke and type 2 diabetes, preventing high blood pressure, increasing HDL or good cholesterol, decreasing risk of cardiovascular disease, managing certain types of cancer, con-trolling certain types of arthritis, sustaining or improving cognitive functioning, decreasing depression and anxiety, and increasing confi-dence and self-esteem, among other medical conditions.

Immune system enhancement is closely tied to nutrition; in fact, the immune system was partially designed to sustain the organism during times when adequate nutrition was not available.[65] Most evi-dence indicates that poor nutrition corresponds to suppressed immune system functioning, yet a preponderance of studies also show that moderately limiting caloric intake actually fortifies immune system function, increasing protection against certain infections and cancers. In contrast, too great of a caloric intake and its results, such as obesity, are associated with compromised immune system functioning.

Antioxidants, vitamins, and minerals are important for immune system support. Antioxidant molecules have the ability to neutralize free radical molecules. Free radicals comprise atoms, ions, or mol-ecules with unpaired electrons. In this instance the "bad" free radi-cals are superoxide and hydroxyl. Free radicals can cause damage to healthy cells and contribute to disease, yet they can also serve a posi-tive function by killing bacteria.

Antioxidants are derived from foods that are rich in vitamin C, vita-min E, zinc, selenium, and beta-carotene. Additional substances that support immune system function include nucleic acids, amino acids, iron, zinc, and magnesium. Absorption of these nutrients is partially dependent upon fluctuation of hormones in the body. For example, insulin hormones secreted by the pancreas exhibit level changes in response to food intake while they simultaneously assist storage of nutrients. Meanwhile, thyroid hormones contribute to a decrease in lipid volume, protein synthesis, and glucose collection. Stress hormones such as glucocorticoids and catecholamines enhance glucose release and lipid metabolization in muscle tissue. Growth hormone influences both an increase and a decrease in glucose and lipids, depending upon the phases of protein synthesis. Like physical exercise and body conditioning, moderation in lipid consumption is key to enhancing immune function. Research shows that while lipids are essential to our diet, immune suppression can occur when they constitute more than 40% of our total caloric intake. At the same time, some lipids exhibit less pro-inflammatory activity.

Before turning to our next section, it seems worthwhile to review aspects of Arnaud Aubert's chapter entitled, "Motivation."[66] On the surface, the concept of motivation can be construed as "...the tendency of an animal to engage in a specific activity at a given time and in certain conditions." Of course the topic is much more complex and dynamic, for motivation also includes "...internal physiological phenomena (i.e., cues such as hunger, thirst, hormones, endogenous rhythms, state of maturation, past experience of the animal) and external signals (i.e., stimuli, releasing factors)."[67] Motivation is variously described as incentive, instinct, need, drive, stimulus, motive, purpose, rationale, impetus, and inspiration. Motivation is also studied by such divergent fields such as business, biology, psychology, education, physics, and religion and philosophy.

Mr. Aubert identifies two perspectives, or stimulus categories, when conceptualizing motivation. The first is behavior that is related to control of physiological homeostasis (e.g., thirst, hunger, sleep, breathing), while the second is behavior that is not related to homeostasis (e.g., play, curiosity, love, career, entertainment). In addition, there are several features of behavior that distinguish a motivational system, including specificity, hierarchy, and flexibility. These categories are used to organize animal research studies. Aubert writes, "Behavioral studies established several psychological and behavioral consequences of inflammation."[68] He continues:

- Common behavioral symptoms of inflammation are not the consequence of a debilitation of infected organisms but, rather, correspond to the expression of a motivational system set up by immune mediators—cytokines—in the brain.

- Inflammation as a motivational system supports recuperative processes and pathogen clearance.
- Inflammation-related behaviors respond to fundamental characteristics of motivational systems with specificity, hierarchy, and flexibility.
- Inflammation as a motivational system is more than a peripheral immune condition but also a central state that influences perception and action.
- This central influence is sustained by emotional and cognitive changes.
- Immune-related behaviors share common mechanisms with other (stress-related) defensive behaviors.
- Inflammation acts as an incentive and interacts with various social motivational systems.[69]

The preceding section examined aspects of psychoneuroimmunology as illustrated by evidence-based research in the following areas: placebo, nocebo, psychological expectations, social engagement, expression of emotion, sleep and relaxation, exercise and physical activity, proteins/antibodies/cytokines, and nutrition. Although empirical inquiry is not always clear or consistent, an overarching trend seems to be that immunological functioning has a reciprocal relationship with healthy lifestyle choices and activities. The significance of exploring this research is to provide insight and empirical validation to connections between psychoneuroimmunology and Joseph Pilates' system of Contrology.

Summary

To achieve a more complete picture of one of Joseph Pilates' primary assertions—that his system of Contrology improves performance of the CNS, immune system function and brain function—it is useful to explore research from chiropractic medicine. There are indeed commonalities between the two disciplines. For example, chiropractic medicine and Authentic Pilates address the fundamental relationships between musculoskeletal structure and functioning as related to the CNS. Similarly, both chiropractic medicine and Authentic Pilates consider CNS activity and immune system activity in relation to overall body functioning. The two disciplines involve systematic spinal variation based upon an integrated set of principles and techniques that preserve and enhance health, emphasizing spinal alignment, spinal conditioning, and optimum spinal range of motion. Finally, chiropractic medicine and Authentic Pilates have a beneficial impact on the interactive functioning between our CNS, immune system, and brain.

It is important to keep in mind that psychoneuroimmunology addresses unity and integration of body-brain systems, rather than specific pathologies or disease categories, although psychoneuroimmunology also gives some attention to pathologies and disease simply as a tool to articulate its primary focus upon health and well-being. The point is that psychoneuroimmunology's primary emphasis is on enhancing the development of knowledge related to physical health, values, and psychophysiological strengths. In addition, psychoneuroimmunology elucidates one of Joseph Pilates' central aims: to sustain and improve immune function by developing, practicing, and teaching the system of body conditioning he called Contrology.

Because psychoneuroimmunology investigates complex interactions among several medical disciplines such as neuroscience, psychology, immunology, medicine, sociology, genetics, and endocrinology—all in the service of understanding, maintaining, and improving health—we find clear parallels with Joseph Pilates' ideas and writings. In his two books, *Your Health* (1934) and *Return to Life Through Contrology* (1945), Pilates explores several areas of inquiry, such as physical and mental conditioning, sociological implications of sedentary living, psychological benefits of maintaining good physical health, the impact of society upon the individual's health, and the importance of maintaining and enhancing one's immune system. Because of his commitment to health and well-being, Joseph Pilates would surely find scientific validation in the modern discipline of psychoneuroimmunology, especially in terms of Jorge Daruna's definition, "...how mental events and processes modulate the function of the immune system and how, in turn, immunological activity is capable of altering the function of the mind."[70] This account of psychoneuroimmunology helps reveal Joseph Pilates' fundamentally holistic system of Contrology, in that the physical benefits of Contrology—improved muscular balance, coordination, strength, stamina, stability, stretching, posture, breathing—are clearly integrated with immunological activity, CNS, and cognitive functioning.

About Peter

Peter began studying Pilates in 1988 and was certified by Romana Kryzanowska in 1998. He continued to train with Romana for many years, then with Kathy Grant. Peter has continued his studies with Jay Grimes whenever possible as well as with other well-respected traditional instructors such as Cary Regan, Anthony Rabara, and Dorothee VandeWalle. Peter loves Joseph Pilates' method of physical and mental conditioning. He is dedicated to teaching and preserving the work. Peter created the ClassicalPilates.net worldwide directory of traditional instructors. Producer and director of the award-winning Classical Pilates Technique DVDs and author of *Discovering Pure Classical Pilates*, he is frequently a guest instructor at training centers throughout the U.S., South America, and Europe. Peter appeared in Romana's first commercial DVD project as well as the DVD titled *Pilates Revealed*, with master teacher Jay Grimes.

REFERENCES

[1] Todd E. Feinberg and Martha J. Farah, *Behavioral Neurology and Neuropsychology*, 2nd ed. (New York, NY: McGraw-Hill Professional, 2003).
[2] Suzanne C. Segerstrom, ed., *The Oxford Handbook of Psychoneuroimmunology*. (New York, NY: Oxford University Press, 2012), xvii.
[3] Jorge H. Daruna, *Introduction to Psychoneuroimmunology*. (Burlington, MA: Elsevier Academic Press, 2004), 1.
[4] Daruna, 7.
[5] Suzanne C. Segerstrom, xvii.
[6] Joseph H. Pilates and William John Miller, *Return to Life Through Contrology*. (Incline Village, NV: Presentation Dynamics, Inc., 1998), 10. Originally Published by J.J. Augustine, 1945.
[7] Joseph H. Pilates and William John Miller, 9-10.
[8] D.S. Goldstein, "Sympathetic Nervous System," *Encyclopedia of Stress*, Vol. 3. (San Diego, CA: Academic Press, 2000).
[9] Joseph H. Pilates and William John Miller, 16.
[10] Adrian J. Dunn, "Interactions between the Nervous system and the Immune System: Implications for Psychopharmacology." (http://www.acnp.org/g4/gn401000069/ch069.html, 2000)
[11] Ilia J. Elenkov; Ronald L. Wilder; George P. Chrousos; Sylvester E. Vizier. "The Sympathetic Nerve—An Integrative Interface between Two Supersystems: The Brain and the Immune System." *Pharmacological Reviews*, 2000, Vol. 52, No. 4 41/865371.
[12] K. King; B. Davidson; B.E. Zhou; Y. Lu; M. Solomonow. "High Magnitude Cyclic

Load Triggers Inflammatory Response in Lumbar Ligaments." *Clinical Biomechanics*, 2009; 25:792-98.

[13]P.M. Fiorentino; R.H. Tallents; J-nH Miller. "Spinal Interleukin-1B in a Mouse Model of Arthritis and Joint Pain." *Arthritis & Rheumatism*, 2008; 58:3100-9.

[14]A. Teodorczyk-Injeyan, and others. "Spinal Manipulative Therapy Reduces Inflammatory Cytokines but not Substance P Production in Normal Subjects." *Journal of Manipulative Physiological Therapy* 2006 (Jan); 29 (1): 14–21.

[15]Steven G. Yeomans, www.spine-health.com/treatment/chiropractic/chiropractic-manipulation, 2009.

[16]J.D. Cassidy; A.A. Lopes, and others. "The Immediate Effect of Manipulation versus Mobilization on Pain and Range of Motion in the Cervical Spine: A Randomized Controlled Trial." *Journal of Manipulative Physiological Therapy*, 1992; 15:570-575.

[17]J.D. Cassidy; Lopes, A.A., and others, 15:570-575.

[18]A.C.J. Terrett and H. Vernon, "Manipulation and Pain Tolerance." *American Journal of Physical Medicine & Rehabilitation*, 1984; 63:217-225.

[19]H. Vernon and P. Aker, and others. "Pressure Pain Threshold Evaluation of the Effect of Spinal Manipulation in the Treatment of Chronic Neck Pain: A Pilot Study." *Journal of Manipulative Physiological Therapy*, 1990; 13:13-16.

[20]P. Shambaugh, "Changes in Electrical Activity in Muscles Resulting from Chiropractic Adjustment: A Pilot Study." *Journal of Manipulative Physiological Therapy*, 1987; 10:300-304.

[21]W. Harris and R.J. Wagnon, "The Effects of Chiropractic Adjustments on Distal Skin Temperature." *Journal of Manipulative Physiological Therapy*, 1987; 10:57-60.

[22]T.A. Tran and J.D. Kirby, "The Effectiveness of Upper Cervical Adjustment upon the Normal Physiology of the Heart." *ACA Journal Chiropractic.* 1977; XI S 58-62.

[23]T.A. Tran and J.D. Kirby, 58-62.

[24]R.G Yates and D.L. Lamping, and others. "Effects of Chiropractic Treatment on Blood pressure and Anxiety: A Randomized, Controlled Trial." *Journal of Manipulative Physiological Therapy*, 1988; 11:484-488.

[25]M.S.I. Dhami and B.A. Coyle, and others. "Evidence for Sympathetic Neuron Stimulation by Cervicospinal Manipulation." in Proceedings of the First Annual Conference on Research and Education of Pacific Consortium for Chiropractic Research, California Chiropractic Association, Sacramento, CA:A5 1-5.

[26]H.T. Vernon and M.S.I Dhami, and others. "Spinal Manipulation and Beta-endorphin: A Controlled Study of the Effect of a Spinal Manipulation on Plasma Beta-endorphin Levels in Normal Males." *Journal of Manipulative Physiological Therapy*, 1986; 9:115-123.

[27]P.C. Brennan and J.J. Triano, and others. "Enhanced Neutrophil Respiratory Burst as a Biological Marker for Manipulation Forces: Duration of the Effect and Association with Substance P and Tumor Necrosis Factor." *Journal of Manipulative Physiological Therapy*, 1992; 15:83-89.

[28]L. Briggs and W.R. Boone, "Effects of a Chiropractic Adjustment on Changes in Pupillary Diameter: A Model for Evaluating Somatovisceral Response." *Journal of Manipulative Physiological Therapy* 1988; 181-189.

[29]Jorge H. Daruna, *Introduction to Psychoneuroimmunology*. (Burlington, MA: Elsevier Academic Press, 2004), 208.

[30]B. Barrett and R. Brown, and others. "Placebo Effects and the Common Cold: A Randomized Controlled Trial." *Annals of Family Medicine*, 2011 Jul-Aug; 9 (4):312-22.

[31]B. Barrett and R. Brown, and others, 9 (4):312-22

[32]B. Klopfer, "Psychological Variables in Human Cancer." *Journal of Projective Techniques*, vol. 21, no. 4. December 1957, 331-340.

[33]S. Cohen; D. Janicki-Deverts; C.N. Crittenden; R.S. Sneed. "Personality and Human Immunity." *The Oxford Handbook of Psychoneuroimmunology* (New York, NY: Oxford University Press, 2012) 146.

[34]S. Cohen; D. Janicki-Deverts; C.N. Crittenden; R.S. Sneed, 146.

[35]S. Cohen; D. Janicki-Deverts; C.N. Crittenden; R.S. Sneed, 147.

[36]S. Cohen; D. Janicki-Deverts; C.N. Crittenden; R.S. Sneed, 150.

[37]S. Cohen; D. Janicki-Deverts; C.N. Crittenden; R.S. Sneed, 153.

[38]S. Cohen; D. Janicki-Deverts; C.N. Crittenden; R.S. Sneed, 155.

[39]S. Cohen; D. Janicki-Deverts; C.N. Crittenden; R.S. Sneed, 155.

[40]Jorge H. Daruna. *Introduction to Psychoneuroimmunology.* (Burlington, MA: Elsevier Academic Press, 2004), 213.

[41]Jorge H. Daruna, 213.

[42]Jorge H. Daruna, 213.

[43]Michael H. Antoni and H. Michael, "Stress Management, PNI, and Disease." *The Oxford Handbook of Psychoneuroimmunology*, (New York, NY: Oxford University Press, 2012) 385.

[44]Michael H. Antoni and H. Michael, 391.

[45]Michael H. Antoni and H. Michael, 396.

[46]Michael H. Antoni and H. Michael, 214.

[47]Roger J. Booth, "Emotional Expression and Disclosure." *The Oxford Handbook of Psychoneuroimmunology*, (New York, NY: Oxford University Press, 2012) 105.

[48]Roger J. Booth, 106.

[49]Roger J. Booth, 106.

[50]Roger J. Booth, 106.

[51]Roger J. Booth, 107

[52]S.D. Pressman and L.L Black, "Positive Emotions and Immunity." *The Oxford Handbook of Psychoneuroimmunology*, (New York, NY: Oxford University Press, 2012), 92.

[53]S.D. Pressman, and L.L Black, 100.

[54]S.D. Pressman, and L.L Black, 100.

[55]S.D. Pressman, and L.L Black, 100

[56]S.D. Pressman, and L.L Black, 214.

[57]S.D. Pressman, and L.L Black, 215.

[58]S. Jain; J. Bower; M.R. Irwin. "Psychoneuroimmunology of Fatigue and Sleep Disturbance: The Role of Pro-inflammatory Cytokines." *The Oxford Handbook of Psychoneuroimmunology* (New York, NY: Oxford University Press, 2012) 321.

[59]S. Jain; J. Bower; M.R. Irwin, 323.

[60]S. Jain; J. Bower; M.R. Irwin, 323.

[61]S. Jain; J. Bower; M.R. Irwin, 323.

[62]S. Jain; J. Bower; M.R. Irwin, 215.

[63]S. Jain; J. Bower; M.R. Irwin, 216.

[64]S. Jain; J. Bower; M.R. Irwin, 217.

[65]S. Jain; J. Bower; M.R. Irwin, 217-220.

[66]Arnaud Aubert. "Motivation." *The Oxford Handbook of Psychoneuroimmunology* (New York, NY: Oxford University Press, 2012) 307.

[67]Arnaud Aubert, 307.

[68]Arnaud Aubert, 315.

[69]Arnaud Aubert, 315-316.

[70]Jorge H. Daruna. *Introduction to Psychoneuroimmunology.* (Burlington, MA: Elsevier Academic Press, 2004), 1.

CHAPTER VI

HISTORY AND APPARATUS

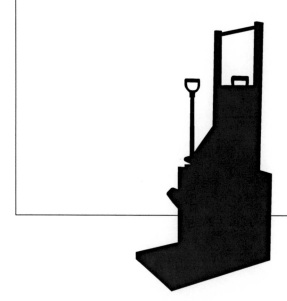

The Inventor

by Kerry De Vivo

...his laboratory was the human body.

Joseph Pilates was an inventor; his laboratory was the human body. He created a vigorous system of body conditioning which necessarily involves mental focus along with physical exertion, called Controlo-gy. Now referred to as Pilates, this integrated system of athletic movement includes over 500 exercises executed on specifically designed apparatus emphasizing uniform development, strength, stamina, balance, breath, precision, stability, concentration, centering, control and flowing movement. Joseph Pilates' apparatus inventions make sophisticated use of simple things, like a studio Mat and springs, that improve the quality and alignment of our bio-mechanical movement patterns as well as our inherent need for intensity, novelty, exertion and equilibrium. With these guiding ideas, Joseph Pilates created an integrated system of exercises that sequentially build upon one another, in addition to diverse studio apparatus that combine to make a unique and comprehensive system. Classical Pilates apparatus and technique exemplify a very high degree of development and expertise in the evolution of body conditioning approaches, even when practicing basic movements. There are scores of wonderful Mat exercises in addition to an enormous range of exercises on apparatus such as the Cadillac, High Chair, Ladder Barrel, Spine Corrector Barrel, Wunda Chair, Magic Circle and Arm Chair.

In present day, Pilates is often presented as the Mat exercises only; but the traditional system requires both Mat and apparatus movement vocabulary as an integrated discipline to mental and physical conditioning. It is widely presumed that Joseph Pilates invented various apparatus to reinforce proper form and articulation of the Mat exercises. Joseph Pilates' studio Mat is an apparatus in its own right. No ordinary mat will do. The studio Mat is raised and has side foot boxes, a dowel rung through both sides for hands to stabilize, as well as a foot strap on the other end. The density and thickness of upholstery has to be precise, enough to support the spine in the many rolling exercises, yet not so plush as to not provide clear sensory feedback. Exercises performed on the Mat can be among the most challenging in the entire system. Deep strength and control are required to perform them correctly.

One of Joseph Pilates' inventions includes the Universal Reformer apparatus. He described the Universal Reformer as "One of the simplest yet most useful pieces of apparatus for all-'round conditioning and corrective work obtainable."[1] Compared to all apparatus, except the studio Mat apparatus, his Universal Reformer is the most widely known; it utilizes springs, a gliding carriage, straps, and a box. The design is simple yet sophisticated, creating a perfect balance between biomechanical science, sport and athletic art form. Early versions of the Reformer had clawed feet; and, like many of his creations, the apparatus was patented. Clearly Joseph Pilates was an inventor and an artisan. A traditional Pilates Reformer provides an opportunity to deepen the Mat work, the foundation of Contrology, through feedback received by the springs and, in some cases, the support of the Reformer carriage. Management of springs, along with concentration, coordination, and precision of each exercise requires a deep sense of physical and mental control as well as practice.

In addition to the Universal Reformer, Joseph Pilates invented other valuable apparatus such as the Foot Corrector, Bean Bag Roll-Up Device, Pedipole, Push-Up Device, Toe Corrector, Breath-O-Cizer, Neck Stretcher, Airplane Board, and many more pieces to support his goal of obtaining physical fitness. Joseph Pilates wrote, "Our interpretation of physical fitness is the attainment and maintenance of a uniformly developed body with a sound mind fully capable of naturally, easily, and satisfactorily performing our many and varied daily tasks with spontaneous zest and pleasure."[2]

Joseph Pilates' studio apparatus provide a wealth of intriguing body experience and conceptually challenging movement in relation to gravity, energy, shape of equipment, balance, stamina, coordination, and so forth. For example, on the Universal Reformer, exercises are performed lying down, sitting up, inverted, prone, rolling on/off, and so on. The physical skill needed in Pilates is evident on the apparatus. Imagine the exercise called Reverse Corkscrew on the Cadillac, or Push Ups (one leg) on the Wunda Chair, Control Balance Step Off on the Reformer, or Jumping Off the Stomach on the High Barrel.

The number of novel and divergent exercises goes on and on. The apparatus and exercises were designed simultaneously, in addition to traditional variations of exercises, making a system suitable for all. Pilates' students had varying physical abilities, and these skill variations are reflected in manifold exercises and divergent apparatus. Take for example the Cadillac, which originated from Pilates' development of the "Relaxor Bed" also called the "Bednasium." Though this piece of apparatus has the versatility to assist those with special needs, it was intended to strengthen and stretch the typical healthy body as well. Similarly tailored to specific needs, the Wunda Chair was created for a client who had a small studio apartment; it converts from a piece of exercise apparatus to a chair.

Contrology "...develops the body uniformly, corrects wrong postures, restores physical vitality, invigorates the mind, and elevates the spirit."[3] To uniformly train the human musculoskeletal system, Joseph Pilates' Method depends upon the ability to guide and control movement. As a result, response to movement impetus becomes crucial, as well as using the will to stabilize certain muscle groups while mobilizing other muscles groups. Control of the apparatus in use, control of breath, and control of the mind are all involved.

Contrology also incorporates oppositional movement, creating a unique dynamics of energy through the body. Utilizing traditional studio apparatus provides important sensory feedback from spring resistance to assist in the discovery and development of oppositional dynamics. This is an excellent means of defying gravity and maximizing the balance of strength and flexibility in muscles. With strong and flexible muscles, it is easier to participate in activities one enjoys: "Constantly keep in mind the fact that you are not interested in merely developing bulging muscles but rather flexible ones."[4]

Most of Joseph Pilates' traditional apparatus utilize springs. Simply stated, springs have two functions: they open, and they close. Muscles also have two functions: they contract, and they release. We can infer the importance of "how" springs are opened or closed, and, how muscles contract or release. This parallel function between springs and muscles is useful to consider. Many people move their bodies through daily tasks and activities without contemplating biomechanics of their movement. For example, from which muscles groups does movement initiate, carry and resolve? Which muscle groups are stabilizing and balancing the body's primary movement being accomplished? How much energy is optimal to accomplish a particular movement, whether it is simply standing vertically from a sitting position, or whether someone is a sports enthusiast who practices swimming, skiing, and playing basketball? By definition, everyone must navigate the body through space on a daily basis, which is a complex endeavor and requires important biomechanical and conceptual skill. We are therefore challenged to constantly learn about, and comprehend, how our bodies move. Classical Pilates occasions us to utilize instinct and critical acuity in the service of coordination. Yet, unfortunately, body and mind can significantly diverge from one another. These challenges make Pilates an exciting discipline that one looks forward to practicing. As improvements in movement patterns, coordination, concentration, and enhanced posture develop, one begins to rely upon Pilates and thrive even more. To sit at a leg press machine and drill repetitions which make muscles contract and release without thought of the depth of movement is a familiar approach to exercise. Pilates challenges us to accomplish far more than isolated muscular movement without actively coordinating all other muscle groups. Throughout the day, nuances of our muscles in various phases of contraction and release find relevance, new energy, and practical usefulness. Pilates challenges us to find length and dynamics in the execution of every action as well as combinations of action. His apparatus assists us to develop our bodies like springs, strong, flexible, articulate, and ideally controlled. Using apparatus with the intentions of Pilates' traditional design preserves the integrity of the work. With sensory feedback from varying amounts of spring resistance, the body gains unique insight about energy, alignment and stretching for intrinsic richness and ability, yet also as applied to specific skilled sports.

Fundamental elements of Contrology can be found in the exercises themselves, the proper relationship to the apparatus, and the layering process of exercises. A traditional lesson should introduce important fundamentals, including the Mat exercises and apparatus exercises. Students learn the proper ways of mounting and dismounting the apparatus; they discover how to initiate from the muscular actions of what Joseph Pilates called our "girdle of strength"; they learn to scoop away from varying spring resistance instead of leveraging peripheral muscles or bones that would replace Powerhouse muscles; they learn that each Pilates exercise is executed for a specific purpose and performed with best effort and few repetitions. We do not repeat an exercise to the point of exhaustion; we do it to the point where we have accomplished its optimal purpose.

The apparatus assists in applying the Pilates principle of centering. Feeling centered and aligned compared to being centered and aligned are not always identical. Traditional studio apparatus, including the studio Mat, provide a symmetrical, balanced, level point of reference for centering and alignment. Most people who practice Pilates find it truly challenging because it reveals their imbalances. As master teacher Romana Kryzanowska would say, "Weakness reveals itself in motion." Working with apparatus makes it difficult to cheat around imbalances. When working with springs, it is quickly apparent when a part of the body exhibits imbalance or less than adequate control.

Consider the principle of centering in relation to initiating movement from abdominals, inner thighs, gluteals, and outer thigh muscles. Take for example, in the Cadillac exercise, Push Through Front. The arms might appear to be the primary working part of the body. However the abdominal engagement moves the spine in the initial rolling back, the arms move in response to the spine, and the Push Through Bar moves in response to the arms. This order of action is maintained throughout the exercise and coupled with oppositional dynamic vs. simple contraction and release of muscles, to maintain control of the apparatus.

To perform the exercises in their intended way, one must focus: "One of the major results of Contrology is gaining the mastery of your mind over the complete control of your body."[5] In addition to achieving new levels of body-brain organization, there are specific ways to position the body in relation to the apparatus for each exercise. For example, there are precise placements of the feet on the footbar on the Reformer, or the hands on the pedal on the Wunda Chair, that are demanded to allow the function of the exercises to be executed correctly and safely. These details require focused attention and intense concentration.

This mind-over-body concept stimulates the nervous system, which in turn aids in repatterning movement and creating uniformity. Working with apparatus requires an intense level of focus. Rules and details must be followed for safety: "The only unchanging rules you must conscientiously obey are that you must always faithfully and without deviation follow the instructions accompanying the exercises and always keep your mind wholly concentrated on the purposes of the exercises as you perform them."[6] The complexity of a Pilates lesson does not permit casual conversation or chatter; this approach cleanses the mind and is a refreshing reprieve in our fast-paced society. It is important to always remember that mind-body control comes from volition, or will, of the participant. As a result, diligent work and dedication breeds empowerment and uplifts the spirit.

How is it possible to create an exercise system for everyone, yet also for each person's needs, idiosyncracies and goals? The inventor, Joseph Pilates, diligently trained in his profession and worked in his laboratory. From a young age, he studied, researched, and experimented with human biomechanics. He designed a system of Contrology that is comprehensive for the typical healthy body, yet the system includes traditional modifications and variations for individuals with symptomatic physical problems. Joseph Pilates described Contrology as a "corrective exercise" system. This system addresses natural physical imbalances for asymptomatic as well as symptomatic individuals. There is a sense in which Contrology can be inherently rehabilitative by providing all individuals with a reliable conditioning system leading toward uniformity and optimal biomechanical functioning. Joseph Pilates' vast collection of Mat and apparatus exercises, in addition to appropriate variations, can help almost everyone improve physical fitness as we can go about our "...many and varied daily tasks with spontaneous zest and pleasure."[7]

About Kerry

Owner of Excel Pilates in Annapolis, Kerry began studying Pilates in 1986 and is a second generation teacher. She was certified by The Pilates Center (1995) and by Romana Kryzanowska at The Pilates Studio (1996). She has a M.F.A. degree in Dance and a B.S. degree in Arts Management. In 1998, she co-founded Excel Movement Studios in Washington, D.C. In 2002, she co-founded Excel Pilates Annapolis. Kerry is co-director of Excel's Teacher Training and Mentor Programs and is co-author of the research study, *The Benefits of The Pilates Method for Shoulder Stabilization in Dancers.*

REFERENCES

[1] Joseph Pilates, How to Look and Feel Like $1,000,000 with the Pilates Universal Reformer. A promotional flyer by Joseph Pilates, (No. 42-Junior Model).
[2] Joseph Pilates and William Miller, *Return to Life Through Contrology*. Edited, reformatted and reprinted (Incline Village, NV: Presentation Dynamics, 1998), 6. Originally published by J.J. Augustine, 1945.
[3] Joseph Pilates and William Miller, *Return to Life Through Contrology*, 9
[4] Joseph Pilates and William Miller, *Return to Life Through Contrology*, 16.
[5] Joseph Pilates and William Miller, *Return to Life Through Contrology*, 9.
[6] Joseph Pilates and William Miller, *Return to Life Through Contrology*, 11.
[7] Joseph Pilates and William Miller, *Return to Life Through Contrology*, 6.

A History of Gratz Industries
By Roberta Brandes Gratz

> *...a combination of "perseverance,*
> *creativity, versatility and luck."*

Gratz Industries, originally known as Treitel-Gratz, opened in 1929 in a small brownstone on lower Lexington Avenue in Manhattan. In the 1930s, it moved slightly uptown to a six-story loft building on East 32nd Street between Lexington and Third Avenues.

The manufacturing and loft buildings on the streets in the East 30s at that time were filled with furniture manufacturers. By the 1960s, an assortment of small manufacturers and esoteric businesses occupied this loft building: a menu printer, bra manufacturer, cabinetmaker, three decorative wood finishers, manufacturer of machines for glove-makers, typesetter, umbrella manufacturer, drapery and slipcover maker, dinette furniture seller, gold stamper, store display maker, and a woman who raised rats. Quite a combination! Some of the businesses worked together on special jobs and were spontaneously and conveniently clustered for the decorating trade. We did metal work for the cabinet-maker and store display maker and used the upholsterer when we needed that work. Everyone did odd jobs for one another. It is difficult to place a monetary or operational value on this kind of synergy.

"By the early 1930s, the company had established itself as the metal shop of choice for, among others, the celebrated industrial designer Donald Deskey,"[1] wrote Charles Gandee in an article about the company entitled, "Heavy Metal" in *The New York Times Home Design Magazine*. Deskey was then doing the celebrated interior furniture for Radio City Music Hall, including the Art Moderne furniture for the office of the great impresario S.L. Rothafel, known as Roxy. Other great industrial designers, like Raymond Loewy with his iconic Coca-Cola machine, George Nelson with his furniture prototypes, and John Ebstein with his toy models for Gabriel Industries, were also customers. The company's history parallels the history of 20th century design.

In 1948, Hans Knoll, a German émigré, wanted to bring the furniture of legendary Bauhaus architect Mies van der Rohe to the U.S. He enlisted the company to engineer and manufacture the Mies line of chairs and tables, now considered classics—Barcelona, Bruno, Tugendhat—all of which were first exhibited at the 1929 International Industrial Exposition in Barcelona. In 1958, architect Philip Johnson turned to Donald for the interior of the Four Seasons Restaurant when it opened in the base of Mies-designed Seagram building on Park Avenue that was also filled with Mies furniture. Johnson was a protégé of Mies and co-architect on the building, and he designed the restaurant interior with Garth Huxtable. That restaurant, a city designated interior landmark, was—and still is—furnished with the classic Mies furniture.

In the 1940s, 50s and 60s, American furniture design was in its heyday. Treitel-Gratz furniture and metal work was going into scores of new office buildings in New York, Chicago, and other cities and suburbs, especially those designed by Gordon Bunshaft of Skidmore, Owings and Merrill.

But aside from the building interiors, Knoll furniture, a line of furniture designed by Nicos Zographos and the industrial design model work, most of Treitel-Gratz's business in the 1950s and early 1960s was actually precision sheet metal for electronic equipment, before that field of work moved to California with the aircraft industry. But as can—and often must—happen in any kind of business, especially manufacturing, as one product line diminishes or moves away, another fills the spot.

This happened for Treitel-Gratz as the art world was transformed in the 1960s. Isamu Noguchi had long been a customer for many of his metal sculptures since the 1940s, but Alexander Liberman was the first of a new group of sculptors who came to Treitel-Gratz not just for its reputation for skillful implementation and metal craftsmanship, but because of its proximity to Manhattan.

People fail to understand the importance of New York City-based manufacturing if they don't recognize the value that industry has to the fields, like art and architecture, for which our city is famous. For designers to be able to implement ideas locally is critical to their craft. Surely it was true for the long line of leading artists, architects, and furniture designers who passed through our factory. We've always been convenient to a subway.

The Changing Art World Changed Us

In the 1960s, Alexander Liberman brought sculptor Barnett Newman to the shop. Newman subsequently brought in a whole group of young Minimalists who were either his friends or protégés, all little known. The Minimalists were changing the nature of contemporary art. Many of them made a big splash with the 1966 Minimalist Show at the Jewish Museum. Donald Judd, Walter De Maria, Sol Lewitt, Robert Rauschenberg, Forrest Myers, Michael Heizer, Robert Indiana, and more. What a cast of soon-to-be stars!

Just as the company history parallels the evolution of interior and industrial design of the 20th century, so does it parallel the evolution of the Minimalist and post-Abstract Expressionist art that emerged in the 1960s, when the center of the art world shifted from Paris to New York. In New York, the art scene shifted from the Upper East Side to SoHo with the new trend in larger and larger artworks and the opening of the Paula Cooper Gallery in 1967. Key artists exhibiting there came to us.

From the 1960s on, office furniture, custom metal work and sculpture dominated. As the field of architecture evolved, so did the content of our production. I. M. Pei, Charles Gwathmey, Robert A. M. Stern, James Polshek, Skidmore, Owings and Merrill and others looked to the company to solve fabrication challenges.

Change is inevitable in manufacturing. One big change with a company like ours can shift the whole picture. In the mid-'60s, Knoll took its business away to its own manufacturing operation in Pennsylvania. At the same time, a new item for production was added. Legend has it that Donald Gratz did some piece work for Joe Pilates before Pilates died in 1967. While no documentation exists to substantiate this idea, the possibility is a good one, since Romana came to Donald not long after Joe's death to make complete machines.

So began a long, productive relationship between Donald and Romana, two people who came to adore one another. The Pilates method was hardly known, let alone the worldwide popular exercise system it is today. Donald and Romana worked out little kinks so the machine produced by Gratz would be precise and perfect. Eventually, Romana refused to train on any machines but those made by us.

In 1955, Donald joined the family custom metal fabrication business, started in 1929 by his father and a partner. Metal fabrication simply means a process by which objects are made out of metal. In the case of Gratz Industries, this means a lot of hand-tooled work. Steel, aluminum and copper, primarily, are bent, drilled, welded, polished and assembled into chairs, tables, architectural elements, Pilates exercise equipment and custom designed objects. None of this is mass-produced. Instead, skilled and semi-skilled workmen individually operate the assorted machines that make up the process. In time, Pilates exercise equipment surpassed custom metal work and furniture as the company's primary product.

Not long after Donald died, David Rosencrans came on as my operating partner. Like many people, he was not familiar with Pilates but learned fast. In fact, he began a regular Pilates workout routine. Ironically, Donald never did. As much as he adored Romana, and as hard as she tried to persuade him to try it, he refused. That did not stop him from recommending that I go to Romana after recovering from a serious car accident in the mid-1980s that left me with some minor but permanent physical disabilities. Reluctantly, I took his advice and was hooked. I have been a regular ever since.

Like many New York manufacturers, our work goes all over the country and abroad. But also, like many local companies, our work is part of the fabric of the city, in homes, museums, offices, building lobbies and in the public realm—Maya Lin's *Eclipsed Time* in Penn Station, the button and needle in the Garment District, the sundial on Staten Island, the Martinelli sculpture on the façade of the UN, the Robert Indiana *LOVE* sculpture at Sixth Avenue and 54th Street, and Bank of America's sculptural logo hanging in the lobby of its new building at 42nd Street and Sixth Avenue. As the city loses businesses like ours, often unnecessarily, the ability diminishes to design or invent and fabricate locally.

The Industrial Network Is Complex

Manufacturers form a complex web of similar and disparate opera-
tors that function both individually and interdependently. The modest
and small scale of most of these manufacturers allows for considerable
flexibility, quick production and innovation. The ability of the designer to participate in the fabrication process can be critical, especially
since so much of local manufacturing is customized work. In 2007 for
example, we fabricated at the behest of Gensler, the national design
firm, a rather complicated floor-to-ceiling bronze screen. Gensler
designers were only a subway ride away to be part of the process.

While "experts" have long been quick to declare manufacturing
dead in New York and other places around the country, many manufacturing companies like Gratz Industries stay very much alive if they
are flexible enough to adjust to changing times and not undermined
by government policies. Too often, industrial districts are declared
"blighted" when many, diversified businesses exist in the seemingly
rundown assortment of industrial spaces.

Few factory buildings or their districts ever look spiffy. Architec-
turally, they range from the design-worthy to the plain. But together they form a comprehensible pattern built over time as industry
evolved. Significantly, industrial neighborhoods contain a mix of scale
that accommodates the large factory or the small job shop with resi-
dential buildings scattered throughout. The mix of buildings and uses
is exactly what sustains the district if not knocked off balance by inap-
propriate rezoning. The uneducated or uncurious observer would be
unaware of what productive businesses exist in such areas that play an
important role in the city's overall economy and social fabric.

To Long Island City

In 1967, Gratz Industries moved across the Queensborough (59th
Street) Bridge from Manhattan to Long Island City, Queens. At the
time, Long Island City, on the east side of the East River, was primarily a manufacturing district, the city's most concentrated industrial
district outside Manhattan. Fully one-third of the district's businesses
had moved from Manhattan. Taking the business out of New York
never tempted Donald. The 32nd Street building was scheduled for

demolition for an Urban Renewal project, and the businesses located in it scattered near and far. The upholsterer moved to Long Island City, too, but several of the businesses from 32nd Street closed for good, years earlier than they otherwise would have. Several left the state. Some would have evolved into a different business, if not fatally disturbed. Undoubtedly, some of them would have disappeared naturally as their markets dried up or they sold out to larger companies but, as can be observed today in similar types of buildings, new businesses would have moved in.

Catherine Rampell notes that many companies manage to reinvent themselves, with a combination of "perseverance, creativity, versatility and luck."[2] She explains that many companies have survived, and some, like IBM, have reinvented themselves many times. Few remember, as she points out, that radio was pronounced dead in 1953 with the advent of television: "But the industry revitalized itself by tapping into new markets," such as "the youth music market, congregating around the car radio...longer-form news and talk radio."[3]

Gratz Industries reflects this pattern, and our production assortment continues to evolve. Some of it stays the same, like the classic modern furniture and Pilates equipment. Some of it continues in a different form; the cast of architects, industrial designers and sculptors changes. New markets open up, like interior work for hotels, high-end retail stores and restaurants in New York and abroad. And who could have predicted a renewed interest in Modernist furniture, giving us an opportunity to again manufacture classic Modernist pieces long out of production? Now Gratz furniture is carried and on display in galleries in New York, Austin, Dallas, Los Angeles, and Chicago. And who could have predicted the global spread of Pilates with our equipment in demand from Sweden, to South America, to Russia?

Some materials, like bronze, or processes, like chrome plating, are too costly to offer easily. And some items are more cost-effective to outsource. But all of these are normal adjustments in any business. Yet, the skills of our 30 workers—machinists, welders, benders, polishers—remain applicable as adjustments come along.

For its 80 years of existence, Gratz Industries has represented the kind of small, individualized manufacturing resource that once sustained New York. The city's once-booming economy was almost entirely based on just this kind of small and medium-size manufacturer. Collectively, the city's manufacturers produced a dizzying and endless array of goods shipped around the globe. Gratz Industries continues this tradition in a robust way and continues to grow and expand the nature of its work. The Pilates equipment, through it all, remains a solid foundation of all of Gratz Industries' production.

About Roberta

Roberta Brandes Gratz, award-winning journalist and urban critic, lecturer and author has published articles in *The Wall Street Journal*, *New York Times*, *The Nation* and others. Her books include *The Battle For Gotham: New York in the Shadow of Robert Moses and Jane Jacobs*, *The Living City: Thinking Small in a Big Way*, and *Cities Back from the Edge: New Life for Downtown*. She was appointed by Mayor Michael Bloomberg to the NYC Landmarks Preservation Commission in 2003 and in 2010 was appointed by the mayor to serve on the Sustainability Advisory Board for PlaNYC. Her family founded and operated Gratz Industries, manufacturers of Pilates equipment.

REFERENCES

[1]Charles Gandee, "Heavy Metal." *The New York Times Home Design Magazine* (April 13, 2003), 153.
[2]Catherine Rampell, "How Industries Survive Change. If They Do." *The New York Times* (November 15, 2008), op ed.
[3]Catherine Rampell.

WORKS CONSULTED

Gandee, Charles. "Heavy Metal." (April 13, 2003). *The New York Times Home Design Magazine*, 153.
Rampell, Catherine. "How Industries Survive Change. If They Do." *The New York Times*. (November 15, 2008), Op ed.

My Journey with Joe

By Richard Rossiter

*He created Contrology for the benefit
and betterment of humanity.*

I was fourteen years old, standing naked in the bathroom, examining my hairdo with the aid of my mother's hand mirror when I discovered a disturbing anomaly. My thoracic spine curved sideways to the right, bent in slightly, then back to the left. I could bend it farther to the right, but try as I might, I could not bend it to the left! At times, I had experienced crippling back pain, but did not know why. Surely this stubborn curvature must have something to do with it, I thought. The back pain came on suddenly every few months. It was so extreme I could hardly breathe, let alone move. I never told my parents about this. It was like a curse that plagued me through my teens, through the military and well into adulthood. In my mid-thirties, I began seeing chiropractors, who finally gave this condition a name: scoliosis. I was adjusted hundreds of times, which helped for brief interludes, but the pain always came back, and with a vengeance. As I grew older, the condition worsened.

In 1966, I joined the military. The war in Vietnam was escalating and the Selective Service was calling upon American men to do their duty. I decided to trump the draft, and volunteered for a six-year tour in the U.S. Army. On August 31, 1966, I arrived at Fort Polk, Louisiana. It was as though I had walked through a door into an alien world: hair cut down to the scalp, rows of bunk bed in a barracks, gas masks, hand grenades, rifles, uniforms, screaming drill sergeants, marching drills. Although I had signed up to be a medic, three weeks into Basic Combat Training, another door opened. On September 24, 1966, I found myself in a small classroom with about ten other recruits selected from other training units. A stern sergeant wearing a Green Beret stood at the front of the classroom.

"Gentlemen, you have been called here based on your performance in your training companies and your aptitude scores. You have been selected to take the Special Forces Test Battery, should you choose to do so. If you pass these five rigorous tests, you may volunteer for Special Forces Training, as well as Airborne School at Fort Benning, Georgia. Most of you will not pass the Test Battery. Maybe one or two of you will go on to complete all the training and those of you who do will wear the Green Beret."

I volunteered to take the exams, passed all of them and went on to Airborne School. I survived sixteen months with Special Forces Training Group, and joined the ranks of the Green Beret. This led me through some wild and bizarre experiences. But here is the point: that damn back pain never let me alone. The demon of my crooked spine tortured me throughout the military. Of course, I never told anyone about it.

It was not until years later that I found lasting relief. During the summer of 1977, I moved to Boulder, Colorado, and became deeply involved in the sport of rock climbing. Eventually, I joined a local gym, Farentinos', and with the help of Bob Farentinos, an Olympic weightlifting champion, I learned to lift weights properly, eventually becoming a personal trainer. This was a case of serendipity or perhaps divine intervention. There, a young man named Stefan Frease was teaching an exercise method called "Pilates" on strange devices he referred to as Reformers. Stefan, a native of Boulder, Colorado, had gone to California to develop a career as a body builder and had been introduced to the Pilates method by Kim Lee, a student of Ron Fletcher. Stefan was deeply inspired by the work, and upon his return to Boulder, convinced Bob to acquire eight Reformers from Current Concepts, Ken Endelman's company. By 1984, Stefan was teaching classes at the gym.

I thought this was a lot of nonsense, but my wife Joyce, a ballet dancer, had heard of Pilates and immediately began taking lessons from Stefan. She lobbied incessantly for me to try it, but I was resistant. When she finally convinced me to give it a go, I found it to be the missing link in my training and understanding of movement. It was deep, powerful and challenging, drawing me into a place of strength and coordination I had not previously experienced. Recognizing its relevance, I continued to take lessons. Among my classmates were Pat Lundgren, Donna McLean, Deborah Robinson and Michael Miller. The five of us flourished under Stefan's instruction, but all good things come to an end. Eventually, he moved on to bigger and better things, taking what he had learned in California to the Aspen Athletic Club. This left Bob Farentinos with a problem. He had a successful Pilates program at the gym and no one to teach it, so he asked Joyce, Michael Miller and me to take over the teaching. Bonnie Von Grebe, another student, became an instructor the following year. We were teachers by default. There was simply no one else who could do it.

There is more complexity to the tale than can be compressed into this telling, so I will give only the backbone. We at Farentinos' Gym came to realize that the Pilates method extended far beyond what we had learned from the now missing Stefan. During the summer of 1988, Deborah Robinson invited Bruce King to Boulder to do a workshop, which I had the good sense to attend. Bruce King was a master instructor who had studied with Joe and Clara and taught at their original studio in New York until 1970. Bruce later opened his own studio at 160 W. 73rd Street, in New York.[1] That weekend, in a gym at the University of Colorado, he introduced us to the advanced Reformer and the Mat repertoire. This was a real eye-opener, as Stefan taught only beginning to intermediate level Reformer.

Mr. King also shared some history of the Pilates method with us. He mentioned that Joe and Clara began teaching in New York about 1926 and that Joe had created many pieces of apparatus to facilitate his system of exercises. We knew so little that an attendee asked if Joseph Pilates was still teaching and if she could take lessons from him. Bruce laughed and said, "Joe is teaching alright…in the big gymnasium in the sky. He passed away in 1967."

He told us that Joe and Clara had trained a number of people who were still teaching the work, particularly Kathleen Grant, Romana Kryzanowska, Ron Fletcher, Eve Gentry and Carola Trier and that we could probably take lessons from them. I decided I wanted to meet these people. At the end of the workshop, we asked Bruce if he would come back to Boulder and teach us more of the work. He responded, "Sure, it just takes time and money." The truth was, Bruce's time was running out and he would soon be joining Joe in "the big gymnasium in the sky."

I continued to teach at the gym, which by 1989 had gone through three owners and as many names, last known as Olympic Health and

Fitness before closing its doors the same year. Joyce became a personal trainer, moved to Crested Butte, Colorado, and opened her own fitness facility called The Gym. Deborah Robinson and Michael Miller went on to a new studio in Boulder called the Pilates Center. Pat Lundgren opened The Centerworks near downtown Boulder. I obtained two of the Reformers from the defunct gym and opened a small studio in the garden-level basement of a friend's house. I never saw Bruce King again and I missed Eve Gentry and Carola Trier for the same reason. They passed away before I could arrange to take lessons from them.

I did, however, go on to study with Romana Kryzanowska, Jay Grimes, Kathleen Grant, Ron Fletcher, Mary Bowen, and Lolita San Miguel, all of whom learned the work from the master himself, Joseph Pilates and his life partner Clara. It was fascinating and enlightening to learn from these great teachers. They each taught the same things, as well as some different things, and enlivened the work with their personalities and unique life experiences. I came to realize that Joe taught his students according to what he felt they needed and according to the potentials he perceived in them. He clearly had his favorites and took some of them farther than others, because he knew they were willing and able to go as far as he could take them. As it goes with human nature, I too had my favorites among these teachers. I would come to wish many times that I could get into a time machine, go back to 1955, walk through the door to the studio at 939 8th Avenue and learn the Pilates method directly from Joe and Clara.

Kathleen Grant, who usually referred to Joe as Mr. Pilates, was among my favorites, and had a profound effect on my understanding of the work and the way I teach it. She could be sweet, hilarious, severe, and ruthless all at the same time. Kathy could have her students laughing, crying and dying simultaneously, executing an exercise so slowly, and holding a position for so long, dying would have been easier. She had a genius for using familiar phrases, situations, imagery, accouterments, and animal behavior to get her students to grasp a movement. Those who were gifted to work with Kathy will be well acquainted with the Green Room, Cats and Kathy's Song (zipper, belt, vest, tape measure). If you didn't know Kathy, you may be thinking, "So what is all that supposed to mean?"

I met Kathleen Grant at the first gathering of the Pilates Method Alliance in South Beach, Florida, 2001, before the PMA was even an organization. It was just an idea. South Beach personifies Art Deco taken to its logical extremes and beyond. I stayed at the Crest Hotel, 1670 James Street in South Beach with other teachers who had come to attend this meeting. My room overlooked the pool, where I spotted an ebullient black lady out on the terrace. That must be her, I thought, so I went out and introduced myself. The lady was indeed Kathleen Grant. We stood face to face, though she was somewhat shorter than I.

I had many questions for her, but I opened with, "What was Joe Pilates like?" Kathleen said, "He was a man much like you, but he had a barrel chest. He was a pugilist, you know." And the conversation developed from there.

From that day on, I went to every one of her workshops that I could arrange to attend. The last time I saw Kathleen was at Pilates on Tour in Denver during the summer of 2007. I taught the opening Mat class for POT, exactly as I had learned it from Romana Kryzanowska. Beth Clark approached me at the end of the class and thanked me for teaching the authentic work. She confided that most of the "Pilates" Mat classes she had attended barely contained exercises created by Joseph Pilates.

Then I went to another room and waited with perhaps 10 other students for Kathleen Grant. I was stretching out on a mat when she walked in. She came right over to greet me. Speaking in part for the others, I said, "Kathleen, it's great to see you again. Thank you for sharing with us. I am so glad to see you." She replied, "I am not so glad, Richard. This may be the last time I do this. I have been teaching for a long time, fifty years. I first went to Joe in 1957. I have done enough."

Kathleen walked to the front of the room and turned to face her students. "I want to start with Cats. Joe always named exercises for animals. Let's do the Weird Cat; he's the new cat in town." We warmed up the shoulders, spine, and hips with Weird Cat, then went on to Restless Cat, Hissing Cat, and Calendar Cat. We did the Hundred with increasingly longer breaths, so that your lungs nearly burst by the end. the Roll Up featured another torture where we had to say out loud our names, addresses and telephone numbers just to roll up, and again to roll down. I had, of course, seen all of this before. Then there was Teaser; just use your imagination. Kathleen asserted, "You have to scare people into alignment!" A more wonderful personality and creative Pilates teacher has never lived.

A Brief History of The Pilates Method

Joseph Hubertus Pilates was born in Mönchengladbach, Germany on December 9, 1883. Recent research[2] indicates that his father was a gymnast or at least had a gym, so the popular stories about Joe being a sickly child with rickets are likely nonsense. He was probably more like my son Raoul, whom I used to take hiking and climbing in the mountains as a youngster. When he was old enough to ride a skateboard, he used to roll around town in a handstand on the board. It was a sight to behold. Joe was undoubtedly more like this than a weakling wobbling around with rickets. Much is now known of Joe's life before he moved to New York in 1926, the details of which are beyond the scope of this essay. It is, however, worthy of note that the various "biographies" of Joseph Pilates are fraught with contradictions and inconsistencies. I give you only the bare bones, a mere outline of the original genius and the resultant teachers, studios and manufacturers from whom I learned the Pilates method, purchased equipment and carried on personal and professional relationships over the last 27 years. Much of the information is from stories told by my teachers, who were students and friends of Joe and Clara. I also gleaned much information from the "Pilates Trademark Trial," *Pilates Inc. v Current Concepts*, June of 2000.[3]

In 1926, Joe opened the original studio at 939 Eighth Avenue, three blocks south of Columbus Circle, at the southwest corner of Central Park, and 23 blocks north of Madison Square Garden (and boxing). The studio was on the second floor, with windows that overlooked 8th Avenue, so that in the summer, with the windows open, there was a lot of noise from the street. There was a small back room that Joe used for rehabilitation and evaluation of new clients. Some of the first generation teachers referred to this as "the sex room." It contained a Wunda Chair and a "Bednasium," later developed into the Cadillac. Joe and his life partner, Clara (Anna Klara Zeuner, born February 6, 1883), lived in a small apartment that adjoined the studio, an easy commute to work. There is good reason to believe that Joe met Clara on a ship called the *Westphalia* during Joe's second trip to the United States in April of 1926.[4] It is documented that Joe had been married twice before in Germany, and had a daughter named Helene from the first marriage. Joe and Clara both declared themselves as single on their naturalization papers. Recent research has uncovered no trace of a marriage license.[5]

As a young man, Joe was keenly interested in physical fitness, especially in gymnastics and boxing. He also had knowledge of swimming, weight lifting, and possibly yoga. He was deeply inspired by the Athenian Ideal, that is, the perfect development of body, mind, and spirit, held in god-like reverence by the ancient Greeks. It is told that Joe traveled with a circus, and had an act wherein he appeared as the "live human Greek statue."[6] He was working as a prizefighter in England when WWI broke out (1914), and being a German national, was placed in an internment camp, first in Lancaster, and then on the Isle of Man. It is here, as a prisoner of war, that Joseph Pilates conceived of and developed, the basic exercise system that he called Contrology, or the Art of Control. With very limited resources, he practiced floor exercises and used bedsprings for resistance training.[7]

The Equipment

The Mat work is the heart of the Pilates method. The uninitiated tend to believe that the Mat is the beginner work, then you move on to the apparatus. This view is perfectly backwards. All of the apparatus was created to support the Mat; because the Mat is so difficult, most beginners can barely perform any of it.

Joe probably built most of the early apparatus himself, including the Universal Reformer, Cadillac, Spine Corrector, Tens-O-Meter (later replaced by the Magic Circle) and the Pedi-Pole. Only minor changes were made to most of the apparatus during the course of Joe's life. The Spine Corrector had wooden side panels with metal handles, very much as it is made today by Balanced Body, though the handles have been replaced by hand slots cut into the side panels. The first design for the Reformer had a very tall frame. A stack of iron plates supplied resistance by a pulley at the footbar end of the frame and a rope attached to the carriage, in the manner of modern weight lifting equipment. This design was abandoned, and probably never built.[8] In its place, the frame was lowered and springs were installed to provide resistance to movement of the carriage.

It is said that he contracted his brother Fred to build the pieces commonly seen in the old films and photographs taken at the 939 Studio. It is known that Joe licensed Atlas Athletic Equipment Company of Saint Louis, Missouri[9] to build the Wunda Chair and the Home Reformer. The latter was a low-slung, inexpensive version of the Universal Reformer, designed for people to use in their homes. A few companies still build the Wunda Chair, which can be used as an actual chair and flipped 90 degrees for exercising. The Home Reformer was re-produced in the 1990s by Stamina Products under license with Pilates, Inc. and was called the Pilates Performer. I.C. Rapoport took some wonderful photographs of Joe at the 939 Eighth Avenue studio in October of 1961.[10] A watchful eye will notice what appears to be aluminum Reformers very similar in design to those built a decade later by Gratz Industries, LLC. Who built these Reformers?

An old film shows Clara sitting in the Wunda Chair, reading a newspaper in the living room of their NYC flat. Joe walks in from the left and bows as though to say, "Excuse me, Madam, it's time for my workout!" Clara jumps up and steps out of the way. Joe then flips the chair, so that the backrest is on the floor, hooks up the springs and launches into a workout routine, while Clara looks on. Why wasn't Clara doing the workout? Most of the first generation teachers say they never saw Clara do any exercises. This is a mystery. Kathleen Grant said, "Joseph Pilates was a man and he created the exercises for men."

So where did all the women come from? Dancers! Professional dancers came to Joe to get help with an injury and to strengthen their bodies. Many of these dancers were women, some of whom went on to teach what they had learned from Joe and Clara. They in turn attracted more women to the Pilates method.

The Tower is another device intended for home use. It was designed as a kit that could be set up in a doorjamb, hence the nickname, "A Gym in a Doorway."[11] The kit consisted of two horizontal bars of 1-inch steel: one fixed to the frame near the top and another that slid along tracks attached to the sides of the doorframe. Resistance for the moveable bar was provided by springs that could be attached to a base plate or the top bar.

Joe had a freestanding version of the Tower in his studio that was set up in a frame made of 2" x 10" boards (the doorjamb) that were held in place by chains bolted to the floor. The overall effect resembled the "Tower end" of the Cadillac separated from the table and made to stand on its own. The significant difference is that the movable bar of the Tower travels along a vertical plane, where the Cadillac's push-through bar travels in an arc. Later versions of the Tower were suspended between two metal rails that ran from the floor to the ceiling and based on its appearance was nicknamed the Guillotine Tower. This is the only version that was ever manufactured commercially. The Tower is an ingenious apparatus with its own repertoire of exercises. Sadly, it is the least known of Joe's important inventions, presumably because it must be affixed to the floor and the ceiling and because only three of Joe's students, Romana Kryzanowska, Jay Grimes and Ron Fletcher, chose to carry on with it. Balanced Body built about a dozen units at the request of Ron Fletcher. I have one of these. Gratz Industries still builds the Tower.

What about those barbells? Many Pilates teachers like to point out that weightlifting is bad for you. "Joe didn't lift weights!" they insist. However, you don't have to be Sherlock Holmes to notice a rack with three barbells backed up against the mirrors in old photos of the 939 Studio. If Joe didn't lift weights, why did he have three barbells in his studio? Maybe they were there just to hold down the carpet! What we do know about Joe is that he taught Contrology. He believed passionately in his work and felt strongly that everyone should do it. He created various advertisements and fliers for his home exercise equipment, complete with instructions for use. His vision extended far beyond the professional dancers who comprised the majority of his clientele. He created Contrology for the benefit and betterment of humanity. "Physical fitness is the first requisite of happiness,"[12] Joe wrote in *Return to Life through Contrology*, published in 1945.

It is known that Joe was mistrustful of government. He had blueprints drawn of his inventions and registered patents for each of them, but he never registered his business with any government agency including the IRS. The 939 Studio had a glass door with black lettering that read, "Contrology, Art of Control, Pilates' Studio, Joseph Pilates" in four descending levels.[13] That was it.

The first business registered under the name Pilates was a nonprofit corporation founded by Ralf Hollander, the Pilates Foundation for Physical Fitness, to which Joseph Pilates granted the right to use his name and equipment in 1964. The foundation was defunct before 1967, but was never dissolved.[14] Joe established a second studio at the Henri Bendel department store in 1965. Naja Corey, who was trained at the 939 Studio, taught at Bendel's from 1967 to 1972, when Kathleen Grant took over, and ran the studio until it closed in 1988.[15]

Teachers and Studios

Kathleen Stanford Grant had an illustrious career as a dancer and choreographer, but suffered a knee injury that cut short her career. She began working with Joseph Pilates in the mid-1950s. Joe called her "Kay" and kept her on the Wunda Chair in the small room to heal her knee injury. She was not permitted to train in the main studio until she had mastered the Wunda Chair. Thus Kathy became known as the master of the Chair. She and Lolita San Miguel were certified by Joseph Pilates to teach his method of exercise as part of a New York State educational program that paid for their training and required a certificate of completion. Joe did not customarily issue teaching certificates. He did train some of his clients to be studio assistants and independent teachers. Some, such as Eve Gentry, Romana Kryzanowska, Bob Seed, Hanna (no one remembers her last name) and Bruce King, taught at the 939 Studio while others opened their own studios. Kathleen Grant taught at Henri Bendel's and in 1988 relocated to the Tisch School of the Arts at New York University. Her studio was on the top floor and was known affectionately as "The Penthouse." She continued to teach at Tisch until her death on May 27, 2010.[16]

Lolita San Miguel has taught the Pilates method for fifty years. She was first certified by Carola Trier and then went on to work with Joseph Pilates himself, by whom she was certified along with Kathleen Grant. Most of Joe's students were dancers and Lolita was no exception. She was a soloist with the Metropolitan Ballet for more than ten years and ballet mistress for the Ballet Hispanico for three years. In 1977, Lolita moved to Puerto Rico, founding the Ballet Concierto de Puerto Rico, where she served as the artistic director and executive director for twenty-eight years. After retiring in 2004, she devoted her time and energy to the teaching of the Pilates method. Certified by Polestar Pilates Education and founder of Pilates y Mas, Inc. in Puerto Rico, she trains and certifies teachers in association with Polestar.[17]

Carola Trier was a professional dancer, acrobat and contortionist who, like nearly all of the first generation teachers of the Pilates method, came to Joseph Pilates with an injury. Joe performed his "magic," quickly healed Trier, as he had done for many others, and she became a believer. She opened her own studio in the late 1950s at 200 West 58th Street, #12B with the approval and assistance of Joe himself. Carola trained many students in the Pilates method up until her death in October of 2000.[18]

Eve Gentry, one of Joe's favorite students, taught at the 939 Eighth Avenue studio from 1938 to 1968. Clara wrote to Eve on December 6, 1968, "I always wished and hoped you could have taken the studio over." She wrote again on March 7, 1973, "How glad I was to see you! Because you, too, belong to the Pilates." (Troy E. R. Gordon, Pretrial Report, Introduction. Charlotte, VT: 2000. p. 4.)

Eve moved to Santa Fe, New Mexico in 1968 and taught many people who went on to become Pilates teachers. Among these was Michele Larsson who began studying with Gentry in 1970 and with her began a teacher certification program at the Eve Gentry Studio. In the early 1990s, Gentry along with Larsson and Joan Breibart formed the Institute for the Pilates Method, which sought to carry on the mission of the Pilates Foundation for Physical Fitness, Inc., bringing together the master teachers Eve Gentry, Ron Fletcher, Bruce King, Romana Kryzanowska and Carola Trier.[19] Eve continued to teach the Pilates method in Santa Fe and around the world until her death in 1994.[20]

Ron Fletcher writes in a biographical sketch dated May 21, 2001, "It's hard for me to imagine how I could begin my life as a boy in Dogtown, Missouri and end up in New York City with Martha Graham and Joe and Clara Pilates as teachers. I think there is a higher power that leads us to our path and that perhaps little is left to random chance."[21] Ron went to New York in 1944 and found a job in advertising at Saks Fifth Avenue. He attended a dance performance by the Martha Graham Company and decided that is where he wanted to be. Martha took him in and he began to practice, rehearse and perform. Before long, he developed knee problems. A fellow dancer suggested he take lessons from Joe Pilates and he did.

Joe put Ron on the Reformer, where he could build supporting strength for the knee and develop the Powerhouse, core support for the pelvis and spine. Ron says,

> "The work (Contrology) was constantly evolving and Joe often used me to try some piece he wanted to see on a body that was beginning to show the Pilates training. I continued working with Martha Graham during this time, treading carefully between these two brilliant visionaries with enormous egos, who were both proprietary about their male students. I learned a lot — not only extraordinarily beautiful movement, but how to perform it correctly from deep within the body, with spirit and with brio, finding my way to an understanding of the concepts and philosophies of these two incomparable teachers."[22]

Ron stayed on with Clara after Joe's death. "There is far to go with this work," she wrote in a letter. "This is just the tip of the iceberg. This work is in your blood. You are the man to create and develop it from this point on. Go and do, just always remember the A, B, and Cs."[23] Ron taught the whole body of the original work, however, a lesson with Ron was a rather different experience from a lesson with Romana Kryzanowska or Jay Grimes. In my opinion, the essence of Ron Fletcher's movements were identical, while the overall picture of the work was quite different.

In 1971, Ron went west and opened a studio on the corner of Rodeo Drive and Wilshire Boulevard in Beverly Hills. It was called the Ron Fletcher Studio for Body Contrology. He was in the right place at the right time and the studio was very successful. Ron went on to teach throughout the United States and worldwide. His work is a synthesis of his time with Joe and Clara, Martha Graham, Yeichi Nimura and his career as a dancer and choreographer. Ron created the Towel Work to stabilize the arms and shoulders during movement and he developed a unique way of using the breath that he calls Percussive Breathing. His teaching on the Pilates apparatus is excellent and is highly choreographed. The classical work is woven throughout his teaching, but it is linked by connecting movements he calls "gozintas" or this goes into that. Ron notes, "I sought to create a piece of movement rather than just a series of exercises."[24] He calls this whole picture The Ron

Fletcher Work. In my opinion, Ron is a brilliant teacher and a wonderful, warm-hearted human being. He often said of his teachers, Joe and Clara Pilates and Martha Graham, "People like this should never die. The world needs them!" I say the same of Ron, who sadly passed from this life December 6, 2011.

Robert Fitzgerald was a student of Joe and Clara. He taught at the 939 Studio, opening a studio on West 56th Street in the 1960s, where he developed a large clientele of dancers. Alan Herdman was among his students.[25]

Bob Seed was a hockey player who trained with Joe and Clara and taught at the 939 Studio along with Romana Kryzanowska, Bruce King and Hanna. Mary Bowen speaks of working with Bob Seed at the 939 Studio, and says that he opened his own studio in Manhattan as did Carola Trier.

Mary Bowen began working with Joe and Clara in 1959. She was a comedienne and actress when she came to study with them. Suffering from a bad back, she began to feel relief after just two sessions. Mary studied with Grant and Kryzanowska, as well as with Bruce King, Bob Seed and Hanna. In 1975, she opened her own studio, Your Own Gym, in North Hampton, Massachusetts.[26] A Jungian analyst, she developed her Pilates plus Psyche system to fuse movement with the unconscious.[27] You can learn more about Mary by visiting her website, or attending her workshops. John Winters was a musician, an organist, who taught at the 939 studio, and is described by Jay Grimes as Joe's "right-hand man."

Jay Grimes was a professional dancer. He worked with Neville Black, Boston Ballet, American Ballet Theatre and eventually performed in Broadway musicals. Jay suffered some imbalances from a mild case of polio as a child. When he took his first ballet class in New York in 1964, his teacher told him he should see Joe Pilates, so he did. Jay went on to dance for eighteen years without an injury, which he attributes to his study of the Pilates method. He worked with Joe through his last years, then continued with Clara until her death, teaching at the original 939 Studio, later moving with the studio to 56th Street, where he taught and studied with Romana Kryzanowska and John Winters.

Jay's clients have included the stars of Broadway, Hollywood, music and opera, as well as politicians, businessmen, Olympic athletes and ordinary mortals. He currently provides continuing education for Pilates teachers and dedicated students around the world.

We were fortunate to have Jay teach a workshop at our studio in Boulder in 2009 and I continue to attend his workshops and take private lessons at his Vintage Pilates studio[28] in Santa Monica, CA. He had much to say regarding the many changes manufacturers have made to the equipment, "Change the body, not the equipment!" The important thing is to, "Get your ass on the machine and move!" He went on, "There is too much pampering and watering down of the work these days. Joe just kicked your ass. He didn't care who you were."[29]

Romana Kryzanowska (1923-) was a professional dancer in New York City Ballet, with George Balanchine as artistic director, and was referred to Joseph Pilates for an ankle injury in 1941. She trained and studied with Joe and Clara until 1944, when she married and moved to Peru. Returning to the United States in 1959, she went right back to the 939 Studio and continued to study and teach with Joe and Clara. Romana is a sage and inspiring teacher of the authentic Pilates method. Joseph Pilates adored Romana and passed on to her all that he could before the end of his life. No one is closer to the original work and no one has had a more profound influence on me as a Pilates teacher than Romana Kryzanowska.

When Joseph Pilates passed away in October of 1967, he did not have a will. After his death, Clara continued to teach at the studio. In 1970, friend and attorney John Steel, a student of Joe and Clara, formed the 939 Studio Corporation, whose purpose was to own and operate the studio and provide support for Clara. Romana Kryzanowska agreed to take over the responsibilities of running the business. In or around 1972, the operation moved from 939 8th Avenue to 29 West 56th Street in New York City. The studio changed its name on June 4, 1973 to the Pilates Studio, Inc. and Romana Kryzanowska became a 50% shareholder. Three years later, Anna Klara Zuener died. From 1979 to 1984, the business referred to itself as the "Pilates Studio for Body Conditioning." On December 8, 1980, Pilates Studio, Inc. filed for a service mark in the name "Pilates" for providing facilities for exercise and physical conditioning. Pilates Studio, Inc. claimed exclusive right and a date of first use of 1923, predating the immigration of Joseph and Clara to the United States! The Pilates Studio, Inc. applied for a second trademark on February 9, 1981 for providing facilities for exercise and physical conditioning. Both registrations were later cancelled.[30]

Pilates Studio, Inc. underwent yet another transformation when Lari Stanton, the principal of Aris Isotoner Gloves, Inc., purchased the assets in 1984, changing the name to "Isotoner Fitness Center." Stanton executed a trademark application requesting a trademark for "Pilates" to protect a method of exercise. The application was rejected and Stanton's attorneys revised the application to read "exercise instruction services" rather than "a method of exercise." Isotoner Fitness Center advertised its product as "STRETCH-ERCISE, a new way of being good to your body, developed at the Isotoner Fitness Center - a Pilates exercise facility." During this time, Romana Kryzanowska was employed to teach there. Within a few years, however, the business was losing money, so Stanton decided to sell it.[31]

Fortunately, a buyer appeared in 1986. Wee Tai Hom, a student of Romana Kryzanowska, purchased the trademarks and complete assets from Aris Isotoner. He formed a company called Healite, whose purpose was to sell specialty foods and other "health-related" products. The studio moved to a new location at 160 East 56th Street, operating under the name The Pilates Studio until 1989. By 1988, Hom created a subsidiary company called "Pilates Studio, Inc."

Healite retained Romana Kryzanowska as an independent contractor and began a teacher training program. Instructors included Moira Stott, Steve Giordano, Bob Liekens, Phoebe Higgins, Cary Regan and others. "The 'test' or final exam consisted of being videotaped by Hom while demonstrating Pilates exercises with Romana as the "instructor."[32] Among the graduates were Sari Pace, Hila Paldi and later the Taylor sisters. Like its predecessors, financial success eluded them. Healite ceased operation, closing its doors "due to financial difficulties" on April Fools' Day, 1989.[33] Hom referred his clients to Sichel Chiropractic, Body Art Exercise, Ltd. and The Gym, setting up a schedule for his instructors to begin work at the latter two facilities. The equipment from the East 56th Street studio was distributed among all three businesses.[34]

Romana Kryzanowska went on to teach briefly at Body Art and in 1989 settled into a more suitable and enduring relationship at The Gym, owned by a gymnastics teacher named Dragutin "Drago" Mehandzic. Romana taught the Pilates method as an employee of The Gym, whose name was later changed to Drago's Gym.[35] It was here that I learned a great deal of what is now called classical Pilates - the original, unaltered method and repertoire of exercises. I traveled to New York off and on from 1997 to 2001 and took lessons directly from Romana and sometimes from her daughter, Sari Pace.

I also took a few lessons and sat in for observation with Alycea Ungaro, who at the time, owned Tribeca Body Work, which became Real Pilates. Alycea was trained by Romana Kryzanowska and is a wonderful teacher who has stayed true to the original work. At that time, the World Trade Towers still scraped the Manhattan sky a few blocks south of her studio. Pausing one day to take a photograph of the towers down Greenwich Street, I had no idea that later the same year they would be destroyed.

Boulder and Beyond

In 1992, Romana and her student/protégé Steve Giordano visited Boulder at the request of Amy Taylor Alpers and Rachel Taylor Segel, "The Sisters." For a short time, Steve was a co-owner with the Taylor sisters of The Pilates Center in Boulder, which opened for business in November of 1990. Romana taught and certified a few students at the Pilates Center on behalf of an entity known as Synergy Exercise Systems, a corporation owned jointly by Steve Giordano and Sean Gallagher. Synergy was in a sense a merger of their previous businesses: New York Institute of Movement Science and Performing Arts Physical Therapy, respectively.[36]

Founded in 1990, Synergy Exercise Systems' primary purposes were the training of Pilates teachers and the manufacturing of Pilates equipment. At about the same time, Gallagher and Giordano established the Pilates Guild, which was to serve as an umbrella organization for teachers certified and licensed by Synergy.[37] Romana was teaching for Synergy as an independent contractor. In June of 1992, Gallagher and Giordano reached an agreement to part company, but Romana stayed on with Gallagher. Steve remained in Boulder, opening his own enterprises to do exactly the same thing: train Pilates teachers and build Pilates equipment under the name Movement Science. He set up the Movement Science studio above the old Harvest Restaurant at 18th and Pearl Street, a few blocks east of the Pearl Street Mall and rented warehouse space to build equipment off of North Broadway, near a topless gentlemen's club called The Bustop. Movement Science used as its logo the Golden Rectangle and Fibonacci Spiral.

Steve Giordano was a substantial craftsman, from whom I purchased several pieces of apparatus between 1993 and 1996. With the equipment sales, he offered Pilates lessons, which I gratefully accepted, finding him to be a skilled and insightful teacher. One day in 1993, I went to his shop to pick up a Reformer. Steve handed me a Reformer Box and led me through the back of the shop, loading the box with pads, straps, foot loops, handles, a three-foot maple dowel, all of the items customarily used with the Reformer. Suddenly he stopped and looked straight at me, speaking low, as though divulging classified information. He said that Sean Gallagher had obtained trademarks for the name Pilates and Exercise Instruction Services and he was planning to file suit against anyone using the name Pilates or teaching the exercises created by Joseph Pilates. Although he and Gallagher had been partners, he confessed the association did not go well, and that was why he did not use the name "Pilates" in his current business ventures.

Steve changed the name of the Pilates equipment business to Solid Woodwork and, in 1996, hired a highly skilled and experienced craftsman, Vic Hart, as his chief builder. He subsequently sold Solid Woodwork to one of his students, Julie Lobdell, abandoned the teacher training program at Movement Science, and went back to New York without graduating a single student.

Julie was a brilliant and experienced businesswoman, who had a far-reaching vision for the company. She brought on Michael Arbuckle, a Pilates equipment manufacturer from Texas, as a partner, retained Vic Hart as chief of manufacturing and proceeded to develop and expand the business under the name Progressive Dynamics, Inc. I always thought the name sounded more like an aerospace company than a Pilates equipment manufacturer, but this was obviously an attempt to ward off the wrath of Sean Gallagher and his attorneys. Julie soon changed the name of the company to Progressive Body Systems and later to Peak Pilates, which was purchased by Mad Dogg Athletics, Inc., the "Spinning" people, in 2009. Hart Wood, Inc., in response to the buyout, began manufacturing its own line of laminated bamboo Pilates equipment under the name Root Manufacturing.

The genesis of Pilates studios and equipment manufacturers is one of continual change, innovation, upheaval, mergers and buyouts. The following news release exemplifies the mercurial dynamics of the Pilates marketplace:

VENICE, Calif. (November 2, 2010) – Mad Dogg Athletics, Inc. announced today that Vic Hart, founder and president of Root Manufacturing and Hart Wood, Inc., will join Peak Pilates as interim president. Hart's appointment follows a longstanding manufacturing relationship with Peak Pilates and Mad Dogg Athletics' recent strategic investment in Hart Wood.

Hart replaces Julie Lobdell, founder and former president, who has transitioned out of the company. Peak Pilates was founded by Lobdell in 1996 and expanded from a local Pilates equipment manufacturer into a worldwide supplier of wood and metal equipment and provider of Pilates education. In early 2009, Peak Pilates was acquired by Mad Dogg Athletics, Inc., creator of Spinning®.

Hart is no stranger to the Pilates industry, founding Hart Wood, Inc. to manufacture Pilates equipment for Peak Pilates in 1996 and introducing Root, the industry's first eco-friendly and sustainable line of bamboo equipment in 2009. With the recent investment in Hart Wood by Mad Dogg Athletics, the Root line of equipment will be exclusively available through Peak Pilates.[38]

Mark Spenard is another Boulder area craftsman who began building Pilates equipment around 1990 and has continued production to the present time. Spenard's company was never a licensee of Pilates, Inc. and is another example of the many pre-existing Pilates businesses that did not want to be regulated and franchised by Pilates, Inc.

The Pilates Trademarks

It would be convenient to avoid any mention of Sean Gallagher's influence on the development of the Pilates method in Boulder, Colorado and elsewhere, but this is not possible. Sean, a physical therapist, was taking lessons once or twice a week from Romana Kryzanowska by 1989 or 1990. Sean, with Steve Giordano, developed a plan that would affect every Pilates teacher and studio in the United States.

On August 3, 1992, Gallagher purchased two trademarks from Healite, Wee-Tai Hom's company, under an asset purchase agreement: one for the names Pilates and Pilates Studio and another for Exercise Instruction Services. Gallagher also acquired the studio's archives, which included photographs, business records, client lists, books, films and other documents dating back to the 1940s.[39]

Gallagher formed Pilates, Inc. in 1992 and in June of 1994, assigned the Pilates marks to Pilates, Inc. He applied to register a third trademark in September of 1992 for the manufacture and sale of Pilates equipment. The application was denied in March of 1994, but Gallagher filed again five months later in response to the PTO denial of the original application. He stated in this submission that the PILATES equipment mark had been used in commerce continuously and exclusively since 1923 and specifically for five consecutive years prior to the registration application.[40] These representations were knowingly and materially false. Gallagher knew, but did not advise the PTO, U.S. Patent and Trademark Office, that Donald Gratz, Ken Endelman, Steve Giordano, and others had been and still were building Pilates equipment without a license from anyone, because no such trademark existed. The Pilates equipment mark was eventually granted in 1995. After purchasing the Pilates marks, Pilates, Inc. entered an agreement with Ken Endelman, under which Current Concepts manufactured Pilates equipment and sold it to Pilates, Inc. for resale. This agreement, however, was of short duration.[41]

By this time, there were hundreds of people across the country, including those trained by Joseph Pilates himself, teaching the Pilates method without a license. Gallagher's plan was to enforce his trademarks, and bring all Pilates businesses under financial obligation and rule of his new enterprise, Pilates, Inc., a Montana corporation with offices at 890 Broadway and 2121 Broadway in New York City. Gallagher soon developed a formal teacher certification program, headed by Romana Kryzanowska, who was employed as an independent contractor in 1993.[42]

Pilates, Inc. began to vigorously enforce its trademarks since it acquired them, and sent hundreds of cease and desist letters to purported infringers and sued for trademark infringement in several cases. The stated purpose for this action was to protect the original teachings of Joseph Pilates from genericide, destroying the value of the marks in bad faith. In 1996, Pilates, Inc. filed suit against Current Concepts, Ken Endelman's company, on three counts of trademark infringement:[43]

> "Plaintiff's theory of the case is that only Pilates, Inc. is teaching the Pilates method the way Joseph Pilates taught it and that everyone else is teaching something different, even dangerous. The facts, however, actually support another theory: that Joseph Pilates never wrote down the proper way to do his exercises or practice his method other than a small book describing Mat exercises (*Return to Life through Contrology*); that Joseph Pilates taught a number of students who went on to open their own studios; that "Pilates" was used by Joseph Pilates and his students to describe a method of exercise, not a brand name of Exercise Instruction Services; and that the plaintiff (Gallagher) is trying to make others speechless by taking away the only word that is used in the industry to describe Joseph Pilates' exercises and method."[44]

Cease and Desist

Pilates, Inc. sent out cease and desist letters to hundreds of Pilates studios and teachers across the country, threatening legal action against any individual or any business using the Pilates Marks.

I received such a letter on a sunny afternoon, October 18, 1996, as I arrived at World Gym, where I had been teaching the Pilates method as an independent contractor since it opened in 1995. This gym was the same place, formerly occupied by Farentinos' Gym, and five subsequent health clubs, which had tried and failed to prevail over the crushing overhead of the retail space at 693-K South Broadway in Boulder.

I went upstairs to the solarium. The Pilates studio was set up in a beautiful room with glass on two sides and part of the ceiling. It housed four Reformers, a Ladder Barrel and a Wunda Chair, all built by Steve Giordano, as well as a Current Concepts Reformer crafted of knotty pine that had survived from the original Farentinos' Gym. The west wall was entirely glass with a door that opened onto a wooden deck. Bear Peak, Green Mountain and the famous Flatirons were just a stone's throw away to the west. When I arrived, no one was teaching. I had the room to myself. The place could impart a real sense of solitude, despite the clanging of weights, pounding of feet on the treadmills and the relentless drone of pop music that flowed up the stairwell from the main floor of World Gym. It was almost quiet with the door closed. Stefan Frease had introduced me to the Pilates method in this same room in 1985.

I sat down on a Reformer and read the letter from Kalow, Springut & Bressler several times. The document consisted of two pages, but it felt like an enormous weight in my hands. Just outside the window, the Flatirons shone in the sun. A few white clouds were suspended in the autumn sky above the mountains. I recalled the moment, three years earlier in Giordano's sawdust covered shop when he warned me of this eventuality.

The law is the law, I thought, but somehow this just doesn't feel right. Pilates is arguably the greatest and most relevant exercise system ever created. It is simply too important to be tethered and monopolized by one person, who in this case, never took a single lesson from Joseph Pilates and who began enforcing his alleged trademarks 25 years after Joe's death.

I was not the only one to perceive the contrived stretch of law behind Gallagher's position: "Any efforts made by plaintiff to police the marks or increase their value was too little, too late and in any event irrelevant."[45] I decided I was not going to just lie down and let Sean Gallagher run over me.

Through the internet, I learned that Ken Endelman intended to fight the lawsuit and had filed a class action complaint against Pilates, Inc. seeking cancellation of the Pilates Marks. So I gave him a call. This was back in the day when Current Concepts, later Balanced Body, was pretty small and you could get Ken Endelman himself on the phone.

Ken confirmed that he had indeed filed a counter claim against Gallagher to have the trademarks cancelled. I informed him that I was planning to open a new studio in Boulder and register the business name as Pilates of Boulder, Inc. Ken advised me to proceed in defiance of Gallagher's legal threats and said that it would serve to strengthen their case when it went to trial. I knew that "The Sisters" at the Pilates Center were also operating in defiance of Pilates, Inc., as was Michael Miller, who had left the Pilates Center and was teaching out of his townhome. Boulder had become something of a mecca for the Pilates method. There were no fewer than fifty people teaching the work and at least two companies building Pilates equipment in the Denver-Boulder area by 1996.

The war was on and the propaganda volume ratcheted up. Much of this drama was documented in *The Pilates Guild News*, *Pilates News*, *The Pilates Trademark Cancellation Newsletter* and an internet forum, list@bodymind.net. *The Pilates Guild News* was Sean Gallagher's publication. The main thrust of the Spring/Summer 1996 edition was to illustrate the great importance of Pilates Inc.'s ownership of the trademarks and of the resultant benefit to the public.

The News went on to boast of Pilates Inc.'s recent legal triumphs:

"The settlement of two trademark infringement suits against The Institute for the Pilates Method of Santa Fe (Eve Gentry and Michele Larsson) and the Joseph H. Pilates Foundation of Rancho Cordova, CA resolves a lengthy dispute as to the right to use the Pilates trademarks. The following people have also agreed to cease and desist using the Pilates marks or have agreed to a court ordered settlement after the commencement of litigation: Carol Amend, Madeline Black, Corefitness, Dance Center Seattle, Denver Physical Therapy, Georgetown Bodyworks, Ballet Arts and many more. The general public is now assured of receiving safe, effective instruction in the Pilates method."[46]

I was not, nor would I ever be, on Sean's list of legal victories.

The other newsletters were focused on the battlefront scenario and the progress of a counter claim to defeat the Pilates trademarks. I read them all with great interest and anticipation of the outcome.

The Pilates Trademark Cancellation Newsletter, Edition Number 2, 1998, stated, "There are three cases happening right now: one in Washington, D.C. between Georgetown Body Works and Pilates Inc.; the second in Los Angeles between Mindy Boehnert (Gallagher's partner!) and Pilates Inc.; and the third in New York between Current Concepts and Pilates Inc."[47]

The latter case evolved into the class action suit against Pilates, Inc.: "The aim of the class action is, as the title of this newsletter suggests, to cancel Gallagher's trademarks and to permit everyone — not just those who pay substantial portions of their income to Gallagher — to use the word Pilates."[48]

Gallagher was a relentless presence on the list@bodymind.net. He appeared to have the law on his side and posed a serious threat to those of us who did not want to march in his parade.

Sean's email address was Mrpilates@aol.com. I wondered what Joseph Pilates would have thought about this use of his name. Responding to his post, I wrote, "If Joe knew that Sean Gallagher was calling himself 'Mr. Pilates' on the internet, I expect he'd storm over to 2121 Broadway and give him a boxing lesson!"

I could clearly see the danger to the Pilates method in allowing "everyone" to call anything they did "Pilates." I did not want to see the Pilates method diluted and mutilated by those who did not know or care about the genius and integrity of the original work. This was, however, a two-edged sword. The authentic Method needed to be protected and faithfully maintained, yet like most contributors to the forum, I did not want to be regulated and franchised by Pilates, Inc. The Pilates name should refer to a method of exercise, not a corporate brand name, I thought. Romana Kryzanowska stated, "Mr. Pilates wanted the Pilates Method to be for the world so that everyone could benefit from it."[49]

In addition to the newsletters, other vehicles succeeded in galvanizing Pilates teachers. The Teachers' Conference on The Method first met in 1997. Organized by Michael Miller, I believe, it was an invitation-only gathering of local Pilates Teachers hosted by various private studios in the Boulder, Colorado area. Attendees included "The Sisters" of The Pilates Center; Michael Miller, Pat Guyton, Mat

Enos, Nancee Wood, Garfield White, another former partner to Steve Giordano; Bonnie Von Grebe and myself, Pilates of Boulder, Inc. Fliers distributed for the gathering never used the name Pilates and the conference had a clandestine, almost subversive feel to it, reminiscent of the secret meetings of La Résistance Française, operating beneath the scrutiny of the Nazi occupation of France during WWII. United by a common cause, teachers and schools who were otherwise enemies in the marketplace shared a real sense of community. The conference was held perhaps ten times in subsequent years.

New York

I first went to New York City during December of 1983 with my wife Joyce to study ballet. It was a real marathon. We stayed in Queens for a week and took the subway into the city every day, spending most of our time at the Darvash Ballet Studio. Joyce referred to Madame Darvash as the "Dragon Lady" and she was! Gabriela Taub Darvash was a world-renowned ballet teacher, coach and choreographer, who had emigrated from the Soviet Union in 1970. Her classes were attended by most of the great dancers in New York City, including such luminaries as Mikhail Baryshnikov and Rudolph Nureyev. Her studio was in a large, sunless room with a resin-dusted hardwood floor and huge mirrors across the front and sides. Narrow windows along the back of the room looked out darkly at a brick wall a few feet away. It seems ironic in retrospect that the Darvash studio was at 2121 Broadway, the same building I would visit fourteen years later to take Pilates lessons at Sean Gallagher's studio.

In the evening, we went to the theater to see performances by the Joffrey Ballet, Pilabolus and a Japanese ballet company, the name of which I cannot recall. We also attended the obligatory New York City Ballet performance of *The Nutcracker*. The next morning, I found myself in class with most of the dancers we had seen on stage the night before at Lincoln Center. I was a comic figure compared to my classmates, despite being a serious student at Ballet Arts in Boulder, under the tutelage of my wife and Barbara Demaree from the Royal Academy of Dance. The woman in front of me at the barre was the "Sugar Plum Fairy." I was in a trance, my breath suspended, frozen in first position with my left hand on the barre. I heard the Dragon Lady's voice, but from a distance, as though she were out in the hallway. Then it hit me like a torpedo, "Ree-shar! Rond de jambe en dehors!"

This was not exactly a holiday vacation in Manhattan. Joyce was the most artistically driven and physically relentless person I have ever known. She was also among the very best rock climbers I have ever known, but that is a whole other story. Joyce is a whole other story. When not at the Darvash Studio, we trekked across town in the ice, snow and frigid air to take lessons from Finis Jhung and David Howard. Our class schedule was grueling.

Joyce was deeply influenced by George Balanchine's vision of the ideal ballerina: "Bones, girl, I want to see bones!" I won't go into her dietary practices, but I can verify that we ate little food—enough to survive the dance classes, but stay as skinny as humanly possible without simply dying. Our diet consisted mostly of bee pollen, figs and dried fruit. Joyce, a strict vegetarian, was also influenced by another maniac—Viktoras Kulvinskas, who wrote the cult classic *Survival Into The 21st Century*. His motto was, "Only the skinny will survive."[50] In rebellion, I occasionally indulged in a hot pretzel that could be had almost anywhere from the ubiquitous street vendors. I would devour the pretzel voraciously, while running down the street from one studio to the next. Joyce regarded this as a profligate indulgence, a sign of weakness, lack of rigor, and general insubordination to the gods of the dance.

At the time, we were unaware of the teachings of Joseph Pilates and of the role his work would come to play in our lives, especially my life. We were in the neighborhood and could have taken lessons from Kathleen Grant at Henri Bendel's, 712 5th Avenue; Carola Trier at her studio, 200 West 58th Street; and Romana Kryzanowska at the Pilates Studio for Body Conditioning, 29 West 56th Street.[51] They were all within a few minutes' walk from each other, just south of Central Park! Hindsight is always 20/20, often giving rise to bitter sorrow. I could just have fits over it now. There I was, right in the cradle of the Pilates method, and I didn't have a clue! It would be two more years before my journey with Joe began at Farentinos' Gym in Boulder, Colorado on Ken Endelman's knotty pine Reformers under the tutelage of Stefan Frease. It was 1996 before I fully realized what I had missed and recognized the need to return to New York.

Several years later, I arranged a trip to Manhattan with one of my clients, Andre Williams, a successful businessman with the physique of a pro football running back. Andre owned a King Air and a passenger jet. The original plan was that Andre would fly us to New York in the King Air, but his personal secretary nixed the idea, pointing out that we could make the trip via commercial airlines five times for less money than one trip in Andre's King Air. We booked a flight on United Airlines, arrived at La Guardia in the afternoon of April 20, 1997 and took a cab into the city. It was a gray, rainy spring day in Manhattan, as we checked into the Helmsley Windsor, 100 West 58th Street, just south of Central Park and a short walk from Drago's Gym.

I had scheduled a private lesson with Romana at 8:00 a.m. and another private lesson with Sari at 11:00 a.m. the next day. Andre and I got up at the crack of dawn, caught the continental breakfast at the hotel, and then hit the streets in search of a flower shop. We found a nice bouquet for Romana and headed straight for 50 West 57th Street. Amy Taylor Alpers at The Pilates Center in Boulder tipped me off that this would be a good strategy of introduction; and it was. Amy said, "Romana is a woman and women love to get flowers." She added, "She also loves champagne!" We had it covered on both counts.

Drago's Gym was located on the sixth floor of an old building at 50 West 57th Street, just two and a half blocks east of Joe's original studio at 939 8th Avenue. The entrance was fairly inconspicuous from the sidewalk and could easily be missed. We took the elevator to the sixth floor and carried our gifts right up to the front desk. Drago, who until that moment had only been a friendly voice on the telephone, was there to greet us. "Good man," he said. "Romana will like this." He placed the bouquet in the middle of the counter, turned it until the arrangement suited him, and then disappeared down a hallway with the champagne.

Drago's was a great place. Romana's Pilates apparatus and Drago's gymnastic equipment shared the main floor. The locker room was down a narrow corridor between the front desk and the Cadillac corner. An "Exit" sign glowed with red letters in the hallway for no apparent reason. The smell of sweat, damp towels and gym socks hung in the air.

I stepped into the main exercise area, gazing out across a sea of mats and varied apparatus. A row of six large windows faced north over 57th Street. Numerous old photographs of Joseph Pilates performing his exercises, in four-frame sequences, hung on the walls and along a partial wall that divided the studio between the entrance, front desk and equipment area. A Pedi-Pole, Ladder Barrel and six Gratz aluminum Reformers were lined up, perpendicular to the wall. Parallel bars, rings and a trapeze bar occupied the space adjacent to the Reformers. A tall corn plant stood in the far corner of the room beside a rack of dumbbells.

The lighting lent a peculiar aspect to the room: gray carpeting, white walls and a black ceiling with fluorescent lighting, offset by the glare from the windows, gave the effect of an underexposed photograph. The apparatus was upholstered in cobalt blue vinyl. The Ladder Barrel, High Chair and one Wunda Chair were painted white, and were from Joe's old studio at 939 Eighth Avenue. All of the vinyl was patched with blue or red plastic tape. Blue mats covered most of the floor, arranged in an upside-down "L" along the east and north sides.

A few apprentices were teaching private lessons on the Reformers and some were practicing on their own. Romana was working with someone on a Reformer toward the end of the row. She turned and smiled as though to say, "You must be the guy from Colorado. You're next." Romana was already a legend in my mind, so that just being there produced a sense of anticipation akin to stage fright. The apprentices had in the meantime surrounded Andre. They had him on the Wunda Chair, Ladder Barrel and Cadillac: Push-Through, Pull Up, Teaser Twist. They bent him and stretched him every which way. He'll be toast by time Romana gets to him, I thought.

It was time. I walked over to meet Romana, who was waiting for me at the third Reformer from the end of the row. She was wearing white pants, tan jazz shoes, and a white V-neck, short sleeved top. She greeted me, "Thank you for the flowers. You came all the way out here from Colorado?" I nodded. "Who trained you?" I told her. I think she was sizing me up. "OK, let's see what you know."

We started on the Reformer. Apprentices with clipboards were seated all around us. Romana said, "Place yourself on the Reformer in one continuous motion for the Footwork. Joe called it the Footwork because it works each part of your foot." She spoke to me constantly, commanding and cueing every exercise, every move. She sometimes stood on the rails of the Reformer to stretch or twist me. We did the complete advanced workout series. I gave it everything I had and more.

At the end, she commented, "Good…better than I expected." Pulling me aside, she said reassuringly, "Well, my newfound friend, you should stay. We'll do Mat later." I had a little Nikon snapshot camera and I asked if I could take a few pictures while she was teaching. She paused and said, "Okay, but don't publish them." Andre had been watching from the sidelines, later commenting, "Man, you were sweating in places people don't even sweat."

Romana's next student was Kathi Ross-Nash. Kathi walked in wearing a two-tone, spaghetti string, unitard with knitted warm-ups rolled down around her waist and black socks. Her shoulders, back and arms were bare. Nearly my height, she was powerful and elegant. I was somewhat awestruck, but I hadn't seen anything yet. As Romana guided Kathi through the same workout I had just finished, I watched every move they both made. It was as engaging and enlightening to watch Romana teaching as it was to watch Kathi's stunning performance. I was amazed at her flexibility, strength and apparent ease in moving through these very difficult exercises. This is how it's done, I thought silently as I moved about snapping photos. This is where these movements are meant to go! I was beginning to understand that Contrology was intended to fulfill the extremes in human potential for length, strength and neuromuscular integration. In this sense, the work never gets easier. It can always be taken deeper, further and integrated more completely as the mind and body are transformed by the work. After Kathi's session, Romana turned to me and said, "This is what Joseph Pilates taught. I change nothing. How could I improve on the work of a genius?"

Romana kept me at her side while she gave a lesson to a man in his 30s wearing a tee shirt, shorts and gym socks. I watched everything she did and listened to every cue. Drago walked in at the end of the lesson with the champagne uncorked and a stack of little paper cups. Romana made a toast to Joseph Pilates and to all of her students. We each had a cup or two of champagne, then spread out on the L-shaped Mat for Advanced Mat Class. Andre really was toast by this time and found a spot at the far northwest corner of the Mats. He was not holding up so well by the time we got to Teaser. Romana called out, "You, over in the corner, stop falling apart!" He bolted upright, drenched in sweat, and managed to pull a little more out of his body. I couldn't hold back a smile.

Our class schedule was not unlike my dance marathon with Joyce in 1983. Andre and I ate lunch at a little restaurant on 57th Street just west of Drago's Gym. After lunch, we pulled ourselves together, walked a few blocks and trained for two more hours at Hila Paldi's studio. The next day was much the same, except that my private lesson was with Sari and after lunch we took the subway south to Tribeca to take lessons from Alycea Ungaro at Tribeca Bodyworks. We stayed in Manhattan for a week and trained like this every day.

Studying with Romana was my primary reason for going to New York, so I scheduled as much time with her as possible. On subsequent visits we worked on the Cadillac, Barrels, Chairs and always the Mat. She talked and spotted me through every exercise. If she felt I did not understand what she wanted, she just got on the apparatus and did it herself. Romana was about 76 years old, but this didn't slow her down any. We were working on the Cadillac one day, doing the Walk Over. I was missing something, so she just hopped up there and performed it beautifully. "Now, try it again," she said. On another occasion she was teaching me how to teach the Mat work, the Roll Up in this case. She stood right over me and said, "Arms up." She took my fingertips and held them straight up, "This is your window. Bring your head through the window. Keep reaching up." Romana was extraordinarily accomplished at assisting and describing exercises. I memorized everything she did and have carried it on in all my teaching to this day.

The Pilates Studio at 2121 Broadway, Suite 201 was another scheduled destination. This was Sean Gallagher's place. Upon entering the studio, my attention was immediately drawn to a large banner tacked above the front desk, displaying the Pilates trademark names and numbers, lest anyone forget Mr. Gallagher was the owner. The studio occupied a large rectangular room with a high ceiling. The front desk and Trademark Registration Numbers were on the left as one entered. A receptionist in workout attire smiled at me from beneath the banners. To the right of her desk, was a row of Mats and Wall Units, set off from the rest of the studio by a makeshift wall that did not reach the ceiling. The wall stopped short of the front desk and allowed access to a larger space with windows that looked out over Broadway. This area contained six Reformers, one Ladder Barrel, three Wunda Chairs, one Cadillac, an "Electric Chair," several Spine Correctors and various smaller pieces. A Guillotine Tower was installed in the wall that divided the studio into separate spaces.

This is the way Joe envisioned it, "A gym in a doorway." Good work, Sean! My first appointment was with Bob Liekens, who kept me on the Wunda Chair for the whole session. I liked working with Bob. He had a charming Belgian accent and proved to be an excellent instructor. I was on an accelerated Pilates learning curve. Like being in love, there was no such thing as too much.

The Trademark Trial

Four years elapsed from the time I received the cease and desist letter from Gallagher's attorneys before the "Trademark Trial" finally went to court. The trial was somewhat long and convoluted, so I offer only the verdict:

PILATES, INC. V CURRENT CONCEPTS

"A bench trial was held by the United States District Court in NYC from June 5 to June 26, 2000... Because defendants did not contest infringement, the central issue at the trial was the validity of plaintiff's marks."[52]

CONCLUSION

"In accordance with the foregoing findings of fact and conclusions of law, the Clerk shall enter judgment for defendants on all of plaintiff's claims. The Clerk shall direct the United States Patent and Trademark Office to cancel Pilates, Inc.'s registrations for the Pilates service mark (Reg. No. 1,405,304, registered August 12, 1986) and the Pilates equipment mark (Reg. No. 1,907,447, registered July 25, 1995).[53]

So ordered.
New York, New York, October, 2000.
Miriam Goldman Cedarbaum
United States District Judge[54]

The Pilates Method Alliance

The creation of the PMA in 2001 was perhaps a sincere response to the fall of the trademarks and to the obvious potential for the Pilates method to become diluted, diffused and adulterated to the point that the original purpose and teaching of the work would be lost forever. Kevin Bowen and Colleen Glenn collaborated to create a non-profit organization dedicated to preserving the essence and value of the Pilates method. They lobbied hard and brought together Kathleen Grant, Ron Fletcher, Mary Bowen and Lolita San Miguel. They also invited Romana Kryzanowska, who refused to participate. Corporate sponsors included Balanced Body, Stott Pilates, and Peak Pilates, who each build Pilates equipment and offer teacher certification programs:

> "The Pilates Method Alliance (PMA) is the international, not-for-profit, professional association and certifying agency dedicated to the teachings of Joseph H. and Clara Pilates. Our mission is to foster community, integrity and respect for diversity; establish certification and continuing education standards; and promote the Pilates method of exercise."[55]

In the spring of 2001, I received an invitation to the first meeting of the PMA. Initially, I was reluctant to attend because I was fed up with being bullied to join, comply, or surrender and did not want to feed a new beast. However, I was forced to reconsider when I learned that Kathleen Grant, Ron Fletcher, Mary Bowen and Lolita San Miguel had agreed to attend. So I went to the first meeting and participated in setting the groundwork for the organization. An important part of the meeting was spent listening raptly to each of the first generation teachers tell their own stories: how they came to meet Joe and Clara, what they were like, their impressions of the studio, the work, the equipment and the other students and teachers who were at the 939 Eighth Avenue studio. It was a unique event that will never happen again.

I stayed with the PMA for six years, attended the annual conferences and gradually lost interest. "Respect for diversity" is a somewhat troubling phrase that allows for the support of programs rather far removed from the original work of Joseph Pilates. My focus as a teacher and school owner is entirely on the original work. Joe had it right. So I had to re-evaluate why I was putting money and time into an organization that seemed to be about everything new and put little emphasis on the original work.

Michael Miller, who was trained by Romana Kryzanowska, never joined the PMA. In 2003, he predicted: "The PMA is going to be a cartel of the equipment manufacturers." At the time, I thought he was wrong. By 2006, I had to reconsider his comment. Its sponsors, the big Pilates equipment manufacturers and the big teacher training organizations, often the same enterprises, control the PMA. Money talks, in business as in politics.

Lolita San Miguel also spoke out against the expanding authority of the PMA: "Joe does not belong to the PMA alone. He belongs to the world." Ms. San Miguel declared, "I fought alongside many others to take Pilates out of the hands of a few people (Pilates, Inc.) who said they owned the Pilates name and everything connected with Pilates and we were successful. I will continue to oppose any attempt to make Pilates the exclusive property of anybody or any organization."[56]

Certification programs, bearing little resemblance to the authentic work, began to appear everywhere, especially on the internet. One notable Pilates school advertised, "Pilates used to be difficult; not anymore!" This statement is truly astounding. Pilates is difficult and it is expensive and for good reasons. The study of Pilates is not akin to becoming a step aerobics instructor or a personal trainer. It cannot be blended with other disciplines, and it cannot be learned in a weekend workshop. It is a comprehensive art of movement, a true science of the body.

Joseph Pilates wrote in *Return to Life*, "Contrology is the complete coordination of body, mind, and spirit."[57] This is a serious proposition. Ron Fletcher echoed the sentiment at a workshop I attended in 2003 with about 100 other certified Pilates instructors from various schools. Ron opened by asserting: "Most of you should leave. You don't really want to do this. This work is too subtle. It is just too difficult. People ask me, 'How long does it take to become a Pilates teacher?' Ten years! It takes ten years to learn how to teach this work."[58]

Classical Pilates

The growth and expansion of the Pilates method has been on a meteoric acceleration curve for the last 20 years. I have often wondered what Joe and Clara would think about it. Could they have imagined in their wildest dreams the international growth, popularity, power struggles and convoluted politics of their humble work? Could they have imagined the "Trademark Trial," Mr.pilates@aol.com, all the equipment manufacturers, the variations, deviations, hybrids and abominations of their work and equipment? Whom would they support? Whom would they oppose? To whom would Joe want to give boxing lessons? Would Joe and Clara be appalled or would they be having a good laugh in "the big gymnasium in the sky?"

As for me, I stick with the original work. I do not make "improvements" or teach exercises that deviate from the work as I learned it from Romana, Kathleen, Jay and Ron. There is an essence, a flow, a main vein that is the Pilates method. All of the exercises created by Joseph Pilates are expressions and extensions of this flow.

"Classical Pilates" refers to the body of work and equipment created by Joseph Pilates between 1926 and 1967. Joe was a genius, an inventor and a visionary. Had he lived another twenty years, would he have kept his work and equipment exactly as it was in 1967? Was it finished? Was it complete?

Clara wrote, "There is far to go with this work. This is just the tip of the iceberg."[59] It is highly probable, considering what we know of Joseph Pilates, that he would have kept creating his work. New exercises, new apparatus, we can only speculate what this would look like.

This perspective creates, at least, the illusion of an opening or opportunity to evolve and modernize the Pilates method. Many self-proclaimed experts have assumed that the original work is dated, unlearned, and that "we know so much more today than Joe knew about biomechanics, body alignment and effective movement that the Pilates method needs to be improved and updated."

Jay Grimes said, "How do they know what was in Joe's mind?"[60] Here is the clincher: Who among us has the intellect, intuition and imagination to expand on this work and hold it within the flow of the original genius? The exercises on the Reformer and Mat are so perfectly linked and sequenced that any attempt at addition or rearrangement feels awkward and contrived. Who could rewrite *Macbeth* and come up with a better play? People change the work because they never properly learned or understood it in the first place.

Romana pulled me aside one day at Drago's Gym, as was her wont, and asked, "What are the five parts of the mind?" I was groping for an answer, staring at photos of Joe doing the Footwork, when she asserted, "Intellect, intuition, imagination, memory and will. Joe liked to ask people this question." I felt at that moment I had none of those qualities, but I memorized her words as usual and wrote them down.

I sometimes imagine Joe walking into the studio, taking a look around, watching the teaching and saying, "Ja, gute Arbeit. Dies ist, was ich wollte." I could not do this any other way.

Proof of Pudding

So what happened to my crooked back? It occurred to me after about three years of practicing the Pilates method that my back had not "gone out" for a long time. I decided to give it the hand mirror test. Stripping down, I took a hard look at my spine. It was straight! I could bend it equally well to the left and to the right. I couldn't believe my eyes, so I stretched a few more times each way into full lateral flexion. I could find no trace of that evil demon, scoliosis.

As Joseph Pilates had written in *Return to Life*, "Fortunately the spine lends itself quite readily to correction."[61] He was right, as he had often asserted, and I was a believer.

Several years later, I unwittingly put the Pilates method's amazing restorative power to the test on a road bike ride in November 2002. My friend Chip Bennett and I met at my place to do a "team time trial" on the rural roads north of Boulder. We were in a big hurry to get started and about a mile from the house I realized that I had forgotten my helmet. We were riding quite fast on Hygiene Road. The sun had set and it was getting cold, so I decided to pull on my gloves. Reaching into the back pocket of my jersey, I pulled on the left glove, then the right. Getting the right glove half on is the last thing I remember. Chip was drafting me and saw what happened or, to this day, I wouldn't know, nor would I be alive.

Four days later, I woke up in the I.C.U. without the slightest clue why I was there. I had needles and tubes in my arms, electronic clips on my fingers, a catheter, and a c-collar. There were unaccountable wounds on my arms and legs. I wanted to go home. I ripped out all the needles, the catheter and tore the collar off my neck. Frantic nurses surrounded me, telling me not to move. They struggled to keep me on the bed, while one of them went for the neurosurgeon.

I was unattended, lying still, when Doctor V walked in and said, "I understand you want to go home."

"Yes," I replied, "I would like to go home now."

"That's fine except for one thing. Dr. V. explained, "You can't walk. You have serious injuries and about eight broken bones. And I want you to know something: you have the worst kind of head injury. It is simply a miracle that you are alive. If you weren't in such good shape, I would have had a different conversation with your family and friends. Your body has not worked against you, but has helped you to survive your grave injuries."

"But what happened?" I asked. At that moment, I believed my car was in the parking lot and I could just get up and drive home.

"You crashed on your road bike." He held a mirror for me, "As you can see, you are still bleeding from your ears, nose and the side of your head. You fractured your cranium," he said, pointing to a place about three inches above my left ear, "down through the ear canal, splitting the basilar bone. You also broke all the bones of your left shoulder, four ribs, which punctured your left lung and you split the top of your femur. I think you should stay here for a while and let us help you."

I could not recall the crash, the ambulance or the emergency room, but the reality of my condition began to sink in. Resigned, I just said, "Okay." It was two weeks before I was allowed to leave the hospital. Then, against the urging of my doctors, I had Bonnie take me home. I was a real handful. The next few weeks were agony. Nothing was pinned or splinted and I could take only Advil because of the head injury. Unable to sleep, get dressed or buy groceries, I needed Bonnie's help with everything. I have called her "Angel" ever since.

I still couldn't walk without assistance, but with a lot of help from Bonnie I set about rebuilding my mind and body on the Pilates equipment at the studio. I was relentless with my own rehabilitation. By mid December, I could run almost two miles without stopping. By the end of December, I was back on my road bike and turned in twenty miles with Chip and my son Raoul. I was really pushing it, but I couldn't just sit around and watch Tour de France re-runs. It was a year before I could do a single Pull Up. It took two years to get my balance back. In three years, I could do most everything, even stand up without falling over. I am stone deaf in the left ear and the ringing in my head never goes away, but this is not a complaint. I can run, ride, climb, do and teach Pilates. I am a lucky man. My point is, the Pilates method saved me again, and I have since had wonderful opportunities to help others come back from horrible accidents and debilitating injuries.

I have been blessed to share the Pilates method in a larger arena. In 1997, Bonnie Von Grebe and I opened Pilates of Boulder, Inc. We moved the studio a few times, trying to find a suitable commercial space and continued to build the business. Sometimes clients confessed, "I love this work. I want to do what you do. How can I become a Pilates teacher?" Quoting Bruce King, I suggested, "Joe trained Romana Kryzanowska, Kathleen Grant, Ron Fletcher. They are all still teaching." "I can't move to New York," the clients argued. "Why can't you teach me?" Eventually, I ran out of excuses and we began a formal teacher education program in 1999.

Bonnie and I learned from Kevin Bowen a few years later that most states require occupational schools to be approved and licensed by the Department of Higher Education. Colorado was such a state. We jumped through a lot of hoops to make this happen and in 2003 we received authorization from the Colorado Department of Higher Education, Division of Private Occupational Schools to train and certify Pilates teachers.

The certification program took on another twist when a U.S. veteran called one day, asking if she could attend our school on the G.I. Bill. I told her we would have to look into it. Winning approval from the Department of Higher Education was trivial compared to the V.A. We re-wrote our catalogue and curriculum several times, filled out a mountain of government forms and revised everything a few more times. With the determined assistance of Mike Harris, Colorado State

Approving Agent for the Colorado Community College System, we were finally endorsed by the state to offer Pilates certification to veterans through the G. I. Bill, paid for by the Veterans Administration. This is a great opportunity and an even greater honor for us. Three U.S. veterans have come through our program to date.

In December of 2010, we changed the name of the business to the Pilates Institute of Boulder, Inc. Our mission is to teach classical Pilates: www.pilatesinstituteboulder. com.

As the business grew, so did my son Raoul. He went from skateboards to gymnastics at Gymnastics Elite Training Center. He became a ski instructor, competitive runner and professional musician. Eventually, he followed in his father's footsteps and became a Pilates instructor. He studied with Michael Miller, Amy Alpers and completed the Comprehensive Teacher Training Program at Pilates of Boulder. He has attended workshops with Kathleen Grant, Jay Grimes, Kathryn Ross-Nash, Edgar Tirado, Brooke Siler, Ron Fletcher and Lolita San Miguel. Raoul has been teaching the Pilates method since 2000 and is an indispensable partner in the Pilates Institute of Boulder.

Joseph Pilates stated in his book, *Your Health*, "My work will be established, and when it is, I will be the happiest man in God's Universe. My goal will have been reached."[62] I, too, share that joy through the revolutionary work of this modern day genius. Thank you, Joe, for your precious gift.

Richard Rossiter

Richard Rossiter lives in Boulder, Colorado where he works as director of the Pilates Institute of Boulder. Richard is devoted to the teaching and practice of Authentic Pilates, and is an avid practitioner of road cycling, running, and rock climbing. He served in the U.S. Army Special Forces (Green Berets) from 1966 to 1969. He earned a B.A. at Western Washington University 1972; M.F.A.: Idaho State University 1977. Richard learned the Pilates Method from Bruce King, Romana Kryzanowska, Jay Grimes, Ron Fletcher, Kathleen Grant, Mary Bowen, and Lolita San Miguel. He is also a PMA Gold Certified Instructor (2005). Richard continues his professional education with Jay Grimes at Vintage Pilates in Santa Monica, California. Richard has written twenty climbing guidebooks, various essays, magazine articles, featured in *Pilates Style*, and is published in *Chicken Soup for The Soul* (2003).

REFERENCES

[1]Gordon E. R. Troy, Pretrial Report, Introduction, *Pilates, Inc. v Current Concepts*, 96 Civ. 0043 (MGC), June 29, 2001, 5.
[2]Internet search, Joseph Pilates: current biographies and articles give varied stories and different dates of birth.
[3]Gordon E. R. Troy, Case Document, *Pilates Inc. v Current Concepts*, United States District Court, Southern District of New York, 96 Civ. 0043 (MGC), 2001, 7.
[4]authenticpilatesunion.com, History, Chasing Joe Pilates, Stacey Redfield.
[5]Public presentations on the life of Joseph Pilates by Ken Endelman, 2010, 2011/ Internet search, Pilates: current biographies and articles.
[6]Sean Gallagher and Romana Kryzanowska, ed., *The Joseph H. Pilates Archive Collection, Photographs, Writings and Design*. Bainbridge Books, Philadelphia, PA, 2000, 34.
[7]Endelman, 2010, 2011/ Internet search, Pilates: current biographies and articles.
[8]Endelman, 2010, 2011.
[9]*The Joseph H. Pilates Archive Collection*, 42.
[10]www.rapo.com, Gallery 2, I. C. Rapoport.
[11]*The Joseph H. Pilates Archive Collection*, 108.
[12]Joseph Pilates, *Return to Life through Contrology*. (Incline Village, NV: Presentation Dynamics, Inc., 1998), 6.
[13]Gordon E. R. Troy, Case Document, *Pilates Inc. v Current Concepts*, United States District Court, Southern District of New York, 96 Civ. 0043 (MGC), 2001, 7.
[14]Gordon E. R. Troy, PC, Pretrial Report, 3.
[15]Gordon E. R. Troy, Case Document, *Pilates Inc. v Current Concepts*, United States District Court, Southern District of New York, 2001, 7–8.
[16]Gordon E. R. Troy, PC, Pretrial Report, 7. Also: www.google.com/search?client=safari&rls=en&q=Kathleen+Stanford+Grant&ie=UTF-8&oe=UTF-8.
[17]Lolita San Miguel, www.lolitapilates.com.
[18]Gordon E. R. Troy, Pretrial Report, Introduction, 3.
[19]Gordon, E.R. Troy, *Pilates, Inc. v Current Concepts*, 7-8.

[20]www.google.com/search?q=Eve=Gentry&ie=utf8&oe.

[21]Ron Fletcher, biographical sketches, May 21, 2001.

[22]www.google.com/search?client=safari&rls=en&q=ron+fletcher&ie=UTF-8&oe=UTF-8. Ron Fletcher, biographical sketch, May 21, 2001.

[23]Clara Zeuner, personal correspondence to Ron Fletcher, March 7, 1973.

[24]www.google.com/search?client=safari&rls=en&q=ron+fletcher&ie=UTF-8&oe=UTF-8. Ron Fletcher, biographical sketch, May 21, 2001.

[25]Stories told by Mary Bowen, Kathleen Grant, Ron Fletcher, Romana Kryzanowska, Lolita San Miguel, Bruce King, and Jay Grimes, 1988 to 2012.

[26]Stories told by Bowen et al, 1988-2012.

[27]www.pilates-marybowen.com/pages/aboutmary.html

[28]www.vintagepilates.com.

[29]Jay Grimes, various lectures/workshops 2009 to 2012, see also www.jaygrimes.com.

[30]Gordon E. R. Troy, Case Document, *Pilates Inc. v Current Concepts*, United States District Court, Southern District of New York, 2001, 7, and www.romanaspilates.com.

[31]Gordon E. R. Troy, Case Document, *Pilates Inc. v Current Concepts*, United States District Court, Southern District of New York, 2001, 11-12.

[32]Troy, Case Document, *Pilates Inc. v Current Concepts*, United States District Court, Southern District of New York.

[33]Gordon E. R. Troy, Pretrial Report, 2001, Introduction.

[34]Gordon E. R. Troy, Case Document, *Pilates Inc. v Current Concepts*, United States District Court, Southern District of New York, 2001, 12-15.

[35]Gordon E. R. Troy, Case Document, *Pilates Inc. v Current Concepts*, United States District Court, Southern District of New York, 2001, 15.

[36]Gordon E. R. Troy, Pretrial Report, Introduction, 12.

[37]Gordon E. R. Troy, Case Document, *Pilates Inc. v Current Concepts*, United States District Court, Southern District of New York, 2001, 16. Gordon E. R. Troy, Pretrial Report, Introduction, 11-12.

[38]Mad Dogg Athletics, internet announcement. No longer available.

[39]Gordon E. R. Troy, Case Document, *Pilates Inc. v Current Concepts*, United States District Court, Southern District of New York, 2001, 17.

[40]Gordon E. R. Troy, Case Document, *Pilates Inc. v Current Concepts*, United States District Court, Southern District of New York, 2001, 70.

[41]Gordon E. R. Troy, Case Document, *Pilates Inc. v Current Concepts*, United States District Court, Southern District of New York, 2001, 17.

[42]Gordon E. R. Troy, Case Document, *Pilates Inc. v Current Concepts*, United States District Court, Southern District of New York, 2001, 17.

[43]Gordon E. R. Troy, Case Document, *Pilates Inc. v Current Concepts*, United States District Court, Southern District of New York, 2001, 17-18.

[44]Gordon E. R. Troy, Pretrial Report, 2001, 2.

[45]Gordon E. R. Troy, Pretrial Report, 2001, 2.

[46]*The Pilates Guild News*, Spring/Summer, 1996, 1.

[47]*The Pilates Trademark Cancellation Newsletter*, Ed. No. 2, 1998, 1.

[48]*The Pilates Trademark Cancellation Newsletter*, Ed. No. 2, 1998, 1.

[49]Gordon E. R. Troy, Case Document, *Pilates Inc. v Current Concepts*, United States District Court, Southern District of New York, 2001, 30.

[50]Viktoras Kulvinskas, *Survival into the 21st Century: Planetary Healers Manual.* (P.O. Box, Wethersfield, Connecticut, Omangod Press), 1975, 37.

[51]Gordon E. R. Troy, Case Document, *Pilates Inc. v Current Concepts*, United States District Court, Southern District of New York, 2001, 9.

[52]Gordon E. R. Troy, Case Document, *Pilates Inc. v Current Concepts*, United States District Court, Southern District of New York, 2001, 3.

[53]Gordon E. R. Troy, Case Document, *Pilates Inc. v Current Concepts*, United States District Court, Southern District of New York, 2001, 82.

[54]Troy, *Pilates Inc. v Current Concepts*, 2001, 82.
[55]www.pilatesmethodalliance.org.
[56]www.lolitapilates.com/lolita-san-miguel-disagrees-with-pilates-method-alliance.
[57]Joseph Pilates and William Miller. Return to Life through Contrology (Incline Village, NV: Presentation Dynamics, Inc., 1998), 9.
[58]Ron Fletcher, workshop, Pilates Method Alliance Conference, New Orleans, 2004.
[59]Clara Zeuner, personal correspondence to Ron Fletcher, March 7, 1973.
[60]Ron Fletcher, workshop, Pilates Method Alliance Conference, New Orleans, 2004.
[61]Joseph Pilates and William Miller, 17.
[62]Joseph Pilates and William Miller, 55.

WORKS CONSULTED

Gallagher, Sean, and Kryzanowska, Romana, ed., *The Joseph H. Pilates Archive Collection, Photographs, Writings and Design*. Bainbridge Books, Philadelphia, PA, 2000, 34.

Kulvinskas, Viktoras. *Survival into the 21st Century: Planetary Healers Manual*. 21st Century Bookstore, 1975.

Pilates, Joseph H., and William John Miller. Pilates' *Return to Life Through Contrology*. Incline Village: Presentation Dynamics Inc., 1998.

Pilates, Joseph H., and William John Miller. *Your Health*. Incline Village: Presentation Dynamics Inc., 1998.

On Springs

By Alycea Ungaro

> *...your spine is spring-like in nature,*
> *your muscles can coil and recoil...*

I feel that now is the time for an equipment renaissance. I want to bring the springs back into the forefront of Pilates, because if there's one thing that's unique about our system, it's that we use springs. Nobody else does that. Somehow our apparatus has taken a back seat to the method as a whole, but I believe it is the foundation of the method and should not take a supporting role. The Pilates apparatus really is the star of the show in many ways.

Nowadays, when people call Real Pilates to inquire about taking lessons or classes, they no longer ask if it's equipment-based. Prospective students usually think they're coming to a kind of yoga studio to take a class with a mat on the floor. As a result, I have taken to saying that we run a dedicated Pilates studio. A dedicated studio means that we practice spring-driven Pilates. I explain that while we teach the Mat work in your sessions, we will always use springs. Many of them are surprised by that.

Springs are what separates Pilates from other body conditioning techniques. We use mats, but yoga practitioners use mats. We use resistance, but a lot of people use resistance. We're the only ones that use springs. I would like to encourage studio owners and teachers to really look at this one essence of Pilates. We open springs; we close them. Yet this fact generates facinating questions: How do we use the springs? Why do we use the springs? What do the springs do? What does it mean to our muscles? We could even talk about teaching with a spring-centric language or developing a curriculum that's more spring-centric.

In the meantime, we should conceptually connect spring action to principles of the work, as well as with the individual's body we are teaching; it's best to describe that connection to our students. Initially, it's visual. I always draw our students' and teachers' attention to the springs: taking the spring out, hooking a spring, demonstrating the tension and recoil of the spring. I always try to visually show clients what is happening. When you move the carriage, the spring lengthens. When you move your straps, you're creating more space between each spring coil. No matter what you're moving, the key movement in an exercise on the Reformer will be movement of the springs. The same holds true for the Cadillac and any other springs you use on the Tower (Guillotine) or Wall Unit.

One of the most significant experiences I have had with springs happened when Amy Alpers was teaching. She came to Real Pilates and taught a workshop. I just happened to be walking by, and she said to the group, "Short Spine?" Amy looked around for a volunteer. Then she said, "Alycea, come here." I lay down on the Reformer to begin Short Spine Massage. She had just given the group a lengthy discussion about the springs and resistance. When I began, Amy actually said, "I need you to take this spring into you." I replied, "I don't even know what that means." But something happened to my body. I had a completely different experience, like an out-of-body experience. When I practiced the Short Spine Massage exercise, everyone applauded. It was bizarre, but I could feel it. I felt that I had become the spring.

That experience got me thinking. I thought, What if I were a spring? What would my muscles do if they were springs? Are they springs? What are the elements of this? So, when I'm training students and teachers, I try to bring up these questions and have them visually connect to the dynamics of springs. Then we try to keep that connection. Romana always said, "Unless the spring is moving, you don't have an exercise." It's true; if the spring stops moving, you don't have an exercise. We keep the springs moving. But I want clients to do more. I ask them to watch the springs and not just look at the apparatus frame, or themselves, or me. They must focus on the spring they're moving. I have to believe that Mr. Pilates, consumed as he was with making all of this equipment, was keeping an eye on his springs. I have to believe it.

Attention to the springs embodies all the principles of Pilates. Properly stretching springs requires precision and flow. They comprise a critical component of control. The first thing we say is, "Don't slam your carriage." If you slam the carriage, you're not controlling your springs. It always comes back to the springs. Recoil action. Opposition. The springs move the way you want your muscles to move in Pilates. The idea that you can use your muscles eccentrically, meaning applying tension while the muscles are stretched, is the embodiment of control.

In order to convey the connection with the spring, and to incorporate it into movement, I often say, "Look at your springs. Can you see all the light and air coming through the coils?" I verbally reference springs and show the client the spring action they create while they feel it, so there is a visual and a physical connection, rather than something intangible. Sometimes people close their eyes, and they just try to feel. But if you can feel it, hear it, and see it, then you've got three points of reference: the visual, the verbal instruction from the teacher, and the tactile. Everything comes together for the student, and they have an "a-ha" moment.

Achieving experiential insight and technique take time. However, I think that the spring can be a wow factor very early on in a student's training. In the very first session with a new client, he learns that springs don't work like anything else. What's so difficult is the release. With dumbbells, resist-a-bands, and tubing you have a moment of letting go, but you can't do that with Pilates springs. You can't turn your muscle off and not lose control or you might catapult across the room. So the springs teach the student by virtue of their properties. I think it's a teacher's job to draw each student's attention to essential properties of springs as the session evolves.

Bringing the student's attention to spring action is more challenging on the Reformer apparatus because the springs fasten underneath your carriage. Until you really understand excercises such as Elephant, Stomach Massage, and Knee Stretches, experiencing the depth of spring resistance is a little abstract. New students can benefit from watching the Roll Back Bar springs, Leg Springs, and more obvious springs. I teach students that the spring is inert; it's passive. It doesn't do anything. All the spring action is based on us. How we move the carriage, how we move our muscles, how we carry movement, how we resolve movement are all reflected in the spring. Springs are so good for you and so not like anything else—that elastic quality of two-way control, two-way strength.

The gift of working with the springs is the ability to translate that feeling when there are no springs. We want to work as though there were springs. I say this a lot to my clients: "Here we are on the Mat, and there are no springs. You're still pulling those imaginary springs out and still stretching them; your muscles are still working. Now you've internalized the spring. Now you've become the spring. On the Mat, you become the spring." Through consistent practice with the apparatus, you can bring that sensation of internal spring resistance to the Mat and enhance your own practice and the quality of the movement which is so inherent to Pilates.

Ultimately, I want people to make connections between the feeling of the spring in the studio and the feeling of the spring in their daily lives. Pilates is for real life. It is critical that people take these connections outside the studio, because at best we have our students three or four hours a week. The rest of their hours are filled with nonspring-like activities. So whether it's a spring in your step, or that feeling of constant opposition and tension, or just a moment when a student can stop in his workday and stand up and do a series at the Wall, the idea that your spine is spring-like in nature, that your muscles can coil and recoil should be present. The act of yawning when you wake up in the morning is a great example. You fully extend. Everything uncoils and elongates, then comes back with control. We talk so much about spiraling in Pilates. Teachers often say, "I'm getting taller. I'm spiraling up." Your muscles, your fascia, wind around. There are lots of natural spirals in the body. But nobody looks at the metal spring and pulls it apart and says, "Oh, look, there it is." It's so obvious. The force is distributed through the spiral of the spring the same way it is distributed through your spinal column and through your body.

It's fascinating to parallel the muscles to the springs, then try to bring all that back together and hopefully, through training with the springs, take those properties into the body. I want my students to feel comfortable moving that way, and to experience the benefit of that connection in their everyday lives. I want them to feel it when they are standing or lifting groceries.

In yoga and many other disciplines, they talk about removing density from the body and bringing in light. I feel that the same idea applies to the core. You want to remove the density. When the core is tightly packed and closed, you can't see any light until you stretch it out. When you hold it open, all the light and energy is released, and the density dissipates.

I imagine that Joseph Pilates was struck by the idea of removing density from the body. He was so consumed with posture and oxygenation. When you add springs into the mix, it just seems obvious that he was trying to pull lightness and airiness up into the body. That is a quality that all Pilates teachers seem to have. They just glide through the room. Hopefully, we impart that to our students. I think we do.

About Alycea

Alycea is the proud owner of New York City's Real Pilates studio. She is a licensed Physical Therapist, the author of six Pilates titles, and the creator of several Pilates props including the Real Alignment Mat. She was formally trained by Romana Kryzanowska in 1993, after a decade of experience in The Method, during which she danced professionally throughout the country. Alycea is as passionate about the business of Pilates as she is about Pilates. She enjoys spending time in the country with her husband and two daughters. You can find her online at realpilatesnyc.com.

Hidden Treasures of Pilates

Epilogue By
José Antonio Ruiz Carretón and Jacquelin F. Drucker

Within the preceding pages are exceptional treasures of traditional Pilates, found both in the people and in the ideas. Some are well-known, some lesser known, and, until now, some nearly hidden. In a way, this is emblematic of Pilates: it is a conditioning technique respected—even revered—throughout the world, yet in many respects, the traditional work can be a relatively unseen, or even misunderstood, treasure. In rehabilitation science, athletic art forms, and sports, the effectiveness of Pilates has been recognized for decades. Yet beyond these professional fields, authentic Pilates sometimes remains unfamiliar to, or misconstrued by, the wider public.

Under the term "Pilates," we find many directions and many departures from what Joseph Pilates created and taught. Even those who are dedicated to the classical approach share responsibility for having created confusion regarding the work, for only a few truly know what is authentic. Many of those who had the honor of working with Joseph Pilates, Romana Kryzanowska and other first-generation teachers show their respect by transmitting knowledge and insight that are faithful to the ways they were taught. Whether through writings, workshops, videos, or simply one student at a time, these professionals help promote awareness of classical Pilates while preventing inconsistencies that, with time, would reshape the Pilates method into something diminished in power and reduced in effectiveness. By following the example of professionals in classical Pilates, many of whom share their knowledge through this book, our community can help ensure the system remains optimally strong, efficient and historically accurate.

Those whose essays fill this book hail from around the globe, and it is heartening to see the rapidly growing presence of Pilates in the international arena. Indeed, Pilates was international in its origins—remaining so in acceptance and recognition—but greater worldwide bonds and networks are forming in the interest of preserving, promoting, protecting, and understanding the work. As this growth continues, an important opportunity arises for the traditional Pilates community to remain connected so we may more effectively share Joseph Pilates' method with all who are interested.

Those of us who value classical Pilates work to promote broader appreciation of its virtues and access to education in the technique. To that end, this book highlights multi-faceted ideas and qualities related to traditional Pilates, thereby shining a bright light on this often hidden treasure. We revel in the insights offered by the gifted professionals whose words appear here, and we know that there are many more individuals who are on the same path of dedication. Let us continue working together to explore and celebrate Joseph Pilates' time-tested approach to physical health, mental fitness and the mind-body connection.

José Antonio Ruiz Carretón

José Antonio Ruiz Carretón discovered the world of body-mind-spirit when he was sixteen years old and began practicing Eutony, which focuses on harmoniously balanced "tonicity in constant adaptation to the state or activity of the moment." Over the years, José immersed himself in different disciplines until he discovered Pilates. In 2002, José moved from his native Spain to New York City to become an independent student of Romana Kryzanowska. He also studied with Sari Mejia Santo and Kathleen Stanford Grant. After completing his certification, José stayed to work at Drago's Gym, teaching alongside Romana, Sari, and Edwina Fontaine for more than four years. Today, José is a widely respected and popular instructor at Pilates Challenge in New York City.

Jacquelin F. Drucker

Jacquelin Drucker is an attorney with a national and international practice devoted exclusively to service as a neutral arbitrator. In authentic Pilates as taught by her primary instructor, Ernesto Reynoso, she discovered an engaging and effective method through which she achieved a level of fitness, strength, and mind-body connection that she never thought possible. Jackie also developed a deep respect for the Pilates community, which she has joined as an owner of Pilates Challenge, located in New York City.